Plague Take It

Also by Jon Peirce:
    Canadian Industrial Relations (Pearson Education Canada, 1999, 2002, 2006).
    Social Studies: Collected Essays, 1974-2013 (Friesen, 2014).
    Love and Love: A Novella (Amazon, 2018).

Also by Ann McMillan:
    Air Quality Management: Canadian Perspectives on a Global Issue, with Eric Taylor (co-editor) (Springer, 2014).
    The New Devil's Dictionary, with Duane Chartier and Irene Agoulnik (Amazon, 2019).
    Naked in Time, with Duane Chartier (co-editor) (Amazon, 2020).

Cover art:
    Loose Cannon Designs
    Painting *The Oceans Are Dying* by Claude Ethier

Plague Take It
A COVID Almanac
By and About Elders

Jon Peirce
Ann McMillan

LIBRARY AND ARCHIVES CANADA CATALOGUING IN PUBLICATION

Title: Plague take it : a COVID almanac by and about elders / Jon Peirce,
Ann McMillan (editors).
Names: Peirce, Jon (Jonathan Charles), editor. | McMillan, Ann (Ann
Constance), editor.
Description: Includes bibliographical references.
Identifiers: Canadiana 20210268719 | ISBN 9781988657288 (softcover)
Subjects: LCSH: COVID-19 Pandemic, 2020——Literary collections. |
LCSH: COVID-19 (Disease)——Literary
collections. | LCSH: Older people's writings, American. | LCSH:
American literature——21st
century. | CSH: Older people's writings, Canadian (English) | CSH:
Canadian literature (English)——
21st century.
Classification: LCC PS8237.C69 P53 2021 | DDC C810.8/03561——dc23

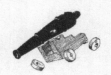

Published by
LOOSE CANNON PRESS

www.loosecannonpress.com

PRODUCTION

Jon Peirce: Co-editor
Ann McMillan: Co-editor
Jany Lavoie: French language editor
Su Mardelli: Technical coordinator
Robert Barclay: Publisher

DEDICATIONS

FROM JON PEIRCE

To Ann McMillan
and Bob Barclay,
my partners in crime

FROM ANN MCMILLAN

To Jeanette Grant
who ended her fight with ALS
on August 15, 2021 and who
showed us how to live
with grace and resilience.
To Jon Peirce and Bob Barclay,
my partners in crime.

CONTENTS

INTRODUCTION

This almanac is a social history about what has arguably been the most consequential, as well as most challenging, time we in North America have known, at least since the end of the Second World War. I stress the fact that it is a social history by way of emphasizing both what it is, and what it isn't. The almanac does not pretend to be any sort of scientific or medical treatise about COVID-19. There is already a plethora of such treatises available, most written by people infinitely more qualified for the task than I would be. No doubt there will be many more by the time the almanac has actually seen the light of day. What it *does* offer is a wide range of material showing what it has been like—and continues to be like—for elders[1] to live their daily lives in the shadow of the worst global pandemic in over 100 years.

All meaningful history is, at its heart, a collection of stories. And all good stories, true stories, stories that we will remember, offer far more than instruction and entertainment. They offer glimpses of their authors' emotional fault lines—lines more readily revealed at a time of great crisis than they might have been in other, less troubled times. It is precisely such stories that Ann and I have sought to collect for this almanac. Any final judgement on how well we've succeeded must be left to you, the almanac's readers. We'd like to think we've given ourselves the best possible chance by using authors from a broad range of backgrounds, from both Canada and the United States and written in both of Canada's official languages, and by choosing stories on an equally broad range of topics, from moving or attempting to obtain health care for problems other than COVID-19 to attempting to continue one's work as a creative or performing artist.

A distinctive feature of this almanac is its use of creative work, in the form of short stories, poems and short plays, in addition to more traditional essays and memoirs. Our approach throughout has been interdisciplinary both as to content and as to literary form. Whether these works illuminate the past, as in Ralph Smith's moving poem about his grandfather, who died in the previous flu pandemic, the present, as in Teresa Patterson's amusing play about an elder's attempt to learn new technology, or the future, as in Ann McMillan's story in the final section, these works offer the kind of insight into what it has *felt* like to live through this pandemic that one might not obtain through a more conventional, all-narrative treatment. In addition, some are truly moving, some are really funny—and a few are both.

It might seem paradoxical to suggest that one could actually have a good time reading about a global pandemic that has sickened and killed so many. Nonetheless, this is nothing more than simple truth, even if the main reason we laugh is to keep ourselves from crying.

Where will we all go from here? What kind of world awaits us once most people have been vaccinated against COVID-19, and we're finally able to resume at least some semblance of our previous 'normal' activities? The truth, as Betsy Hoffman suggests, gently if pointedly in the short poem with which the almanac ends, is that we simply don't know. Rather than racking our brains speculating about what may or may not happen, it seems to me the better part of wisdom to simply accept the fact that we don't know, and then to go to work, to the best of our ability and limit of our strength, to try to create the kind of future world we'd like to see and inhabit, whether that entails political or environmental activity or involvement of a more personal kind through the creative and performing arts, or through volunteer work in one's home community. For now, the field is wide open. There's all sorts of interesting, useful and important work to be done by people of good will. In the meantime, it's Ann's and my fervent wish that this almanac will offer readers inspiration, a laugh or two, and a bit of hope, by showing how a broad range of people have managed to cope with and adapt to the pandemic, often quite successfully.

Merci et bonne chance à tous! Stay healthy and keep laughing!

J. P.
Gatineau, Quebec
July, 2021

---

[1] For the purposes of this almanac, we have defined 'elders' to mean anyone over the age of 60, or with a serious disability.

SECTION 1

Plagues from the Past

The current COVID pandemic is far from the first such pandemic we have experienced. In all likelihood, it won't be the last. We offer this glimpse at pandemics from the past with the hope that knowing a bit more about those earlier events will enhance our understanding of our own situation today.

Elizabeth Hoffman, Jeanette Grant and Ann McMillan begin the section with an historical overview of plagues and pandemics from ancient Greece right through to the misnamed 'Spanish' flu pandemic of 1918–20. This is followed by Ralph Smith's epic poem, 'Graveside Thoughts Upon the Spanish Flu,' in which the central character is the grandfather Ralph never knew, because he died of the flu. The section concludes with Paul Pickering's aptly-titled play, 'Long-Term Perspective,' in which a centenarian long-term care home resident, a survivor of the 1918 flu pandemic, discovers some interesting connections she has to her male nurse, who's young enough to be her great-grandson.

Lessons from History
Elizabeth Hoffman, Jeanette Grant
and Ann McMillan

According to Merriam-Webster, a pandemic is 'an outbreak of disease that occurs over a wide geographical area… and typically affects a significant proportion of the population' (Merriam-Webster, n.d). Without a doubt, COVID-19 meets the definition. It is not the first outbreak to do so.

COVID-19 was one of the biggest stories in the entire world for 2020 (Cowen, 2020). No weapon in any country's armament had the power to stop it as it rampaged from east to west and to every corner of the earth. It paused the economy of the planet as humankind hid at home awaiting the pandemic's next move. None of us could see it with our naked eye, but we knew it was out there waiting to kill and injure. World news spurred by UN agencies such as the World Health Organization (WHO) alerted us to COVID-19's potential in early 2020 and scientists sent its characteristics throughout the world (WHO, 2020). Health departments everywhere became aware of the possibility of pandemic as the virus moved. Our century had the advantage of scientific knowledge and the support of medical experts and facilities to care for the ill and learn about the disease that older civilizations did not. But have we learned what we could from the previous pandemics we have experienced? Are there lessons that we could have learned to improve how we have responded? Our response has often been linear and predictable, and raises some questions for planners of future pandemic response (Kolata, 2020; Ratliff, 2020; Schmidt and Undark, 2020; and Shiller, 2020).

We know that there were prehistoric pandemics from evidence of fossils and burial sites in Africa and northern Europe. We are fascinated by our Neanderthal ancestors who lived during the period 30,000 to 50,000 BCE. We had thought that Homo Sapiens somehow swept in and eliminated the Neanderthal. Recent evidence shows, however, that most of us with non-African ancestors have Neanderthal genes. Further, there is evidence that COVID-19 is less prevalent with more of those genes. It is possible that the Neanderthal succumbed to a disease that did not also decimate Homo Sapiens. In fact, pandemics have played a more defining role in our history than we generally credit them with (Jarus, 2020; Wade, 2018; Zhang, 2018).

For as long as humans have shared space with animals, they have shared similar germs and diseases. Bubonic plague, measles, smallpox, cholera, yellow fever, malaria and influenza, all major sources of pandemics, can be traced to interactions between humans and animals and their wastes and infestations. Mosquitoes, fleas, ticks, monkeys, rodents, deer, horses, humans and now bats can all be vectors of transmission (Kahn and Burdeau, 2021; McMillen, 2016; Owen, 2020; Rosenwald, 2021).

The earliest evidence of a particular disease-causing mass death is provided by DNA taken from burial sites in Sweden and China from about 3,000 BCE. It provides the first evidence of the bubonic plague bacteria, *Yersinia pestis*, which would cause havoc many centuries later. *Yersinia pestis* may have been associated with a decline of settlements as the Stone Age gave way to the Bronze Age, as well as the mass migrations that accompanied that transition. We do know that the rise of settled agriculture brought Homo Sapiens and their domestic animals closer together, as they tended to live together and exchange diseases (Callaway, 2018; Szalay, 2016; Wade and Zhang, 2018).

There was a series of Egyptian Plagues, described in the Bible. Ten plagues are reported in Exodus, but most scholars agree that this isn't a historical account. However, it is difficult to separate the fact from the myth (Green and Symes, 2014; Jarus, 2020; Rosenwald, 2021).

The first well-documented plague occurred in Athens, Greece, in 430 BCE (Kahn and Burdeau, 2021). Athens at that time was at its height, a city of over 250,000 souls. Warriors returning from battles abroad brought the plague home. Ethiopia, Egypt, Libya and the territory of the Persian King were hit, but nowhere, according to Thucydides, an Athenian, was the effect greater than in the heat of summer in the crowded hovels of Athens.

War had broken out in the Greek world with Athens and her allies in one camp and the Peloponnesian city of Sparta and her allies in the other. Athenian strength was mainly sea power while the Peloponnesians excelled with land forces. With the coming of summer, the Peloponnesians, under the command of the Spartan King, Archidamus, invaded Athens. They set about devastating the countryside in the traditional manner (Mackie, 2020; Szalay, 2016; Thucydides, c.400 BCE).

Pericles, the Athenian general who was in charge of the war strategy, had built walls down to and including the port of Piraeus. These walls allowed the Athenians to withstand enemy land attacks since food supplies came in through the harbour, so ravaging the fields did not compel the residents to go forth and battle in the plains as with previous wars. Farm animals were shipped to the island of Euboea and all the country people of Attica crowded into Athens, which was already crowded. For the newcomers from the country there was no decent housing. The streets were narrow and hygienic conditions deteriorated as the numbers grew. The wealthy fled, but the poor were crowded tightly together so that disease was easily transmissible. (Huremović, 2019; Littman, 1969; Jarus, 2020; Mackie, 2020; and Thucydides, c. 400 BCE).

Then, men who had returned from battles in Egypt brought the plague into Piraeus, from whence it quickly spread into the upper city. Thucydides wrote:

> People in perfect health suddenly began to have burning feelings in the head; their eyes became red and inflamed; inside their mouths there was bleeding from the throat and tongue, and the breath became unnatural and unpleasant. The next symptoms were sneezing and hoarseness of voice, and before long the pain settled in the chest, and was accompanied by coughing. Next the stomach was affected with stomach-aches and with vomitings of every kind of bile that has been given a name by the medical profession, all this being accompanied by great pain and difficulty. In most cases there were attacks of ineffectual retching, producing violent spasms; this sometimes ended with this stage of the disease, but sometimes continued long afterwards. Externally the body was not very hot to the touch, nor was there any pallor: the skin was rather reddish and livid, breaking out into small pustules and ulcers. But inside there was a feeling of burning, so that people could not bear the touch even of the lightest linen clothing, but wanted to be completely naked, and indeed most of all would have liked to plunge into cold water. Many of the sick who were uncared for actually did so, plunging into the water-tanks in an effort to relieve a thirst which was unquenchable; for it was just the same with them whether they drank much or little. Then all the time they were afflicted with insomnia and the desperate feeling of not being able to keep still. In the period when the disease was at its height, the body, so far from wasting away, showed surprising powers of resistance to all the agony, so that there was still some strength left on the seventh or eighth day, which was the time when, in most cases, death came from the internal fever. But if people survived this critical period, then the disease descended to the bowels, producing violent ulceration and uncontrollable diarrhea, so that most of them died later as a result of the weakness caused by this. For the disease, first settling in the head, went on to affect every part of the body in turn, and even when people escaped its worst effects, it still left its traces on them by fastening upon the extremities of the body. It affected the genitals, the fingers and the toes, and many of those who recovered lost the use of these members; some, too, went blind. There were some also who, when they first began to get better, suffered from a total loss of memory, not knowing who they were themselves and being unable to recognize their friends?'
>
> (Thucydides, 1954 translation, chapter 2, pp 49 and 52)

Even with the clear descriptions of Thucydides, we do not fully understand what disease caused the Athenian Plague. Various researchers support smallpox, measles, bubonic plague, typhus, Rift Valley fever and ergotism (Huremović, 2019; Littman, 1969; Jarus, 2020; Mackie, 2020). Any of these would have been made worse by the cramped conditions.

From all the deaths, moral decay and hopelessness in Athens there came one small benefit. The Peloponnesians left Attica earlier than they had intended because they were afraid of the infection. Still, never again would Athens rise to such heights as leader of an empire as she had occupied before the onset of the plague (Kagan, 2003). Later, as the Roman Empire grew in population and influence, there were several plagues. The Antonine Plague of 165 to 180 AD, during the reign of Marcus Aurelius, was caused possibly by smallpox (Watts, 2020). It was preceded by a Chinese epidemic and was brought by armies and traders returning from Asia. Physician Galen, the most revered medic of his time, recognized the importance of hygiene to health. He described five million deaths in total, as many as 2,000 per day (Flemming, 2019, and Littman, 1973).

This pandemic is viewed by some as the beginning of the end of the Pax Romana and the Roman Empire. It is also thought to have contributed to the spread of Christianity. While there were few Christians at the start of the plague, they cared for patients and shared their faith while preaching about the existence of an afterlife, an appealing thought at the time (Rosenwald, 2021, and Zinsser, 1950).

The Cyprian Plague of 249 to 262 AD was similar to the Antonine Plague and was described by Saint Cyprian. It was characterized by dysentery, loss of motor skills and fever, and bleeding from all orifices. Its origin is still debated, but may have been either influenza or a hemorrhagic fever like Ebola. It moved from Asia to Alexandria and from there across the whole empire (Harper, 2017 a & b; Rosenwald, 2021).

The Justinian Plague of 541 to 542 AD followed. It was named for Emperor Justinian, who survived it. This plague moved across the Asian Steppes and killed 35 to 100 million people, about half the combined population of Europe, the Middle East and North Africa. It was the bubonic plague, spread primarily by rats and fleas. Substantial depopulation of townspeople and farmers throughout the Mediterranean, Europe and Eurasia resulted. It is seen as a harbinger of the Dark Ages (Rosenwald, 2021; Zeigler, 2016). Recent research indicates that the bubonic plague became endemic in European mountain marmots at this time (Green and Symes, 2014).

The Black Death of 1348 was also bubonic plague, spread by rats and fleas. It started in China in 1331, with half of the population dying of it. The Mongol empire established by Genghis Kahn, who had died in 1227 AD, began to decline as a result. The plague spread along the Silk Road, which linked the Middle East and Asia to the western world and Mediterranean trade routes. Fleas could live in bolts of textiles such as silk or wool. Marmots were the source of the 14th century fur trade and the fleas could live in their furs as well, long enough to survive transport along the Silk Road. Once unloaded and spread out, the fleas would leave the textiles and furs to feast on local black rats that lived with humans. One of the first signs of a new infection was the death of large numbers of rats, followed by the fleas biting humans (Green and Symes, 2014; Lawler, 2016; and Szalay, 2016).

The pandemic spread by transition to a pneumonic form, spread by coughed droplets, like today's coronavirus. There were other forms as well, including septicaemic and gastrointestinal. Approximately 75 to 200 million people, or one-third to one-half the population of Europe, died with some large cities experiencing 70% mortality (Green and Symes, 2014).

One contributing factor to the severity of the Black Death was the worldwide cooling temperatures in the late 13th and 14th centuries. This created a favourable environment for plague propagation in the central Asian high plateaus where the plague was endemic. This cooling also contributed to sudden harvest failures in Europe, which impacted people's diet. Cooling temperatures continued and are now referred to as the Little Ice Age of 1303 to 1830 (Green and Symes, 2014).

Deaths of that magnitude caused major social and economic upheaval. Peasants died in larger proportions than the nobility, who could flee. That led to a labour shortage, giving the peasants greater economic power. Land became cheaper than labour and sheep substituted for row crops. Still, feudal lords tried to impose their will on peasants (Cantor, 2014; Kahn and Burdeau, 2021; Rosenwald, 2021; and Tuchman, 2011).

In Britain, the economic effects of the plague worried the government, and in 1351 Parliament ratified the Statute of Labourers, which set up a rigorous system of wage and price fixing to prevent servants from charging excessive wages. A wide range of labourers were prevented from charging more than the pre-plague prices for their goods or work. They were also committing a crime if they did not serve those who required them. As demand for workers grew, the law quickly became unworkable. Ambitious and wealthy villagers began to dress smartly and affect the appearance of their betters. Parliament approved a re-issue of the 25-year-old sumptuary laws in an attempt to preserve a visible distinction between the classes, restricting the wearing of furs or the popular pointed toe shoes, and also restricting what the lower classes could eat (Jones, 2009).

Peasants revolted in the 1370s, and then migrated to towns where they could be free. This cadre of newly free people contributed to the decline of the Feudal system and supported the flourishing of science, art and literature and the eventual 15th century Renaissance (Cantor, 2014; Lambrecht, 2019; Tuchman, 2011).

The spread of disease became associated with trade, while pressure increased to find an alternative to the Silk Road by sailing west to what we now know as the West Indies, or south along the west coast of Africa, in hopes of finding an alternate route to India and China. Both Columbus' first voyage to what became known in Europe as the New World, and the Portuguese voyages around the Cape of Good Hope, were undertaken in search of better trade routes to Asia (Newitt, 2005).

During the 16th and 17th centuries, the population of the New World was wiped out by plagues. It is estimated that 80 to 95% of the indigenous population of North, Central and South America died due to smallpox, influenza and measles. Measles was highly contagious, affecting 90% of people exposed, and deadly in a population that had never been exposed and had no herd immunity (Huremović, 2019; Daschuk, 2019).

According to a 2010 paper in the *Journal of Economic Perspectives*, 'Historian and demographer... David Cook estimates that, in the end, the regions least affected lost 80% of their populations; those most affected lost their full populations; and a typical society lost 90% of its population' (Cook, 1998; Nunn and Qian, 2010).

This depopulation may have been a reason that Europeans were first welcomed at Plymouth and Jamestown. It may also have encouraged Europeans to settle farther and farther west (Daschuk, 2019). Finally, the slave trade began because the natives were dying and the conquistadors needed labour. Also, free European immigrants could become landowners themselves, which increased the demand for labour to develop and work plantations (Cook, 1998).

The plague hit Alghero, Sardinia in 1582, brought by travellers, probably from Marseilles. It reportedly killed 60% of the city's population. A doctor named Quinto Tiberio Angelerio stepped forward to help; he had come from Sicily, where there had been a plague epidemic in 1575. When plague patients came forward to him, he pushed hard to quarantine them. Eventually, with the support of the viceroy, a triple sanitary cordon was set up around the city to prevent outsiders from trading. Although the death toll was high in the city, the disease did not spread to surrounding regions. In the booklet *Ectypa pestilentis status Algheriae sardiniae* he described his approach. All meetings and entertainments had been forbidden, only one person per household could go shopping, and citizens were advised not to leave their houses. Six-foot-long canes were to be carried so people would keep their distance. Rails were added to shop counters to maintain distance. Angelerio even understood the possibility that the disease could be transmitted on the surfaces of items, and instructed that houses be disinfected, whitewashed, and ventilated. Suspect textiles were disinfected by smoke. Finally, Angelerio assigned specific tasks such as digging graves to those who had survived the plague, since these were known to be high-risk jobs (Gorvett, 2021).

From 1665 to 1667, Oxford and Cambridge closed due to the plague. Sir

11

Isaac Newton was a student at Cambridge and while home from the quarantine he did much of the research on gravity, calculus and optics that became his magnum opus, *Principia* (Fara, 2018). He referred to 1666 to '67 as his Year of Wonders, the title of a fictionalized account by Geraldine Brooks of the town of Eyam, which became infected by the plague as the result of a tailor ordering bolts of cloth from London. Encouraged by two ministers, one Puritan and the other Anglican, the residents of Eyam voted to quarantine themselves for the duration of the plague to prevent spreading the disease to other villages. They even held church services and other meetings outside when the weather permitted. The Earl of Devonshire agreed to provide provisions if the town enforced its quarantine. About half of the residents of Eyam died (Brooks, 2002). Clearly, people then understood the basic nature of disease transmission and how to control its spread through distancing and isolation.

By 1720, the city of Venice, Italy, had set up a quarantine program involving all of the port cities around the Italian peninsula, including Marseilles, France. A ship known to be carrying the plague left Lebanon, stopping in Cyprus and Greece, before heading to Italy. Venice alerted cities and harbour-masters to turn the ship away or burn it in the harbour; there are letters in the Venetian archives demonstrating compliance with this advice. When the ship reached Marseilles, it was first quarantined in the harbour and was about to be turned away or burned. But Marseilles was suffering from famine and people clamoured to at least unload the grain. Merchants wanted the silks and cloth aboard. As a result of the decision to unload the ship, 50,000 people died in the city, as did another 50,000 from surrounding cities and towns. Finally, a virtual wall was erected around the city and countryside and leaving the city was made punishable by death (Cippolla, 1981). This incident confirmed the understanding of disease transmission and the measures that would be necessary to control the spread.

By the 17th and 18th centuries, the underlying cause of the plague was still unknown. Most educated people, however, knew that bolts of cloth and transported grain spread the plague. They knew that quarantines and social distancing helped to prevent spread. They also knew that face coverings helped to prevent spread, since they helped to contain the pneumonic form of the plague, which accounted for pandemic spread (Cippolla, 1981; Green and Symes, 2014).

The last bubonic plague epidemic started in China in 1855, and spread to India, Hong Kong in 1894, Hawaii in 1899, and finally San Francisco in 1900. It caused 10 to 15 million deaths, mostly in India. During this plague, the bacterium (*Yersinia pestis*), which causes plague, was finally discovered in 1894 by Alexandre Yersin, working in Hong Kong (Achtman, *et. al.*, 2004). The knowledge of the source of the infection has led to effective controls which, along with the discovery of antibiotics, have essentially eliminated the threat of this disease (Achtman, *et. al.*, 2004; Green and Symes, 2014).

In addition to the bubonic plague, there were pandemics of cholera, typhoid fever and yellow fever in Europe and the Americas in the 18th and 19th centuries. Both cholera and typhoid fever are spread by dirty drinking water; thus, sewers and safe water supplies virtually eliminated cholera in North America and Europe (Harvard, c.2020; Marineli, et. al, 2013). Yellow fever was brought to the New World by the slave trade. It is endemic in Africa and spread by mosquitoes there. Draining swamps and eliminating a particular African mosquito vector (*Aedes aegypti*) in North America eliminated the threat (Prinzi, 2021). However, yellow fever caused a major epidemic in Philadelphia in 1793 with nine percent of the population dying (Fenn, 2001).

The Spanish Flu was so-called because only Neutral Spain reported on it during World War I. This flu was actually caused by the H1N1 type-A influenza virus with pneumonia and bacterial infection complications. While the initial source is disputed, it was spread rapidly by troops moving and then returning home from World War I. The 'Spanish Flu' was made worse by malnutrition and wounds of war, so young men and pregnant women suffered the highest mortality from it. Eventually, about 500 million people around the world were infected, which was about one-third of the world's population. Estimates of death range from 17 million to 100 million, making this one of the deadliest pandemics in history. The flu came in four waves: Spring, 1918; Fall, 1918 (the deadliest wave); Spring, 1919; and Spring, 1920. Fall, 2018 coincided with Armistice Day, November 11 (Bristow, 2012; Porter, 1965; and Taubenberger and Morens, 2020).

Philadelphia did not cancel a Liberty Loan parade on September 28, 1918 and 200,000 people attended. More than 12,000 people died in the next six weeks. St. Louis did cancel and had only 500 deaths. This was another difficult lesson about the necessity to isolate and socially distance to avoid spreading disease (Barro, 2020).

And what about today? Do we need to fear the diseases that have caused pandemics in the past? Smallpox, measles, cholera, yellow fever, typhoid fever and the flu all have vaccines that are effective against them. Arguably, the development of vaccines has been one of the most significant contributions of medical science to the health of populations, since they limit the spread of our most contagious diseases (Snowden, 2019).

The plague is now better understood, and although a few cases occur world-wide each year they are treatable with antibiotics. Also, with modern hygiene and avoiding touching dead animals and being bitten by fleas, cases are rare (Green and Symes, 2014).

There are a number of similarities amongst all the pandemics discussed. Rapid and efficient disease transmission was a factor in the seriousness of the outbreak. The wealthy could often escape to second homes or to the homes of family members who lived in less densely populated places where they could socially distance. The poor, the infirm, the malnourished and marginalized, and those who could not escape high densities were usually hit the hardest (Rosenwald, 2021; Snowden, 2019).

People hate quarantines and will violate them if possible. During the London quarantine, plague houses were nailed shut, while during the Marseilles pandemic people would be killed if they tried to leave. Some people comply, some believe rumours and false information, some blame the 'Other', some throw caution to the winds, and some join religious cults… every time! (Cippolla, 2012; Green and Symes, 2014; Johnson, 2006).

Back in the time of the Athenian plague, Thucydides observed that:

> The catastrophe was so overwhelming that men, not knowing what would happen next to them, became indifferent to every rule of religion or of law. All the funeral ceremonies which used to be observed were now disorganized, and they buried the dead as best they could.

He continued:

> [There began] a state of unprecedented lawlessness… It was generally agreed that what was both honourable and valuable was the pleasure of the moment and everything that might conceivably contribute to that pleasure. No fear of god or law of man had a restraining influence. As for the gods, it seemed to be the same thing whether one worshipped them or not, when one saw the good and the bad dying indiscriminately.

(Thucydides, c. 400 BCE)

This behaviour was also common in later accounts of plagues, and we can see similar tendencies today as rules about isolation and societal closures have tightened.

Most programs developed to control the spread of COVID have been based on past history and on science. Isolation and quarantine have been common elements, as have distancing and preventing droplet spread. While in the time of COVID-19 we have had conspiracy theories surrounding the virus to challenge the health experts, most of us believed what facts were given us by government leaders. 'No-mask' groups march but most of us play it safe and cover our faces. Partying is seen as not a good idea when public records show how the disease spreads in these venues, and public exposure shames party goers. Both knowledge and shaming have mainly eliminated licentiousness.

In much of the world medical and health experts have been heard and respected. While, as in many past pandemics, the exact nature of the disease being fought was at first not known, uncertainty was reduced as the pandemic progressed. The tried-and-true approaches: restrict movement, isolate, maintain distance and wear masks, and adapt workers have worked well.

With vaccines on the scene in 2021, hope is returning to the world. The isolation that has kept many of us alive will end. Health officials broadcast improvements daily through the news media. Memories and stories of COVID-19 will fade, just as all the others have done, until the next pandemic drags it back into the present. We should try to remember that there will be a next time, and make sure that we continue to be careful in indoor settings, particularly those involving large numbers of people, so that the 'next time' will be later rather than sooner.

References

Achtman, M., G. Morelli, P. Zhu, T. Wirth, et al. 2004. 'Microevolution and History of the Plague Bacillus, *Yersinia pestis*,' *Proceedings of the National Academy of Sciences* 101, no. 51: 17837–

Barro, Robert J. (2020), 'Non-Pharmaceutical Interventions and Mortality in U.S. Cities during the Great Influenza Pandemic, 1918-1919, NBER Working Paper #27049, available at: https://www.nber.org/papers/w27049

Bristow, Nancy K. (2012), *American Pandemic: The Lost Worlds of the 1918 Influenza Epidemic.* New York: Oxford University Press.

Callaway, Ewen (2015), 'Bronze Age Skeletons were Earliest Plague Victims', *Nature*, October, 22, 2015, available at: https://www.nature.com/news/bronze-age-skeletons-were-earliest-plague-victims-1.186

Cantor, Norman (2014), *In the Wake of the Plague: The Black Death and the World It Made*, Simon and Schuster.

Cippolla, Carlo (1981), *Faith, Reason, and the Plague in 17th Century Florence*, W.W. Norton.

Cook, David (1998), *Born to Die: Disease and New World Conquest, 1492-1650.* New York: Cambridge University Press, 1998.

Cowan, Lee (2020), CBS, *The year in review: Top news stories of 2020, month-by-month*, CBS News, December 27, 2020, available at: https://www.cbsnews.com/news/2020-the-year-in-review-top-news-stories-month-by-month/

Daschuk, James (2019), *Clearing the Plains: Disease, Politics of Starvation, and the Loss of Aboriginal Life*, University of Regina Press.

Fara, Patricia (2018), *Isaac Newton at Woolsthorpe Manor, National Trust*, Aylesbury.

Fenn, Elizabeth A. (2001), *Pox Americana: The Great Smallpox Epidemic of 1775-82*, Hill and Wang.

Flemming, Rebecca (2019) 'Galen and the Plague,' Caroline Petit (ed.) *Galen's Treatise Περὶ Ἀλυπίας (De indolentia) in Context*: Brill Publishing, pp. 219–244.

Gorvett, Zaria (2021) 'The 432-year-old manual on social distancing,' BBC, January 8, 2021, available at:
https://www.bbc.com/future/article/20210107-the-432-year-old-manual-on-social-distancing

Green, Monica H. and Symes, Carol (2014) 'The Medieval Globe 1 (2014) - Pandemic Disease in the Medieval World: Rethinking the Black Death,' *The Medieval Globe*, Vol. 1, No. 1, available at:
https://scholarworks.wmich.edu/tmg/vol1/iss1/1

Harper, Kyle (2017a), 'Solving the Mystery of an Ancient Roman Plague,' *Atlantic*, November 1, 2017, available at;
https://www.theatlantic.com/science/archive/2017/11/solving-the-mystery-of-an-ancient-roman-plague/543528/

Harper, Kyle (2017b), *The Fate of Rome: Climate, Disease, and the End of an Empire*, Princeton University Press.

Harvard University Library Curiosity Collection (Harvard, c. 2020), 'Cholera Epidemics in the 19th Century,' *Contagion: Historical Views of Diseases and Epidemics,* available at:
https://curiosity.lib.harvard.edu/contagion/feature/cholera-epidemics-in-the-19th-century

Huremović, Damir (2019), 'Brief History of Pandemics (Pandemics Throughout History), *Psychiatry of Pandemics,* May 16, 2019, available at:
https://www.ncbi.nlm.nih.gov/pmc/articles/PMC7123574/

Jarus, Owen (2020), '20 of the worst epidemics and pandemics in history,' *Live Science*, March 20, 2020, available at: https://www.livescience.com/

worst-epidemics-and-pandemics-in-history.html

Johnson, Steven (2006), *The Ghost Map: The Story of London's Most Terrifying Epidemic—and How It Changed Science, Cities, and the Modern World*, Riverhead Books

Jones, Dan (2009), *Summer of Blood: The Peasant's Revolt of 1381*, Harper Press.

Kagan, Donald (2003), *The Peloponnesian War*, New York: Viking.

Kahn, Robert and Burdeau, Cain (2021), 'Plagues and Humanity,' *Courthouse New Service*, July 25, 2021, available at: https://www.courthousenews.com/plagues-and-humanity/

Kolata, Gina (2020), 'How Pandemics End,' *New York Times*, May 4, 2020, available at: https://www.nytimes.com/2020/05/10/health/coronavirus-plague-pandemic-history.html

Lambrecht, Eric (2019), 'How did the Bubonic Plague make the Italian Renaissance possible?' *DailyHistory.org*, January 12, 2019, available at: https://dailyhistory.org/How_did_the_Bubonic_Plague_make_the_Italian_Renaissance_possible

Lawler, Andrew (2016), 'How Europe Exported the Black Death,' *Science*, April 26, 2016.

Littman, R.J. and M.L. (1973), 'Galen and the Antonine Plague,' *American Journal of Philology*, Vol. 94, No. 3 (Autumn, 1973), pp. 243–255.

Mackie, Chris (2020), 'Thucydides and the Plague of Athens—What It Can Teach Us Now,' *Pocket Conversation*, available at: https://getpocket.com/explore/item/thucydides-and-the-plague-of-athens-what-it-can-teach-us-now

Marineli, Filio, Tsoucalas, Gregory, Karamanou, Marianna, and Androutsos, George (2013), 'Mary Mallon (1869-1938) and the history of typhoid fever 26(2),' *Annals of Gastroenterology*, 26(2), pp. 132–134, available at: https://www.ncbi.nlm.nih.gov/pmc/articles/PMC3959940/

McMillen, Christian W. (2016), *Pandemics: A Very Short Introduction*, Oxford University Press.

Merriam-Webster. (n.d.). 'Pandemic.' In *Merriam-Webster.com dictionary*. Retrieved July 25, 2021, available at: https://www.merriam-webster.com/dictionary/pandemic

Newitt, Malyn D.D. (2005), *A History of Portuguese Overseas Expansion, 1400–1668,* Routledge.

Nunn, Nathan, and Qian, Nancy (2010). 'The Columbian Exchange: A History of Disease, Food and Ideas,' *The Journal of Economic Perspectives* 24, no. 2 (2010) pp. 163–88.

Porter, Katherine Ann (1965), 'Pale Horse, Pale Rider,' in *The Collected Stories of Katherine Ann Porter,* Harcourt Brace, originally published as a stand-alone story in 1939.

Prinzi, Andrea (2021), 'History of Yellow Fever in the U.S,' *American Society for Microbiology,* May 17, 2021, available at: https://asm.org/Articles/2021/May/History-of-Yellow-Fever-in-the-U-S

Ratliff, Evan (2020), 'We Can Protect the Economy from Pandemics. Why Didn't We?' *Wired,* June 16, 2020, available at: https://www.wired.com/story/nathan-wolfe-global-economic-fallout-pandemic-insurance/

Rosenwald, Michael S. (2021), 'History's Deadliest Pandemics, from Ancient Rome to Modern America,' *The Washington Post,* February 22, 2021. Available at: https://www.washingtonpost.com/graphics/2020/local/retropolis/coronavirus-deadliest-pandemics/

Schmidt, Charles and Undark (2020), 'Coronavirus Researchers Tried to Warn Us,' *Atlantic,* June 13, 2020, available at: https://www.theatlantic.com/health/archive/2020/06/scientists-predicted-coronavirus-pandemic/613003/

Shiller, Robert J. (2020), 'Why We Can't Yet See the Economic Effects of the Current Pandemic,' *New York Times,* August 4, 2020, available at: https://www.nytimes.com/2020/05/29/business/coronavirus-economic-forecast-shiller.html

Snowden, Frank (2019), *Epidemics and Society,* Yale University Press.

Szalay, Jessie (2016), 'Plague: A Scourge from Ancient to Modern Times,'

Live Science, June, 2016, available at:
https://www.livescience.com/55259-the-plague.html

Taubenberger, Jeffery K. and Morens, David M. (2020), 'The 1918 Influenza
Pandemic and Its Legacy,' *Cold Spring Harb Perspect Med*, available at:
http://perspectivesinmedicine.cshlp.org/content/10/10/a038695.full.pdf+html

Tuchman, Barbara (2011), *A Distant Mirror: The Calamitous 14th Century*,
Random House.

Wade, Lizzie (2018), 'Did a new form of plague destroy Europe's Stone
Age Societies?' *Science*, December 6, 2018, available at:
https://www.sciencemag.org/news/2018/12/did-new-form-plague-
destroy-europe-s-stone-age-societies

Watts, Edward (2020), 'What Rome Learned from the Deadly Antonine
Plague of 165 A.D,' *Smithsonian Magazine*, April 28, 2020.

World Health Organization (2020), *Novel Coronavirus Situation Report 1*,
January 1, 2020, available at:
https://www.who.int/docs/default-source/coronaviruse/situation-
reports/20200121-sitrep-1-2019-ncov.pdf?sfvrsn=20a99c10_4

Zeigler, Philip (2016), *The Black Death*, Horizon, New World City.

Zhang, Sarah (2018), 'Ancient DNA Is Rewriting Human (and
Neanderthal) History,' *Atlantic*, June 13, 2018, available at:
https://www.theatlantic.com/science/archive/2018/03/ancient-dna-
history/554798/

Zinsser, Hans (1950), *Rats, Lice, and History*, Boston: Little, Brown and
Company.

Graveside Thoughts Upon the Spanish Flu
Ralph Smith

Parish Priest
God's hand clapping down
on this table of parched land,
tell me Father
what have we done
or not done?
So many of our parish
levelled,
buried in blankets of sand,
is it penance for the Great War?

They believe it a Spanish invasion
and not Your armada come.
They proclaim it a new church
built on the rock of science
and not the world
of my boyhood in Ireland,
green with valleys of death,
shepherd watching over us.
Now . . .
last words must be spent,
spittle to the wind and sand—
for Frank Smith, late of our parish—
so that he may flourish tomorrow
in the company of martyrs
from the new Spanish war.

And then . . .
move along,
there's more burying to do.

The Reeve
Webb 1914 to 1918:
ten killed in action and
this year
Archie Fletcher, Dan Mozoski
Emma Braun, Lena Geisbert, Alex what's-his-name,

Ina Propp, Freddy and Wilbur White
(twins for god's sake),
all in their prime
wiped out by flu.
Soon only old-timers left
to look after the kids,
you have to be young and peachy
or wrinkled pruney
to keep going here.
You must hunker down in your shack
with prairie sand and clay
coming through the chinks
blowing off this hungry graveyard—
seems we can't feed it enough.

I passed a few words
with Frank Smith,
farm dirt all over him,
quiet except when fuddled
with homebrew.
Sad there's not a penny
left in the village purse
for this poor woman and so,
donations?
No, Anglican though she be,
dad and boys R.C.,
most folks here don't go with that
and their church
so I'm told
is flat broke.

But I'm showing up gravely for the village,
price to pay for public office.
I just wish there was no
darned sand swarming up
from all those fresh graves
and me breathing in bits of flu.

Maude, Wife
Oh he could sing lovely
Irish tunes when he left off
the horse and the plough,
gave himself to a glass

21

or two of poteen
of his own making
but
who will mind the still now?

My husband's Irish temper
and I have felt the back of his hand,
that same hand that caressed me
gave me comfort in our poverty.
Why did he go out so soon
to the land?

He was over the worst,
and I had just washed his thick hair
when he said he was going out,
no woman could keep him longer
indoors
he was called out to the land
and brought shivering back by his brother,
Frank with his fever again.

My poor Ralph staring at a gravestone,
your father no longer your pal.
My poor Raymond, red and crying
in my arms,
the green of your father's days
will not lighten your way.
But my boys
you will hear of my English past,
you descend from Blood.

While your father's father and his father's father
were wild and angry,
my family quietly powerfully
ruled.

Joseph, Brother
Jesus Joseph and Mary
shite on this hole,
may Plague take
houses   whores
cows   cousins
mules   mothers

wheat   winters
guts   gophers
and   each
and   everyone
but

in fine flesh
deliver brother Frank back
to where we would climb
wind-worn rocks
long shanks down
into fiery foam
brawny breakers
a smell like semen and
fiery fathoms down where
whales and worlds were
ours for hours.

We didn't come here for this
you kept back from the war
with your flat feet and
me conscripted then
meandering back minus one leg
and our allotments dry,
only a few cents to be wrung out of them,
a waste of seed and horseflesh.

That English bitch Anglican witch
besotted you Frank
and she shall not
raise those boys:
me and our brothers
in Ireland
will see it done
in the name of father.

Ralph, Oldest Son
'...live in your presents'
What's the priest saying?
I can't think while Uncle Joe
keeps pushing his hand down
on my shoulder like he's holding
me up when it's t'other way round.

Ralph Smith

Gopher hiding over there by a stone,
could he be from down
where the coffins are stuck in muck
chewing in through the rotten wood
helping himself to a meal?

Last summer dad and me
right by here shooting gophers
wait and wait hardly breathing
the smell of his sweat
smooth match stroke on box
puffs of smoke out his nose
me with the twenty-two trained on a hole
hot finger on cold trigger
then, a crunching behind me
and I fire, raising a little brown cloud
turn and uncle's loping over
leaning on that stick of his
'Waste of good ammunition!'
He's cross, words come out his mouth
like he was spitting tobacco juice.

Dad gives him a look.

'Next year I'll take the boy deer hunting,'
he says.

Mrs Austen, Mother In-Law
Maudie my only daughter
you lapped up my tales like they were Devon cream
while steaming over the ocean
and even here
watching my husband Archie out the window—
his whole life a store clerk in Holsworthy—
now trying to be a farmer
and oh we would laugh at the old boy
and I promised a prince of true blood
would come to enchant you away.
Instead came Frank
with his peasant Irish song
and yet—to do him justice—
he was kind to me after Archie passed.

24

That first night when you took me in
I went out in the dark to pee
fell into the ice cellar—
you left off the top my dreamy forgetful daughter—
and I'm dazed, literally seeing
more stars than there were at sky's tunnel
cold, revulsed by animal stink
I reach and feel something hard
grab and pull
a whole load comes down
beast's sinewy sticky skin
hoof like a devil's
I scream and scream.

A light like second coming
bearded face beaming down
bearing a lantern
me down there dancing with
a deer's shank

Frank with a ladder
down he climbs
don't cry mom
lifts me out.

Raymond, New-Born
Sailing in my vessel
I heard once
then again again
songs from land ahead,
rhythms that matched
two heart beats
mine and yours.

That was before the
sea rose with urgent straining
and I was storm-gulfed
ropes ripping, wind whirling
twisted tossed tormented
then came brightness that blinded
and a labored launch
soft words of the singer, your pained shouts
and opening my mouth what came out

25

was my first cry, a lament
an exorcism of dry land.

Now cradled in your breasts
I may be safe in port
but it is cold for all that
and the voice of the singer
is replaced by babble –
this is weird
as they suppose I babble!

Your heartbeat now my only song
it is fast, strained,
it is my other self
and so . . .
is it the pain of another birth?

Frank, The Dead
In the beginning there was void
and the body was all.

There were fever-fled flesh and bones
microbes dismounting
and yet
feeling was given
yes, a sense of touch
and no vision or hearing
smell stoppered, thank god
and names have flown away
like frightened flocks of birds
yet there's weight pressing down
from the ground above
a circle
but not joined
hearts not beating together.
Flesh memories:
rain and wind on hair
rough fingers on child's feather-soft palm
horse muscles pulsing inner thighs
woman skin sliding on man skin.

Weight lessening now
and movement is outward

something above ending
and circle expands
on flat fallow land
rolls away like iron wheels
spreading, shaking
expanding ocean to ocean
then shakes two rough terrains
and gently rocks prairie and emerald isle
with touch light as goose feather
then finally
lifts off.

The 'Parish Priest' verses of this poem were first published in *The Prairie Journal*, issue Number 61, 20.

Long-Term Perspective
Paul Pickering

CHARACTERS

MAUDE JENNER: an extremely old woman, quite positive, and she tends to speak slowly. Maude is dressed well, if in a slightly outdated style. She wears a colourful mask around her neck.

RANESH: a male nurse, youthful, somewhere between 25 and 35, of Indian background. Ranesh wears a standard nurse's outfit. He wears a standard blue medical mask around his neck.

SETTING

A care facility, bedroom; mid-morning. There is a simple bed by the wall, a chair and a side table. There is a box of tissues on the table next to a framed photograph of an old man, and a clock turned away from the audience.

COVID19 has spared this facility thus far, by a combination of luck and the facility's engaging in progressive precautions.

TIME

It is October 2020.

SCENES

SCENE 1: Mid-afternoon

SCENE 2: Mid-morning, the next day

As the play starts, Maude is sitting up, in her bed, squinting, reading a book. Every 10 seconds or so she glances at the clock and after the 4th time, puts down her book and rolls her eyes.

SCENE 1

MAUDE

(*Impatient*) Where *is* that boy? (*Maude looks down further on her page and frowns. Then suddenly smiles at the door, as Ranesh enters. She pulls on her mask*)

RANESH (*Crosses to Maude's bed, carrying a crossword puzzle book, a glass of juice, and a pair of glasses, all of which he arranges on the table. His mask is around his neck. He gives her a big smile, and sits in the chair next to her*)

RANESH

Hi Maude, how is my favourite resident this morning?

MAUDE

(*Looking at Ranesh with caution*) Ranesh, why are you not wearing your mask? I've not lived this long to die of something silly.

RANESH

(*With a big smile, he leans forward a little*) Maude, I'm staying on-site; I am in your bubble. I tell you every day. (*He pulls up his mask to his mouth*) Have you been outside? Do you want me to put it on?

MAUDE

(*Smiling a little*) Just checking. If you've been on-site that's fine. You really ought to stay with your husband, though——he will find a replacement for you if you are never there! (*Pause*) I worry!

RANESH

(*Drops his mask with an open-handed gesture and a smile*) Serge and I are fine. We Zoom every day. I see our children, we smile, we hug, we kiss. (*Kisses the air*) They know how important my work is, and they know it's not forever.

MAUDE

Just keep reassuring me, OK? You are a dear boy. I feel so very attached to you, but your own family is terribly important.

RANESH

Of course, Maude. (*Hands her the glasses and the crossword*) I don't know how you can read without these, but I'm sure you want them back. They were in the reading room. And I brought you a new Times crossword collection.

MAUDE

(*Takes the crossword and smiles. Puts her hands to her eyes and realizes her glasses are not there. Looking at her glasses, Maude shakes her head and closes her eyes a moment*) Again!

RANESH

(*Leans back a little*) The world's gone crazy Maude. You'd think wearing a mask or keeping physical distance would be a no-brainer for everyone. Serge says he gets bad looks and comments whenever the kids are with him on walks, and it's actually worse when they wear masks. Worst pandemic of modern times, and people forget how to behave properly.

MAUDE

It was worse last time.

RANESH

What do you mean, Maude?

MAUDE

The pandemic after the war. More died, and people wanted to behave normally—just like they do now. But we got through it, and life goes on. We'll get through it again. Well, you will. (*Smiles at Ranesh*) I might not last that long! Your kids will just have vague memories of it, kind of like I do.

RANESH

(*Leaning forward, looking at Maude*) Maude, are you talking about the Spanish flu? After World War I? You were alive then?

MAUDE

(*Looking a little amused, and smiling*) Well, what else? Of course, I was alive. And don't blame the Spanish for that one. No one deserves that kind of blame.

RANESH

Oh my. (*Pause*) I had no idea. (*Looks at Maude as if seeing a different woman*) Maude that was 1918. How old were you?

MAUDE

(*Deep sigh*) Ranesh, it was a long time ago, and it hurts to go there. But I do care for you, dear boy, and you ask for the right reason, so give me a moment. (*Closes her eyes, takes a couple deep breaths, and settles into herself. When she opens her eyes, she sees Ranesh and smiles, and looks somehow stronger*) My father was a soldier in the Great War, as we now call it. He somehow came back in one piece. Well, physically anyway. He lost part of himself of course. He had awful dreams. (*Pausing, as in reflection*) That was common. (*Pause*) My uncles didn't come home at all. I was the youngest: three years old when Poppa came home. That was my first memory really: Poppa coming home and Momma crying. (*Smiles*) We were happy for a while. But then Poppa and Momma started acting upset and scared. We children had to stay inside and my older brother didn't go to school anymore. (*Takes a deep breath*) Momma got a cough, and then my brothers got it. All three were coughing, and then they were just gone. (*Pause*) Poppa couldn't stop crying. (*Pause*) It was just me and Poppa for a while. Then he got the cough and he was gone too. The flu took them all. My aunts and cousins too. *(Maude takes a deep breath, and takes a tissue and blows her nose. Ranesh looks stricken)*

(Maude smiles at Ranesh, takes a tissue and daps her eyes with it) Do you mind if I keep going? Somehow, I feel you should know this.

RANESH

(Takes a tissue and lightly blows his nose, pauses, and blows it again) Only if you want to, Maude. I had no idea. *(Speaks softly and leans a bit forward, looking at her)* I do want to hear this.

MAUDE

(Giving Ranesh a queer look, she then smiles and shakes her head) Your behaviours do sometimes puzzle me. It's as if I know you more than I do. *(Looks past Ranesh for several seconds, remembering. Then slowly starts speaking)* I was such a small girl, and had no family. I had no idea what was going on around me. I could have ended up anywhere, but one of my father's war buddies came to get me and adopted me. We moved here to Hamilton, and life began again.

RANESH

There was no other family?

MAUDE

Not that I ever knew. But Poppa Matthew and Momma Lilah became my family. I was their only daughter. They were as good to me as they could have been to any child. We were not typical, of course, and everyone knew that by looking at us.

RANESH

How would people know? You can't tell by looking... unless the children are... *(Stops talking and looks surprised)*.

MAUDE

Like yours? Adopted? Of a different background? *(Gives a lovely smile)* Ranesh, that was us! Poppa Matthew and Momma Lilah looked like you. They were born here, but their families were from India. It was pretty unusual in those day for Indian-looking parents to have a girl who looked like me.

RANESH

(Speechless. Long pause) Tell me more please, Maude. I can't quite believe all this.

31

MAUDE

I grew up with them. I always knew of my first family, of course, and I always knew I was fully loved by both. I grew up in a wonderful community and my parents were such amazing people. Poppa Matthew could not have children because of the war, so I was their only child. I thought my life would end when Poppa Matthew and Momma Lilah died. But I was an adult by then, and life does go on.

RANESH

How did they die, Maude?

MAUDE

(*Speaking a bit softer, exhales slowly*) They had moved to Florida for work. They co-ran a shipping company. It was after I was out of school—it was a great success for them, and they loved it. The Homestead Hurricane it was called, 1945, they both died in their home during the storm. (*Pauses, and sees her juice for the first time. Takes a long slow sip. Visibly shaken, puts the juice back and smiles weakly. Dabs a tissue to each eye*) Such sad days when I think of them.

RANESH

(*Looks very sad*) I should let you rest. (*Stands*) You've told me quite a story, and I'm really thankful. You have had a full life.

MAUDE

(*Nodding, and then puts up her hand to stop Ranesh*) No, Ranesh. Wait. My life is not a tragedy and I want to finish with something more joyful.

RANESH

Maude—it's enough, I don't want you to get overtired. We can talk more tomorrow if you want.

MAUDE

(*Smiling*) No, it's important. You have other things to do, but you will be talking to that lovely, caring man of yours this evening and I expect you'll want to tell him something I have told you. I'm the storyteller today, so let me talk a few more minutes. (*Pauses. Then speaks playfully*) What else would I be doing today?

RANESH

(*Sitting back down in his chair*) Well, you are fascinating, and lovely as always, and I am not sure about this, so promise me you will not overtire yourself.

MAUDE

I promise, dear boy. (*Pause. Puts a firm hand on her juice and takes a sip, while looking at Ranesh*) When I was about 20, Poppa Matthew and Momma Lilah decided that I was going to work out OK. Or so they enjoyed telling me. (*Pause*) They said they had the chance to extend our family, so they spent the next few years sponsoring one of Momma Lilah's cousins and his family, from India. I remember it so well. It was all colonial then, of course, and the family was able to get to England easily enough. The city they went to had a funny name, but I forget it now. Getting to Canada was difficult, though. By then we had been through the Depression of course and the war years were starting. A lot of people were trying to find better places to live. We didn't have as much money as we were accustomed to, but Poppa Matthew and Momma Lilah said this was essential, so we cashed in everything we could. We got them here, and they became family. (*Pause. Takes a sip of juice. Smiles*).

(*Ranesh sits very still and watches Maude, enraptured*).

I watched their children grow up, get married, and have their own children. My husband and I were so blessed to be part of their lives, and after I lost my parents, I guess we became the centre of the family. (*Pause*) Such wonderful memories. (*Pauses and looks at Ranesh as if from a distance*) Those wonderful cousins have all passed on, and even many of their children have. There are so many grandchildren and great-grandchildren I am afraid I have lost track of them, and they of me, but they had such brave and kind grandparents I know they are making the world a better place. (*Leans back in her bed, with a big smile*).

RANESH

(*Speaking softly and looking at Maude tenderly*) Before COVID, you weren't getting many visitors. I didn't realize you had a family.

MAUDE

Well, two of my children have died, and the other two live so far away. They don't like to travel, and can't now, of course. We do talk from time to time.

RANESH

Tell me about your family, Maude.

MAUDE

I was married to such a lovely man. We met when he moved to Hamilton after getting his engineering degree from Waterloo. I finished my own

33

studies and we had a few years of working, and then started on our four children. There were cousins everywhere it seemed, no matter where we were. It was glorious. Everything for me goes back to what I learned most from Poppa Matthew and Momma Lilah. Family is essential.

RANESH

(Tearing up, and reaching for another tissue) Maude, that's beautiful. Thank you. *(Pause. Looks at her carefully. Speaking slowly)* Maude, what were the names of those first cousins? The ones who came from India?

MAUDE

(Surprised) Their names? Samuel and Rita. Why?

RANESH

(Catches his breath a little) I'm wondering about something. What was your husband's name?

MAUDE

(A little pleased, and a little confused) My husband's name? Luke. Luke Jenner. *(Smiles at her memory of Luke)* What makes you ask?

RANESH

(Pause… speaking carefully.) I'm just wondering about something. *(Speaking normally)* Maude, you've been amazing with your story, but I have to insist you rest. I'll be back tomorrow. You have given me so much to think about, and yes, to tell my family about. *(Picks up the glass, and heading towards the door speaks very softly and thoughtfully)* I'll have some questions to ask them, too.

MAUDE

(Settling back into her pillow) Well, I am glad to tell you—you are such a wonderful listener.

(Ranesh exits, with the empty glass).

SCENE 2

MAUDE

In bed, looking to be asleep. Lying flatter than the day before. Her glasses are on the table, and the crossword book is on the floor. Ranesh comes in with a glass of juice. Seeing her, he puts down the glass in a hurry and leans over to Maude.

RANESH

Maude? *(Waits. With some urgency, and a tad louder)* Maude?

MAUDE

(*Opens her eyes and smiles at him*) Hello dear boy. I'm still here. Just enjoying my memories. It's what I have these days. (*Looks more carefully at Ranesh, and smiles*) How's the world?

RANESH

Still carrying on, I guess. (*Smiles*).

MAUDE

(*Sitting up a little, carefully and slowly*) So, what are we talking about today? I covered a lot of territory yesterday.

RANESH

Yes, you did. I want ask you a few things, if that's OK.

MAUDE

(*Reaching her hand to his arm, happily*) Of course it's OK. What do you want to know?

RANESH

(*Looking at her carefully*) Maude. The town in England your cousins went to first, after India. You said it was an odd name. Could it have been Slough?

MAUDE

(*Sitting up more*) Why, it might have been. Let me think. (*Closes her eyes for a few seconds*) It could have been, yes! I think it was. (*Big smile*) Why would you say...

RANESH

(*Cutting her off, and getting excited*) And Maude, those cousins, 'Samuel' and 'Rita.' They were coming from India. Could they have been 'Sami' and 'Ritu?'

MAUDE

Well yes, I think they were, but this was the 1950s, they wanted to fit in more, so they changed... Ranesh, what is this about?

RANESH

(*Takes a very deep breath, and looks about to cry and to burst*) Maude. I think your cousins, the ones who came first, were my great-grandparents! (*Takes a tissue to wipe both his eyes*).

35

MAUDE

(*Looking in wonder*) Ranesh?

RANESH

(*Blows his nose*) Maude, one last question. Your husband. Was Luke Jenner his given name?

MAUDE

(*Distracted. Not hearing Ranesh*) What?

RANESH

Was Luke Jenner the name your husband was given at birth?

MAUDE

(*Quietly*) His birthname? (*Breathing quickly, and reaching for a tissue*) No, he was born Lokpriya Jena. It's a Sanskrit name. He changed it to Luke Jenner. It's what so many people did to fit in. He was born in Rajasthan, India, the same region as Momma Lilah's cousin. But... How? (*Wipes her eyes with tissue*).

RANESH

(*In great excitement*) Oh, Maude! Your Poppa Matthew and Momma Lilah, to me, were great-uncle Matias, and great-aunt Laylah—they brought my great-grandparents here! My parents told me stories of how 'Aunt Mada' and 'Uncle Loki' helped my whole family to settle and succeed in this country, after Mada's parents died. You are my great-aunt Mada! (*Very emotional*).

MAUDE

(*Holds out a hand for Ranesh to take. Also very emotional*) 'Mada.' I've not heard that name for so long. It feels wonderful to hear it again. (*Sits fully up in bed and puts an arm out to touch his shoulder*) I look at you and I can see Sami and Ritu. And now look at you; making the world a better place. (*Smiling, with a few seconds pause*) Dear boy. You have taught me something so very important today. You've reminded me how essential family is! I thought all I had was my past to enjoy, but it seems I have a bit more of my present as well.

Lights dim. . .

Notes

ON STAGE

Maude Jenner:
> Born 1915, Canada.

Ranesh:
> Born between1987 and 1997, Ontario, Canada.

MENTIONED

Maude's husband: Luke Jenner/Lokpriya Jena:
> Born 1910 Rajasthan, India, died 2003, aged 93.

Maude's father:
> Born 1891, married 1910, died 1920, aged 29.

Maude's mother:
> Born 1893, married 1910, died 1919, aged 26.

Maude's first brother:
> Born 1911, died 1919, aged 8.

Maude's second brother:
> Born 1912, died 1919, aged 7.

Matthew/Mathai:
> Maude's father's friend/adopted father, born 1898, married 1919, died 1945, Homestead, Florida, hurricane, aged 47.

Lilah/Laylah, Maude's adopted mother:
> Born 1900, married 1919, died 1945, Homestead, Florida, hurricane, aged 45.

Ranesh's mother:
> Born in Ontario, Canada in the 1960s.

Ranesh's father:
> Born in Ontario, Canada in the 1960s.

Ranesh's great-grandparents, Sami and Ritu:
> Arrived in Canada from England, in the 1950's, born in Rajasthan, India, having departed about 1940.

SECTION 2

The First Wave

*T*he first selection, taken from my lengthy Journal of a Plague Year, *shows how the shutdown began in Nova Scotia—one of the earlier provinces to enact comprehensive shutdown regulations although it was among the last to experience confirmed cases of COVID. Some of the measures described in the following passage were not enacted in other provinces, particularly in Western Canada, until weeks later. Readers from other Canadian provinces or the U.S. may find it interesting to compare Nova Scotia's shutdown process with the shutdown processes used in their jurisdictions.*

The second piece describes the reopening process that took place in Nova Scotia, as in most other Canadian provinces, during the late Spring and early Summer of 2020. I found that the process bore some surprisingly strong resemblances to the Soviet Union's 'thaw' period under Nikita Khrushchev during the late 1950s and early 1960s, which I had read about when I studied Russian history at Dalhousie some years back. Just as Khrushchev's relaxation of many of Josef Stalin's strictures inspired a feeling of relief among Soviet citizens, so did Premier Stephen McNeil's relaxation of the strict lockdown measures that had been in place from late Winter through mid-Spring. At the same time, it's important to remember that, as had been the case under Khrushchev, the relaxation under McNeil was far from total. Many lockdown restrictions remained in place, most notably those affecting the performing arts, such as theatre and dance. It is also worth noting that universal mask requirements were first imposed not during the height of the lockdown, but smack dab in the middle of the 'thaw' period. The thinking may well have been that so long as people had to wear masks to the grocery store, drugstore, and bank, they would not likely become too complacent about COVID.

Nova Scotia Shuts Down
Jon Peirce

Sunday, March 15

(My late mother's birthday as well as the Ides of March). As of Friday, March 13, pretty much everything in life is on a wartime footing, owing to the Coronavirus pandemic crisis. One can't go a day, or even an hour or two, without learning of more cancellations of ordinary, everyday events. While some events from prior cycles have been allowed to go forward to complete the cycle (e.g., last night's performance of *Jitters* at Bedford Players, the cast party for *A Tribute to Broadway*), the new cycle, going forward, will be radically different from the previous ones, or indeed, from anything we have seen in the past 100 years, since the 'Spanish' flu epidemic and the Halifax Explosion.

Even during World War II, churches still held services, and professional sports leagues like Major League Baseball and the National Hockey League continued to operate. MLB and the NHL both announced the suspension of their seasons earlier this week. On Friday, the city announced the closing of all municipal pools and recreation centres, and the non-book operations of public libraries. The latest suspension is that of Mass by the Roman Catholic diocese. Masses can be conducted today, but they are being suspended as of tomorrow (Monday, March 16).

Seeing all these cancellations, in rapid succession, is like seeing lights going out on a Christmas tree, or store lights going out in a storm, or guests leaving a party at midnight.

As I believe that this time of plague will mark a watershed and will be a time of fundamental change in our attitude to life and in our strategies for coping, both individually and as a society, I am launching this journal in order to record these critical changes, as well as to note the effect that all these changes have had and will have on me, my family, and my close friends. The suspension of Masses is certainly an escalation in the enclosure of our lives to protect against the plague. If, in addition, we see complete closure of the public libraries and (God help us) suspension of public transit, we will know that we are in a battle for our collective lives. The suspension of public transit would cost many workers their jobs and put many businesses out of business.

Monday, March 16

Service at St. Margaret's yesterday—an eerie feeling, as we could all sense this would be the last time we would see each other at a live service for some time. If the Catholic Church was going to be suspending masses, could the Anglican Church be far behind in suspending its live services? Already there were some restrictions in place, including a ban on the traditional 'Peace' and the offering of communion in one kind only (bread). There was also no coffee hour after the service. The choir, of which I am a part, still sang, and there was congregational singing.[1] But the entire service (including the singing) went forward in extremely subdued fashion. I left the church to drive home wondering if I would ever see some of my fellow parishioners again—those in infirm health, in particular, who might not live through the pandemic or might be afraid to venture out again even after its first phase was over.

Checking my internet this morning, I wasn't at all surprised to learn that our Bishop, Ron Cutler, had indeed followed the lead of the Catholic Church in ordering a halt to all live services and church gatherings effective this week. While the initial suspension is only through April 3, I expect it to last much longer.

Aside from the suspension of church services, the main development of note is the closing of the Dartmouth Sportsplex, effective tomorrow morning. I shall try to get over there for one final walk around the track before the closure. Also hope to see my friend Theresa at the little restaurant there. In addition, all three of the bridge games I've been taking part in have been cancelled. Hardly a surprise, as a game involving a large number of people handling the same cards in an enclosed indoor space would be a breeding ground for the disease. As with church and singing, it will probably be a long, long time before I play bridge again.[2]

Since writing this, I've learned that all Metro Halifax libraries are closed for at least three weeks, effective today, and that VIA Rail is cancelling its overnight Montreal-Halifax trains for three weeks.[3] And—this one is a real shocker—all dental offices in Metro Halifax have stopped providing non-essential services; they are open for emergency services only.

Went last night to the Celtic Corner pub for their 'fish and fiddles' night. Danced up a storm for over an hour. At the next table, one little girl, only 3, started dancing up even more of a storm than I was, and another kid, a little boy just learning to walk, 'accompanied' us on some percussion blocks which served as a sort of primitive drum. In between, ate pan-friend haddock with the fixings and drank 1½ pints of Guinness. If one is to maintain one's sanity, it's important to have as much fun as possible while one can, so I'll keep on doing this as long as the pubs stay open. So far, I have not heard of restaurant or pub closures in Metro Halifax, though there have been some in Sydney and other parts of Cape Breton. Still, I have the feeling that this will be the last 'Fish and Fiddles' evening for a long, long time.[4]

After returning from the pub, took in the Biden-Sanders debate for the Democratic presidential nomination on TV last night. The major focus was on the COVID crisis, which took up at least the first half of the two-hour debate. To my great surprise, Biden, who has been pitifully weak in the debates up to this point, came up with many practical ideas for dealing with it, whereas Sanders did not have much to offer beyond the need for single payer health care and radical overhaul of the whole health care system. I agree with him on these points, but a President must be able to look to the near term as well, to deal with immediate crises. Here Biden far outshone his more left-wing opponent. A Biden nomination now appears a foregone conclusion. I *cannot* believe I am now supporting Joe Biden, having been a hard-left Sanders-Warren supporter for years and having long despised Biden on almost every count. But we have to remind ourselves that wartime elections (and presidencies) are different—and that this really is wartime even if no one is firing any weapons. Biden is zooming so far to the left, adopting ideas like Warren's bankruptcy plan, that by the time of the nomination we probably won't recognize him. Perhaps having few fixed principles isn't always a bad idea; it makes it easier to abandon what principles one has than would be the case for someone like Sanders who has all sorts of fixed principles, but sometimes seems to find it difficult to live in the moment.

Meanwhile, I'm starting to lay in critical supplies, but relatively gradually. I'm trying not to hoard anything. Yesterday, in need of a thermometer, I made the creative move of buying an ovulation thermometer at Shopper's in the nearby Dartmouth Shopping Centre, after going to three or four other stores and coming up empty-handed. This proved somewhat more expensive than the conventional device, but at least I now have a thermometer. My only remaining necessity is a surgical mask. Hand sanitizer would be highly desirable but is not absolutely necessary, as I won't be travelling much and it is almost always available when one goes out.

My move back to Ottawa, which was originally going to happen June 1 with a house-hunting trip in early April, is on hold for one month while I assess the situation. Before the end of April, I'll make an assessment of how long it seems likely to be before community transmission of the virus has ended. Right now does not, to say the least, seem an opportune time to be making a house-hunting trip. My view is that if one's business is not essential (e.g., visiting a sick or dying relative), one should not travel.

Tuesday, March 17

Restaurants and bars have all closed, except for take-out and delivery, in Ottawa. It's probably only a matter of time before the same thing happens here, though the bars are open today for St Patrick's Day. And the Democratic presidential primary in Ohio has been postponed by order of the Health Commissioner. A potentially frightening prospect for democracy, though at this point it doesn't really matter in terms of the results. Biden's nomination seems all but a foregone conclusion.

Am trying to have my personal grooming attended to while I still can. So, yesterday I got a haircut. The haircut and sideburn trim were okay, but the stylist couldn't trim my moustache because it is on my face. This leaves me with the unsavoury option of letting it grow longer or cutting it myself. If I do that, it will probably *look* as if I'd cut it myself. Of course, I could also shave it, but it is an important part of me and shaving it is the last thing I want to do right now. Today I'm having a pedicure. My nails are frequently getting stuck in my socks and I simply can't reach them all. In their masks, the pedicurists look as if they were part of a space crew. This will make the experience less relaxing than it might otherwise be. But I do need it.

Meanwhile, my anxiety disorder appears to be kicking in, big time. I thought my chest congestion was the aftermath of a little bug I caught during the last days of *A Tribute to Broadway*, the musical I was in as a chorus member earlier this month. But the congestion has lasted longer than it should have, and even past the near-end of the accompanying nasal congestion. I suspect that what I'm seeing is the 'racing heart' symptom of anxiety disorder.

The worst effect is my inability to sleep. Only slept about five hours last night, and another 45 minutes in an afternoon nap. Two days ago, I only slept an hour in an afternoon nap even with a Clonazepam pill. It's dangerous to keep going on with this little sleep. If I don't get more sleep, and soon, I'm sure to get sick. Have tried St. John's Wort, but so far, to little avail. Also did quite a bit of deep breathing in bed. It helped, but only a little. It looks as if I am going to have to go back on Paxil, which I gladly gave up three years ago, for the duration of this crisis. Now the trick is to find someone to prescribe it for me. If my former psychiatrist can do it, fine. But if he can't or won't, it could be a long loop through to someone who can help. This needs to be addressed *now*. Maybe it's also time to hit the cannabis store on Clyde Street to get more spray, oil, etc. to tide me over until I can get the Paxil.

Worried about my sister Mary, 74, in assisted living in Brewer, Maine. If she got really sick, it could be very difficult for me to go and see her, though as a U.S. citizen (still) I could probably get across the border. Getting back into Canada might be another matter. Also worried about my friend Ruth (80) who lives here in Dartmouth in her own house, but is having increasing mobility and vision issues and is due to have a major eye treatment on Wednesday.

Later today, I'll be getting in touch with my church to see what I can do to help them in the crisis, and will also be writing a letter to my MP and the Minister of Sport urging them to work to cancel the upcoming Olympics. Such a spectacle would be a veritable breeding ground for pestilence of all kinds, and could well lead to a repeat of the horrific 1918 'Spanish' flu epidemic, undoing all the good work we have been doing, at great sacrifice, to distance ourselves from other people to avoid spreading the virus.

Wednesday, March 18

Thankfully, my old psychiatrist phoned in a prescription for Paxil for me, which I picked up yesterday. It has three renewals, which means I won't have to worry about contacting him again.

New closures today include bars and restaurants (except for take-out), which will be closed as of tonight. These closures parallel those already made in other jurisdictions, so I find I am no longer shocked or startled. It was all quite predictable.

People are starting to exhibit some of the hoarding behaviour characteristic of wartime, particularly with regard to toilet paper, hand sanitizer, wipes, alcohol, thermometers, and surgical masks. The toilet paper one is the least comprehensible, as the disease has only one minor intestinal phase, leading to diarrhea for two or three days in some (but by no means all) patients. People have nonetheless been panic-buying the stuff, leading to shortages which need not have happened. The hand sanitizer shortage may be of a different nature. I suspect that in this case, most of the available supplies may have been commandeered by businesses needing them to remain open. Not altogether a bad thing. But all of this demonstrates the need for a rationing system of some kind. If the stores can't enforce one, the government will need to step in. So far, there don't appear to have been any food shortages, and the government and store chain presidents claim the supply chain is robust and there should not be any shortages. We'll have to wait and see if this is actually the case.

Going to give blood today. The Canadian Blood Services said on their web site that they are facing shortages, particularly of certain blood types, as many of those who had previously made appointments to give had cancelled owing to the crisis. It makes me feel good that there's something I can do.

I must say that Nova Scotia is probably about the best place in the world to be doing my plague time. The things that in 'peacetime' aggravate me most about the province—the conservatism, the social control, the conformity— are precisely the qualities that are needed to get everyone through a wartime crisis. Everyone, pretty well, is of a like mind. We are unlikely to have criminally insane outliers like Trump supporter Kid Rock keeping his Nashville bar open through the plague. And people here are kind. Truly kind. Not a formula for growth, but definitely a formula for security, turning once again to Maslow's hierarchy of needs. And security, now, is first and foremost. Growth cannot take place without a firm foundation of security underneath it. So my growth period, regrettably, will have to wait until it is safe for me to move to Ottawa/West Quebec.

Friday, March 20

Changes in the past two days. Hair and nail salons are now closed—a good thing I got in to both when I did. Hours have been shortened at banks, grocery stores, and the liquor stores (not sure how long the latter will remain open, but if they are closed, it's an interesting and perhaps scary question how alcoholics will get their fix). While Canadian Tire is still open, we're getting pretty close to an essential services model, pretty much the same in all jurisdictions, comprising drug stores, grocery stores, banks, gas stations, and, perhaps, hardware stores and car repair places. Not sure about laundromats and dry-cleaning establishments, but I should think that the former, at least, would qualify as an essential service.

Finally got a return call from my Anglican parish priest, Charles Bull, responding to my offer of help during the crisis. I was, he explained, the 18th call on his list for the day. He then allowed as how he was exhausted. I can relate. I have been feeling exhausted myself these past few days. In addition to the sheer volume of work both of us have been doing, there's the matter of future shock, or rather reverse future shock. It is as if we are being far too rapidly catapulted back into a past era, when quarantines were about the only strategies communities had for dealing with mass outbreaks of infectious disease. Excessively rapid change, whether of a forward or reverse nature, *is* exhausting. One has barely re-established one's footing when, bingo, new stuff happens and one must again re-adjust and reshape one's perspective.

While the weeks ahead will certainly be very difficult, I'd like to think that we are nearly finished this first part of the crisis. By now, it seems, we at least know what we are facing. Almost all jurisdictions in North America are now operating on pretty much the same essential services model, with the most minor of inter-jurisdictional variations. There are not many more services that can be cut… the liquor stores, perhaps, or possibly even public transit, though that would work massive hardship on many and is, I am sure, a last resort. I expect that the next two or three weeks will show whether the measures already taken here, including the now-familiar social distancing, have in fact been enough.

Blood donation proved quite the adventure. When I went for what I thought was my originally-scheduled appointment, at 11:00 Wednesday, the clinic was locked up tight as a drum. A sign on the door said its hours that day were 3:00 to 7:00 p.m. What the hell? After some angry rapping on the door on my part, a woman opened up and I told her what the situation was. She checked the system and said that my appointment had been for 11:00 *Tuesday. WTF?* It was past that time when I called to make the appointment. The woman apologized for the screw-up. If it had been anything other than a blood donation, I'd have walked out the door and not come back, but given the importance of giving blood, I steeled myself to more wasted time. With some difficulty, I was able to get an appointment for 5:20 that same afternoon.

Arrived a bit after 5:00. After some preliminary questioning at the door, designed to reveal whether I had some contagious illness, I was given a temporary donor card and sent to one of several laptops to take a detailed medical questionnaire. The questionnaire, comprising some 60 to 70 items, asked about things as varied as my medical history, my travel and residence history, and the prescription drugs I was currently using. Having 'passed' this—I assume that if there'd been a glitch, I wouldn't have been allowed to finish—I sat in a chair opposite the room where the actual bloodletting was going on, cooling my heels for 40 minutes or so before a technician called me into a side room for a few more questions and a haemoglobin and blood pressure test and temperature-taking. Then I waited another 20 minutes or so in a chair in the bloodletting chamber itself, before I was finally allowed to take my place in a reclining seat. It didn't please me that I had to remind the technician that the seat hadn't been cleaned following the previous donor's departure. Surely it should be a matter of course for the technician taking the equipment out of the donor's arm to clean the chair immediately upon his or her departure. *This* was a reminder of one of the things I *don't* like about Nova Scotia—the frequent technical incompetence and lack of attention to detail (as manifested also in the botched appointment scheduling). While the newly-cleaned chair dried, I munched some pretzels and drank a large cup of water.

Finally, around 6:40 p.m., a full hour and a half after my arrival, the apparatus was installed and the donation itself began. When, not long after that, the apparatus was removed, by a different technician than the one who'd installed it—another thing I found strange—she said that the actual donation had taken just under 7 minutes. I seem to remember its having taken longer than that the only previous time I'd given blood, in 1976 when I was a grad student at Dal. For reasons not at all clear to me, I had to stay in the chair for about five minutes after the apparatus was removed, hoping all the while that my anxious bladder didn't lead to an accident! Having relieved that anxious bladder, I was then directed to a small recovery room, where there was juice, tea and coffee, and an assortment of cookies. Over the shortbreads and apple juice, had an interesting conversation with the technician supervising the room about, of all things, painting, which she had just recently taken up, in middle age. Encouraging her to keep up her painting, I finally took my leave about 7:15—two hours after my arrival on the site.

Yesterday (Thursday), having experienced fairly serious difficulties getting into both Facebook and the internet, I decided it was time for a full-scale computer cleanup, something the machine hadn't had for a little over a year. Called up Geeks on the Way, my service provider, to try to book an appointment with my trusty, tried-and-true techie, Brent Rowley. At first the customer service rep balked, saying I should try to get the work done online, but after he proved unable to explain at all clearly how such a cleanup could in fact be done online, he relented and said Brent could come if he was willing to. At 5:00 he came and started a cleanup that lasted a little over an hour. He was his usual affable self and, as always, taught me something new about my machine, showing me the panel that controls the time at which updates can be done. (Evidently those updates were the major source of my problems, as they had left, Brent said, some eight gigabytes of unnecessary stuff on my hard drive.) I was grateful enough for his having gone out of his way to help me out that I gave him a $20.00 tip, something I'd never done before. Hopefully it won't be necessary for me to call on him again before the move to Ottawa, but in case I do need to, I now have his card.

The number of confirmed and prospective cases in the province stands at 14: five of one and nine of the other. (I don't remember how many of each.) It's interesting to observe that Nova Scotia has been enacting the same kind of controls, with its 14 cases, at about the same time as other Canadian jurisdictions like British Columbia, with about 200 confirmed cases, and even American jurisdictions like New York and California, which have had many times more cases than that. It's also worth noting that many businesses have been doing more than the law requires, either by shutting down when their type of business wasn't required to do so, or by shutting down earlier than required. Along similar lines, my landlord, Killam Properties, has also 'gone the extra mile,' by posting a notice on the front door requesting that all those whose business in the building is not essential not enter. Entry is now restricted to outside people providing essential care or building staff proving essential services. I rate my cleaning lady, Colette, as falling into the former category, as I could not possibly keep up with the cleaning by myself at this point, and the risk of harm (including disease) from not having the place properly cleaned would in my view far exceed that from having her enter the building, do her business in my apartment, and leave promptly. I doubt that anyone will question me or her, but should they do so, that is precisely what I will tell them.

Given how far ahead of other, far more heavily affected jurisdictions (especially those containing large cities) we are here in Nova Scotia, I'm cautiously optimistic that we'll be able to avoid major carnage. Of course, all bets are to a degree off when the students return from March break in the States—some such students living in Toronto contracted the disease earlier this month, according to what I've read on the Internet—but hopefully there aren't that many of them and airport screening will catch them. There was little or no airport screening of the early returnees to Toronto, according to one in-person account by a COVID patient living there.

In the good deeds column, I've volunteered (to my church) to read or sing over the phone to anyone wanting such a service.[5] Given the closure of the libraries and bookstores, there might well be some demand for such a service. I also told my Anglican priest, Charles Bull, that I'd be available to sing as a chorister in a virtual service (once the choir director gets over the nasty cold he had last Sunday, at our final pre-shutdown service), to coordinate volunteer efforts, or to put out a newsletter.

Dartmouth, Nova Scotia
March, 2020

Notes

[1] Though I would see most of my fellow parishioners again, as the church resumed live services in June and most were willing enough to attend, March 15 would be the last time we would sing together as a choir and the last service with congregational singing at least through late August, when I would leave the province. I don't know what the current situation is with regard to music in church services in Nova Scotia.

[2] I still have not done so. Some of my bridge-playing friends appear to have switched to online bridge, but I have no interest in that. There were also some sporadic efforts, during the Summer 'lull' in the cases, to resume in-person duplicate bridge. But I took no part in those efforts, not regarding the situation as safe even during the Summer 'lull' period. Needless to say, I've played no bridge since moving to Quebec.

[3] This cancellation has since been extended twice, first to May 1, and later to November 3.

[4] Celtic Corner did reopen for food and beverage service in June—but alas, the wonderful fiddler never returned, at least during the rest of my stay in Nova Scotia.

[5] I did provide this service once, on a Sunday morning, to a retired United Church minister, singing several Anglican hymns from our hymnal and one folk song to her. It was, I think, a rewarding experience for both of us. Regrettably, no one else thought to avail themselves of my offer, which continued my long Nova Scotia tradition of being able to do almost anything once but very few things more than once.

Recovering from the First Wave: The Mid-Cycle 'Thaw'
Jon Peirce

Saturday, April 25 was the first time I began to think about the possibility of reopening. Bear in mind that Nova Scotia was then still in full lockdown mode, as was virtually all the rest of the country. On that day, I heard on CBC Radio News that Prime Minister Trudeau would soon be meeting with provincial premiers to draw up a jointly agreed set of guidelines for the reopening of the economy. Whether those guidelines were ever drawn up, let alone put into effect, I don't know.

What I do know is that by this time, a number of provincial premiers were actively discussing their reopening plans. For example, in Saskatchewan, Premier Scott Moe had the day before announced a five-stage reopening plan, to begin May 5 with the opening of parks and outdoor facilities such as golf courses. And on that same day, New Brunswick Premier Blaine Higgs announced his province's multi-stage reopening plan, the first phase of which involved a two-household bubble, with members of one household free to visit those of another, but no one else.

Lost in all the fanfare around reopening was the April 25 announcement, by High-Liner Seafoods in Lunenburg, that it would be introducing mandatory masks and screening for its 300 employees. Through the early stages of the pandemic, masks, about which many public health officials, including Canada's chief public health officer, Dr Theresa Tam, had been openly skeptical, had played a relatively minor role. I owned only three or four, and wore them only to doctors' and optometrists' offices. The four Atlantic provinces got through the pandemic's first wave in relatively good shape pretty well without masks, relying almost entirely on strict lockdown measures and social distancing to hold COVID in check. Neither I nor most of the other people I knew, with the exception of those with a history of autoimmune disorders, wore masks to the grocery store, the drugstore, or the bank. Nobody I knew would even have thought of wearing a mask outside. But as the recovery period progressed, universal mask-wearing in all public indoor places would become pretty much the norm. By the end of July, most Canadian jurisdictions had adopted some kind of formal mask requirement. Evidently a universal wearing of masks would come to be considered a sort of quid pro quo, the price citizens would have to pay for the reopening of the economy. As this gradually became the norm, I started to see an increasing number of people wearing masks outside as well as inside, though a bare face would remain the norm out of doors, at least in Nova Scotia.

In any case, by the beginning of May, pretty much all the talk, both on the Internet and on CBC Radio News, was about various provinces' reopening plans. At the same time, we learned that New Zealand was planning a major reopening, possibly to include even bars as well as restaurants. Given that country's amazing record, of only 21 deaths on a little over 1000 cases, I felt that New Zealanders had more than earned the right to celebrate.

Reopening proceeded at about the same speed as the arrival of Spring: that is to say, slowly and circuitously.[1] In Nova Scotia, the first step was the reopening of provincial and municipal parks, announced by Premier Stephen McNeil on May 1 to take effect the following day. In addition, Nova Scotians were again able to go to their cottages (though they were advised to stay there if they did go again), golf courses could reopen for maintenance, or to open their driving ranges, and recreational boating and fishing were also allowed.

To say that Nova Scotians responded enthusiastically to the parks' reopening would be to understate. When I went to Dartmouth's Leighton Dillman Park, near my apartment, for a walk on Sunday afternoon, May 3, I found the parking lot nearly full. Rarely had I seen as many as a dozen people during my eight years of walking there. But on this day, there were many dozens—probably well over a hundred—and walkers and kite-flyers had taken to the park's grassy slopes as well as its many paths. For the first time that I could remember, this little gem of an urban park was being fully appreciated and utilized by Dartmouth residents.

Nor was Leighton Dillman the only park drawing an unusually large crowd on the first day of reopening. Evidently all the parks were busy, at least around Metro—busy enough that the *Chronicle-Herald* published a front-page story about it on Monday morning, May 4. There were big crowds, so I read, at Point Pleasant and several other of the better-known municipal and provincial parks. But despite the crowds, it appeared that the vast majority still respected social distancing. I was very glad to see that, because if that hadn't been the case, the parks would again have been closed up tight as a drum. Nova Scotians' social conformity and near-timidity in the face of authority, qualities which in normal times I had tended to find seriously irritating, were serving them and the province well in this instance.

Much of the U.S. was taking a far different course. On April 25, in the presence of medical advisor Dr Deborah Birx, who shamefully said nothing, President Trump suggested injecting disinfectant as a way of combating COVID. Within the next few days, about 100 poison control centres in the U.S. had reported cases resulting from people having injected or ingested some kind of disinfectant, pursuant to Trump's advice. While a few courageous Governors, generally Democrats on the East or West coasts, like New York's Andrew Cuomo, did stand up for public health and safety, these voices of reason were few and far between.[2] Far more typical was the state of Georgia, whose Trumpite Governor, Brian Kemp, allowed bowling alleys, hair salons, and tattoo parlours to open on April 27. While the Democratic Mayor of Atlanta refused to allow the reopening to happen in that city, such courageous municipal officials were again few and far between. It was not without irony that the U.S. would pass the one million mark in cases on April 28. Meanwhile, north of the border, provinces such as New Brunswick and Prince Edward Island had not seen any new cases in over a week.

In states (again, generally those with a Democratic governor in office) which did maintain some kind of restrictions on business, there were strident, not infrequently violent protests against the continued closures through much of May. Around May 19, by which time Nova Scotia's recovery rate had topped 95% of non-fatal cases, pictures of drinkers packed into Milwaukee bars cheek-to-cheek on their bar stools went viral on the Internet. The bars reopened after right-wing Republicans sued to overturn the Democratic Governor's order keeping them closed, and the state Supreme Court went along with the suit. The anti-lockdown protests would accelerate in the last week of the month. That week, those protests included the hanging in effigy of the Democratic governor of Kentucky, and the sending of armed men to storm the Capitol in Michigan, where Democratic governor Gretchen Whitmer, then considered a possible vice-presidential nominee, had put in place some of the country's toughest lockdown measures. On the Internet, there were large numbers of photos of half-naked bathers, packed wall-to-wall, from beaches in Kansas, California, Texas, and various other states.

While all this was going on, the Nova Scotia provincial government was relaxing restrictions on pharmacies, again allowing them to dispense up to three months' supply of medications at one time, providing the medications in question were in adequate supply. Earlier in the month (on May 9), home-based midwifery and pet adoptions had been allowed to resume. More significantly, New Brunswick had on May 11 gone to full second-stage reopening, with libraries and museums allowed to reopen, along with non-essential businesses such as bookstores, and restaurants—at 50% of capacity. But it's important to remember that by this time, New Brunswick had had virtually no active cases for some weeks. To all intents and purposes, the pandemic's first wave had been wrestled to the ground, something that had happened in very few U.S. states, and certainly not in the southern and southwestern states that were the quickest to reopen.

Ontario, which had more cases than the Atlantic provinces but many fewer than most American states, undertook its own major reopening on May 16. On that date, retail stores located outside of indoor malls and with a separate street-front entrance could reopen, providing they maintained social distancing. Libraries could reopen for pickup and delivery service, and elective surgeries and diagnostic procedures were able to resume, as well as in-person psychological and other mental health services. Domestic services such as housecleaning and grounds maintenance could also resume, as could individual sports such as tennis where social distancing was possible. Various media services such as technical services and publishing were also able to resume, but not activities involving the gathering together of performers, such as live filming. And veterinarians and pet grooming services were allowed to reopen, as well as marinas, boat clubs, and public boat launches. So too could golf courses, although clubhouses could open only for washrooms and their restaurants could open only for take-out. Given the number of ongoing cases in Ontario at the time, these were considered fairly bold measures for a Canadian province, though they'd have been regarded as timid half-measures by most American standards.

Ontario Premier Ford's continuing, fairly cautious approach to the pandemic is suggested by the fact that on May 21, about a month before the normal ending of the school year, he announced that the public schools would not reopen until September. One of the few provincial premiers to proceed aggressively with school reopening was Quebec's François Legault, who in early May had ordered elementary schools outside of Montreal to reopen May 11, and those in Montreal on May 19. What was noteworthy about Legault's aggressive stance toward school reopening was that at the time, Quebec had by far the highest rate of COVID cases and deaths and lowest COVID recovery rate in the country, with over half of Canada's cases and deaths despite having less than a quarter of the country's population. Legault did eventually give in to intense public pressure, allowing schools in Montreal to remain closed through the Summer. But even then, he ordered Montreal's day care centres to reopen on June 1, and schools in the rest of the province reopened as scheduled.

In fairness, some of the same rambunctious behaviour by young people cavorting on American beaches did make its way into Canada late in the Spring. Specifically, in Toronto on May 22, the reopening of parks and some unusually warm weather led to a mob of half-clad young people, some considerably less than six feet from each other, in Trinity Bellwood Park—a situation aggravated by the fact that public washrooms had *not* been reopened, causing many to be forced to relieve themselves in the open, and resulting in intense criticism from public officials the next day. But the situation was clearly an anomaly for Canada. While there continued to be occasional incidents of this type throughout the Summer both in Ontario and in Western provinces like British Columbia, such events remained the exception—thankfully.

The beginning of June saw the ever-cautious Premier Stephen McNeil of Nova Scotia finally announce a major reopening for that province. Effective June 6, restaurants and bars could reopen, at 50% of capacity. Hair salons and nail salons could also reopen, as could non-essential businesses and dentists and eye care establishments. While McNeil waited some time to reopen the province, his was arguably the most comprehensive reopening of any Canadian province. Interestingly, each business would take its own path toward reopening. The owners of some were clearly champing at the bit to get started again; these stores posted signs in their windows days before the actual start of reopening, saying 'Reopening Soon' or something to that effect.[3] Others, particularly some of the restaurants, proceeded more cautiously, letting their customers know that it would take a few days for them to 'get up to speed' in the new regime. One business that took its time reopening was the Celtic Corner, in downtown Dartmouth, which had been one of my favourite pubs prior to the pandemic.

In fairness, it should be noted that when the restaurants did reopen, there were many changes for both restaurant staff and their patrons. Overall capacity was strictly limited, and tables were now at least six feet apart from each other. Customers were required to sign in on entering, leaving a phone number where they could be reached, presumably in the event that a COVID case was found in the establishment. And customers were also asked to apply hand sanitizer on entering. The number of people allowed to sit at any one table was also strictly limited.

When outdoor patios reopened, restrictions on gathering size were somewhat relaxed, making it possible, for example, for me to have nine people at my farewell party at Celtic Corner in late August. But the check-in and hand sanitizer rules were still in effect, and we were also expected to sit at least six feet apart from each other. These restrictions notwithstanding, we were all glad to get our restaurants back—or mostly back. The live music which had been a feature of some (including the Celtic Corner) and the jukebox music which had been a feature of others (including the Ship Victory, my other favourite local pub) would not return, at least not during the rest of my stay in the province.

Whether the jukeboxes and live fiddlers have come back now, I simply don't know. In any event, one additional requirement would come into effect in late July. With the advent of the provincial mask requirement for all indoor public places, restaurant patrons were expected to wear masks at all times while in the restaurant, except when actually eating or drinking. Restaurant staff were also expected to wear masks when working. Enforcement of this edict was not uniformly strict in Nova Scotia eateries—no doubt in large measure because the province continued to have very few new or active cases throughout the Summer. Indeed, its case numbers would remain low into the Fall, and indeed, even in the pandemic's second wave, Nova Scotia would not record as many new cases as it had during the first wave, and (thankfully) no new deaths.[4]

Evidently the first phase of reopening had gone well, because on June 26, Premier McNeil announced a new phase of reopening, effective July 3. Restaurants and bars could operate at full capacity and remain open until midnight. Public swimming pools could reopen, and so could movie theatres. Events such as concerts could also go forward. Permissible gathering size was increased from 50 to 200 or 250, depending on who was sponsoring the gathering, except for private home gatherings like family barbecues where the limit remained 50. In Halifax and Dartmouth, Saturday morning outdoor farmers' markets reopened, on a new basis. Church services could again be held 'live,' though there was still no choral singing or congregational singing. While this might at first glance seem like an odd restriction, choir rehearsals had been identified, early on in the pandemic, as among the leading 'super-spreader' events for the disease. One such rehearsal, in Washington state in March, involving about 100 choristers, had led to several dozen cases of the virus and, most regrettably, to two deaths.

All in all, this was about as close to a full return to 'normal' life as any Canadian province would experience. In my view, the broad reopening was fully justified by the minuscule number of cases in the province at the time. Hard though this may be to believe now, in February of 2021, days, or occasionally even weeks would go by without any new cases being reported.

It may or may not have been coincidental that just at the time Premier McNeil was announcing the province's broad reopening, on Saturday, June 27, I experienced my first social event since mid-March—a sing-along and potluck on the balcony of a private house. And I also witnessed my first handshake since mid-March—one man shaking another's hand near the Lido Pool at the Waegwoltic Tennis Club in Halifax. Speaking of the Lido Pool, a cold-water colossus whose waters I had enjoyed for over a decade, I had my first swim of the season there on June 20.

During the Spring, I'd been unsure about rejoining the Waegwoltic, given that I knew I would be leaving the province sometime during the Summer. But my decision to hold off on my move until the end of August, combined with the broad provincial reopening in June, made another Summer's membership seem like a good idea after all.

Initially both tennis and swimming facilities opened under tight restrictions. Tennis was limited to singles, and that only in 30-minute stretches, soon increased to 60 minutes. But before too long, doubles as well as singles would be allowed, doubles courts could be booked for up to 90 minutes, and private lessons resumed. Swimming underwent similar liberalization. At first, swimming was only in the warmer 'Main' pool, only by reservation, and only for 30 minutes at a time. An intricate series of ropes delineated permissible ways of entering and leaving the pool area.

With the reopening of the Lido during the week of June 15, the club's swimming capacity was greatly increased. Members didn't need to make reservations to swim in the Lido. Soon, with demand for the Main Pool reduced by the reopening of the Lido, reservations were not necessary in that pool, either. The ropes would soon disappear, to be replaced by arrows indicating which way swimmers should proceed up and down the staircase to and from the aquatics locker rooms. By July, swimming lessons and other youth programs, including day camps, had resumed. By July, as well, the club's excellent, newly-refurbished dining facilities had reopened, and Friday night steak and salmon barbecues had resumed. The bar did not reopen, but it was possible to order beer or wine with meals, which was more than enough for me.

All in all, the Waegwoltic delivered a huge dose of normalcy at a time when I, along with many others, was sadly in need of it. By mid-July, aside from the requirement of a mask in the dining room (except when actually eating or drinking) and in indoor club facilities generally, and a request that members check out as well as in, the club was operating pretty much as it always had during my decade-plus of membership. While enjoying a long, leisurely swim in the Lido, I would feel in touch with both nature and my body. After the swim, there was generally an opportunity for a bit of pleasant banter with other older men in the locker room, which relaxed me and contributed to the overall feeling of near-normalcy. If I did indeed manage to stay sane through my move, the Waegwoltic deserves much of the credit.

The Dartmouth Sportsplex, near my apartment on Wyse Road, reopened the week of June 22, not too much later than the Waegwoltic had. But whereas the 'Waeg's' reopening had proceeded quickly, that of the Sportsplex would be slow, cautious—even cumbersome. Its pool, for example, would not reopen until July 22, a full month after the beginning of the facility's general reopening.

When it did reopen, the Sportsplex was a totally different place than the friendly, only lightly regimented facility where I had prior to the pandemic enjoyed Chair Yoga classes and power walks around a track, followed by tasty lunches in its small café. The café would not reopen, at least not during the rest of my time in Nova Scotia (until the end of August). And the building itself would be locked. One could enter only by prior appointment, to engage in activities such as walking, skating, or, later, swimming, at pre-arranged times. Simply dropping in for an hour of exercise was no longer an option. There were also severe restrictions around the use of the locker rooms and showers, including, for a time at least, a requirement that those wishing to swim shower at home before coming to the Sportsplex—a requirement that seemed to me pretty sure to backfire, big time.

I'm all but certain that the new strictures and requirements greatly reduced Dartmouth residents' use of the facility. One doesn't always know in advance whether, or when one will be free for exercise two or three days hence. Give the large size of the walking-running track and of the Sportsplex's main pool, as well as the minuscule number of active COVID cases in the province by this time, quantitative limitations on users, of the sort initially used at the 'Waeg,' would have seemed more than adequate to protect members and staff against COVID. And the locked entrance doors were a complete turnoff, at least to me, making the facility seem almost more like a jail than a sports centre where people came to play. Due in large measure to these many restrictions, I would never again use any of the facilities at the Sportsplex after the start of the pandemic in March.

A key element of the mid-cycle 'thaw' in the Atlantic provinces was the 'Atlantic Bubble,' which allowed residents of all four Atlantic provinces to travel freely within those provinces without being subject to the usual self-isolation rules. In addition to allowing freer travel within the region, the Bubble was designed to help bolster the region's struggling tourist trade. The Bubble came into effect on July 3 and was very popular with Atlantic Canadians. One survey found that over 80% of Atlantic Canadians approved of it.[5]

The Bubble didn't directly promote travel to more western parts of Canada (e.g., Ontario or Quebec), but it did make such travel easier to accomplish by allowing travellers to stop overnight (e.g., in New Brunswick), instead of requiring them to drive straight through with stops only for gas, meals, and the calls of nature, as had been the case prior to the Bubble.[6] In addition to making life easier for travellers, this aspect of the Bubble arguably helped bolster the sagging hotel business in New Brunswick and Nova Scotia.

The Bubble remained in place through the Summer and early Fall of 2020. In November of 2020, however, rising Atlantic case levels prompted its indefinite suspension, with Newfoundland and PEI withdrawing from the Bubble on November 24, and New Brunswick following suit two days later. While some officials from the region have suggested that the Bubble might reopen, no concrete actions along those lines have yet been taken.[7]

The two areas that benefitted least from the province's reopening in the late Spring and early Summer were intercity transit and the performing arts. By early Summer, Metro Halifax's transit service was pretty well back to pre-pandemic levels, with service frequency pretty much the same as it had been prior to the pandemic. The only real difference was the mask requirement, which took effect on the city's busses and ferries in July, shortly before it would take more general effect in all indoor public spaces. Given that most passengers didn't (and don't) have to stay on a bus or a ferry for all that long at one time, the requirement was not particularly onerous.

Intercity and interprovincial transit services were sharply curtailed as a result of the pandemic. Marine Atlantic ferries continued to operate, and (Maritime Atlantic) bus service continued to run between Halifax-Dartmouth and Truro, Moncton, and the South Shore of Nova Scotia. But service was far less frequent than it had been; in many cases, it appeared people were simply afraid to board the busses, even with a mask on. Outside of the region, intercity bus transit was faring even worse. On May 11,

Greyhound Lines announced the suspension of all remaining service within Canada, having already drastically reduced its services earlier that year. At this writing, I don't know if Greyhound Lines has as yet restored any of those suspended services. A recent[8] announcement that the former Ottawa Greyhound station site will be sold to the Brigil real estate company, who plan to launch a major redevelopment of the site starting in March, does little to inspire confidence as to the future of intercity bus service in Canada.

Passenger train service to the Maritime region was completely curtailed as of mid-March. No VIA Rail trains have entered or left the region since then. While the suspension of train service was initially for a period of three weeks, it has since been extended several times and would now appear to have become indefinite. At this writing, I simply don't know when or even if passenger train service to the region will be resumed.[9] As a long-time train rider, I hope that the pandemic does not become an excuse for eliminating such service entirely. That would be bad for the region and its citizens, and, beyond the very short term, bad for the environment as well.

As for air travel to, from, and within the region, it has been all but gutted. While it is still possible to fly from Halifax to central Canadian cities such as Montreal, Toronto, and Ottawa, service to smaller centres such as Moncton and Sydney has been drastically reduced if not completely eliminated; service within the region generally is but a mere shell of its former self.[10]

The creative and performing arts sectors were hit perhaps harder than any other, as COVID would make live dance, theatre, and music performances and even rehearsals a virtual impossibility for many months, and perhaps even longer. While both individual artists and arts companies have adapted heroically, going among other things to virtual performances and streaming of live performances,[11] the situation has remained dire both for many artists and for many arts organizations, with the ongoing cancellation of music festivals, concerts and concert tours, and dance and theatrical performances. I have no firm data on the extent of economic devastation suffered by creative and performing artists, but anecdotal evidence suggests that a great many have had to more or less abandon their art to find other ways to support themselves and their families.

Among the most enlightened and sensitive responses was that of Germany, whose government in late March announced a comprehensive relief program, to the tune of some 50 billion euros ($54 billion) to the country's creative and cultural sectors, including the media. The aid was for self-employed individuals who are self-employed as well as small businesses, and would extend to artists and small cultural business. In addition, social security (including unemployment insurance) was made available to freelancers—including artists—for a period of six months, with expenses provided for housing to ensure that 'everyone can stay in their own home.' To this end, the government injected another 10 billion euros ($11 billion) in support. The sum offered by the German government dwarfed the totals offered by most other countries. Britain's arts council has announced a package of $190 million in support to the arts. And in the U.S., while Metropolitan Museum of Art called on the government to give U.S. museums a $4 billion bailout, the final *total* for arts initiatives in the Senate stimulus bill is less than 5% of that—this in a country with several times Germany's population.[12]

In Canada, while comprehensive data are not yet available, it appears that supports for the arts and artists has been more generous than in the U.S. or the U.K., but far less generous than in Germany. A December 9 statement by the Canada Council, 'COVID-19 and the Arts Sector,' noted that the federal government's November 30 Fall Economic Statement had stated that funding would be provided 'to help ensure that more artists, arts groups and arts organizations [could] continue to create work and deliver their programming digitally during the COVID-19 pandemic.' Earlier (by May 4, 2020), the Council had advanced funds, amounting to 35% of their annual grants, to core-funded organizations. And on May 8, the federal government invested $500 million 'to help alleviate the financial pressures of affected organizations through the COVID-19 Emergency Support Fund for Cultural, Heritage, and Sport Organizations.' Phase 1 of this initiative saw the Canada Council distribute $55 million to arts organizations severely affected financial by the pandemic, while Phase 2 saw the Council distribute $7.8 million in emergency support to Indigenous and equity-seeking groups and organizations. While such initiatives have undoubtedly helped some artists and arts organizations survive, the need for a comprehensive approach to arts relief remains.

In any event, on August 28, I drove my more than fully loaded 2010 Camry out of Nova Scotia for my move to Gatineau, in West Quebec. I suspected that when I arrived in Gatineau, I would find much tougher COVID regulations, given the far greater number of cases experienced in Quebec as compared to any of the Atlantic provinces. For the first month or so of my residence here, this wasn't the case. Providing I wore a mask, I could go to restaurants, shop in stores, and use public facilities such as parks and libraries in the same way as I had in Nova Scotia.

This all changed on Thanksgiving weekend. Following a fairly sharp rise in new cases in late September and early October, Quebec Premier Legault closed the restaurants in Gatineau and throughout the Outaouais, and put new, much stricter limits on gathering sizes in both private and public places, restrictions announced to the public through a harsh official blast sent to all functioning cell phones in the province. The mid-cycle thaw was over. We would all need to adapt ourselves to a second, probably longer and very likely harsher (as indeed it turned out to be) wave of restrictions. The war against

COVID had resumed, full bore. God only knew when we might expect to return to some semblance of normalcy once again.

Gatineau, Quebec
February, 2021

Notes

---

[1] On Mother's Day, it would be a balmy +2°C in the heat of the day, at high noon.
[2] Cuomo, on April 14, had said he would refuse to reopen his state's economy if he thought doing so would put public health and safety at risk.
[3] A modest but interesting manifestation of reopening occurred on June 9, just a few days after the first reopening became effect. On that day, I found no security guard posted outside the No-Frills store I patronized in the Dartmouth Shopping Center, for the first time since late March.
[4] Based on data from the CBC Virus Tracker, as of February 9, 2021. Regrettably, the previous low case numbers did not continue during the third wave, in the Spring of 2021.
[5] Source: Wikipedia entry on Atlantic Bubble.
[6] For more detail on how the Bubble helped facilitate my move from Nova Scotia to West Quebec in late August, see my 'Farewell to Nova Scotia,' which has also been included in this almanac.
[7] As of February, 2021.
[8] In the February 15 CBC online news.
[9] While I can understand the suspension of overnight train service, which would certainly pose potentially significant health risks, I can't understand why the region cannot at least have daytime service between centres such as Halifax and Moncton, or, for that matter, between Halifax and other cities and towns in Nova Scotia and New Brunswick. This would not be any riskier than ongoing VIA service between Toronto and Montreal, or Toronto and Ottawa, which has thus far proceeded largely without incident.
[10] A December 9 *Travel Week News* article by Kathryn Folliott, 'Air Canada advises more service cuts in Atlantic starting January 11,' details draconian cuts to Atlantic Canada's airline service, including both those already undertaken and those about to be undertaken. Those cuts include the complete removal of service from Sydney, Nova Scotia and Saint John, New Brunswick, as well as the suspension of routes to Charlottetown, Fredericton, Deer Lake, and Halifax. Previously, in late June, Air Canada had discontinued service to Bathurst, New Brunswick and Wabash, Newfoundland, while cutting many other routes across the region. For its part, Westjet had on October 14 announced a reduction of 80% of its Atlantic capacity. All information in this note is drawn from Folliott's article.
[11] See among others Harold Tausch, 'COVID, Technology and Me.' Tausch's essay appears in the technology section of this almanac.
[12] Kate Brown, 'Germany Has Rolled Out a Staggering €50 Billion Aid Package for Small Businesses That Boosts Artists and Galleries—and Puts Other Countries to Shame,' *Art Net News,* March 25, 2020.

SECTION 3

Health and Dying

*H*ealth *(or the lack thereof) and dying are at the core of the COVID experience. The nine pieces in this section describe a broad range of personal experience, from living with a family member who has COVID and recovering from a stroke during the pandemic to seeing beloved family elders die of the disease and being helpless to do anything about the situation.*

The section begins with John Allen's moving account of living with a spouse with COVID; a spouse who had previously been something of a COVID-denier, if you please. Next comes Jackie Amable's memoir of her mother, a truly extraordinary woman who survived Prairie droughts, frequent moves through northern Ontario and even an encounter with the fearsome Hurricane Hazel, only to die of COVID in an Ontario long-term care home at the age of 105. This is followed by Jeanette Grant's surprisingly philosophical, even at times upbeat account of what it's like to be suffering from a terminal illness—in this case, ALS, or Lou Gehrig's Disease—during the COVID pandemic, and by Ian Johnson's saga about recovering from a stroke during the pandemic. Not without a touch of black humour, Ann McMillan's poem, 'Aged Lament,' places COVID at the end of a long list of complaints to which elders are subject, ranging from wrinkles, crinkles, and keratosis to gonorrhoea, bursitis, and chlamydia. What next, indeed?

Trying to be with, and to care for, aged relatives confined to long-term facilities has, for many, been among the greatest challenges of the pandemic. Susan Mills' story about watching her mother deteriorate through the window of a nursing home will resonate with the numerous Canadians who have been faced with such a situation. So too will Jany Lavoie's brief memoir about her 100-year-old mother, 'Ma mere, centenaire de la COVID.' And Teresa Patterson's short story, 'Life Support,' a gentle but powerful protest against COVID-deniers from the perspective of an elder whose nurse daughter is dying, will move anyone who doesn't have a heart of stone.

On a related subject, my own essay-memoir, 'COVID and Mental Health,' has sought to show how ill-equipped the already battered Canadian mental health system was to deal with the serious mental health consequences arising from pandemic-induced lockdowns. Finally, Jim Petrie's ultimately upbeat memoir about giving up drinking during the pandemic is a prime example of someone using a time and an experience most would have considered extremely difficult to achieve major positive change in his own life.

When They Come Back
John Kevin Allen

It is 7:00 a.m. on this early Spring morning. I glance outside our kitchen window; frost hugs the ground behind our house and the woods dance in a wind that has picked up. I've started a morning pot and so the coffee maker sputters and clicks while I step outside and crunch through the grass to spread small piles of dried corn from our feed bins. I pause to enjoy the peach and rose hues sneaking up the horizon to the east as early sunlight pokes through the trees, but I have visitors waiting and so I come back into the warmth, into a kitchen full of nutty aroma. I pour a cup, station myself at the window, and wait for my daily ritual to begin.

Four whitetail deer emerge from the woods looking this way and that, their steps tentative, their ears high. Three adult does and one juvenile, maybe a male, make a dark trail through the grass to the golden piles. They each bend down to take mouthfuls of corn and rise up to chew, stray kernels falling from their mouths as they scan the house windows. I raise my cup to my lips; one doe gazes up at me and cocks her head. If she senses danger, she will stamp her foreleg to alert the others, but that leg never moves. She swallows, then bends over for her next mouthful. I lower my cup. The early morning ballet continues, graceful necks down for the mouthful, up for the crunch and swallow until the piles are gone. The deer nuzzle the ground to gather up stray kernels and one by one return to the woods.

Thirty minutes later, my wife shuffles down to sit at our kitchen table. She doesn't like mornings and so I have to wait a little to share my news. I finally do and she blinks as I describe the three does and the baby. Each visit from the deer is a harbinger of good things ahead. They are a shooting star, a long-lost heirloom found. The deer came, I tell her. What a great day it's going to be. She nods, eyes still bleary from sleep. She tolerates my excitement at this early hour, but even morning fogginess is not enough to quell her sarcasm, the spice in our relationship. 'Well, how nice for you,' she smirks and sticks out her tongue.

My excitement was born of absence. Six months earlier, the deer had stopped coming. Golden piles of corn remained long after I put them out, reduced a little by squirrels and rabbits. A few blue jays fluttered down squawking and ate the kernels one at a time, but those piles never disappeared. I wondered if a neighbour had erected a fence at the other end of the woods or if the deer had been culled by the wildlife people concerned about some wasting disease. Maybe the corn was too uninviting and I needed to try another brand. So, my wife and I had gone to the local farm and feed store to find alternatives. At the farm and feed store, I paused at the entrance to put my mask on. I pointed to the 'Please Wear a Mask' sign at the entrance.

'You should put yours on,' I said, the words out before I could stop them. The fuse was lit.

'You know what you are,' she said. 'You are a mask-hole. No one has the right to tell me what I can and can't do. You and all the other lib sheeple get right in line when the government tells you to.'

Public health is politicized in our rural county and my wife is among the many who, if they wore masks, would wear one with the yellow 'Don't Tread on Me' flag of the American War of Independence. As we entered, we saw many walking around maskless, shopping with a hint of swagger that said, 'Don't tread on me with your liberal jackboots. You do and you'll get more than you bargained for.' The War of Independence lives on in the farm and feed store.

I did my best to laugh her out of her outrage. I made a joke about the mask police taking her away to have one permanently sewn to her face, which provoked a grin, but she returned to railing against the evil of governmental overreach. In the past, I had responded to these give-me-liberty-or-give-me-death moments with humour, but it was becoming harder to do. She knew I was a chaplain at a hospital that treated dozens of COVID-19 patients, many immobilized by the disease, entangled in respirators doing the work their bodies could no longer do for them. She knew the stories I was hearing from my fellow chaplains working on the COVID units, of patients' bodies hijacked by this aggressive disease, of families in anguish as the virus outpaced the hospital's interventions. And yet she still insisted the pandemic was an overblown conspiracy and those patients were outliers.

'They all came in with underlying health issues,' she told me when we returned from the feed store. 'Really, it's no more destructive than the flu,' she insisted, emphasizing the rarity of anyone previously healthy developing full-blown COVID-19.

I responded with the story of the 25-year-old woman with no previous health issues who had come into my hospital with typical symptoms: a persistent cough, loss of taste and smell, a lingering fever. The virus had taken her with terrifying speed, leaving her medical team helpless as the disease filled her chest with concrete. Two weeks later, she lay unconscious and dying. The attending physician called her parents to tell them they should come quickly. It was nighttime and one of my fellow chaplains met them in the hushed lobby, took them through dark hallways to their daughter's ICU room and explained that they could not enter, but could only see her through an observation window. She also explained they could only stay an hour due to the hospital's restrictive visitor policies. The parents, both in their late fifties, stood at the window… their daughter was unrecognizable through the tangle of tubes and wires that enclosed her like a cocoon. They huddled there in the quiet and as the hour came to a close, her father reached up and placed his fingertips on the window and held them there until it was time to leave. Five misty rings of longing remained as the chaplain walked the parents back to the lobby, saying the doctor would notify them when their daughter had passed away. The couple did not sob or moan or sniff. They were quiet, said thank you, and held hands on their way to the parking garage. This chaplain, a woman who has witnessed more death and pain than anyone I have ever met, blinked back tears as she told this story.

My wife nodded but remained unconvinced. 'It's sad, but still, not that many people die from it. More people die from the flu each year.' I wanted to tell other stories, but stopped. This was like talking to a brick wall. Besides, I was a mask-hole, a discredited witness, a liberal stooge. To persist would be pointless.

Weeks went by and the deer still didn't come. I went to the kitchen window each day as Fall gave way to Winter to see if the piles of corn had disappeared in the night. They had not. One morning, I was craning my neck to look for hoof prints in the snow when my wife began to cough from our upstairs bedroom. This was not unusual—her lungs have flared with asthma now and again—but this cough was different. It rattled her chest in a way I had heard once a few years ago when she'd coughed so hard that she couldn't draw a breath. When she finally did, my sassy, spicy wife whimpered that she was scared. I was terrified. That terror formed in the back of my throat as I took the steps two at a time to our bedroom where she was sitting up, coughing, wheezing, one finger held up at me: wait, wait. I could not and went to her, but the wait finger insisted I give her space. She pulled an albuterol inhaler from her bedside table, took a long hit and breathed. Crisis averted.

'I'm fine,' she croaked, eyes red and watery.

'Are you sure?' I was edging toward the door, ready to run back downstairs and grab my cell phone to call the hospital as I had the previous time.

'I'm fine,' she insisted and shooed me out of the bedroom, but the cough persisted that day and for days after. I moved out of our bedroom to the guest room next door to give her the freedom to cough in the night as I'd done the time before, but it was really a quarantine for us both. I sensed what was coming.

Fever arrived, accompanied by blistering headaches and an inability to smell or taste. Her edgy snark dimmed to a dull lethargy. One morning, she sat slumped across from me at the kitchen table, hollow-eyed and coughing. She was not fine. I insisted that she go with me to the local health clinic to get looked at. She agreed without a fight.

We arrived at the clinic entrance and met the 'Masks Required' sign. I glanced at her, expecting daggers and a frosty look, but got none as she slipped a plain surgical mask on without a word. We sat in the waiting area, where there were many masks for sale in a display area. I make jokes about their placement next to the adult diapers. Cough too hard and you'll soil yourself. She offered a smile with her tired eyes, but I could tell even this was an effort and so I stopped. The nurse called her in and I waited. An older woman with a cane and a foot boot sat and stared straight ahead as another woman four seats down coughed from behind two masks. A man sitting across from the coughing woman stood, stretched, perused the mask display and sat down in a chair further away. The pandemic had created a caste system separating the infected from those not infected. I wanted to offer a look of empathy to the coughing woman to let her know that I was Above All That, but she stared at the floor.

When my wife reappeared, the nurse confirmed that she probably had COVID-19. She could get tested when she felt better, but it would be best to quarantine herself over the next 10 days. If the fever did not break in a day or two, she should go to the hospital. But even if the fever broke, the fight would be far from over; the virus could always reassert itself. We'd need to watch and wait.

The fever did break a day later, but the virus left its muddy boot prints in her lungs. Every night, I cringed with each cough, each gag from her bedroom. Whatever self-righteous 'I-told-you-so' *schadenfreude* I'd harboured crystallized into guilt. I had been vaccinated due to my work in healthcare, but she had not. I was on a life raft while my wife flailed adrift, coughing and sputtering in the turbulent sea of this pandemic, the sharks getting closer. I was helpless to help my wife, who had developed a shuffle, and was exhausted from too much coughing, lifeless from too little air in her lungs.

Please God, I prayed each night, don't let her be cocooned in that ICU room and leave me standing outside. Please don't make me leave my finger-prints on that window.

Every day, I texted her from work. Coughing made phone calls difficult, but our texts were just as listless as our conversations.

- How are you feeling?
- Fine.
- Are you sure?
- Yes.
- Can I get you anything on the way home?
- No.

I distracted myself with visiting patients on the mental health floors where I served as chaplain. Many of these patients had flailed in the roiling sea of the pandemic, horrified as the sharks took everything and everyone they loved. One woman had been notified by e-mail that her career of 23 years had been sunk by 'pandemic-related adjustments.' Days later, her aging mother died of complications related to COVID, followed by her father. Then her brother had shot and killed himself, overwhelmed with grief, isolation, and alcohol. She told me that she could no longer see any light; the virus had taken it all away, leaving her in shadows that whispered despair in the long nights. I heard her story repeated in room after room, each telling accompanied by a haggard emptiness. The pandemic had touched none of these patients' bodies, but it had maimed their souls with its dead-eyed indifference.

I didn't realize how overwhelmed I was with my patients' despair and my own until I lost my composure at a department staff meeting. We were doing our pro forma how-are-you-doing check-ins, when I shared that my wife was struggling 'but she's getting there.' My voice caught and I began to curse... and immediately apologized. It was not all fine. It was not all good. My hand was balled into a fist jammed in my lap. I shared with the group the fright that I dared not share with my wife. My colleagues, all chaplains, nodded quietly. Some reached out to me with their hands, others with their eyes. All of them were kind. They had heard this story, heard these emotions many times on their floors among the families of COVID patients. The chaplain who'd accompanied the quiet couple asked me how she could help and I asked her to pray for my wife. Just pray, I asked and I felt better, a bit of steam released from my pressure cooker. I realized that I was not alone.

Weeks went by. Although my wife did not get dramatically better, she didn't get worse, and so we settled in for a recovery marked by accommodation. We adjusted to the demands that the virus had made on us like some uninvited house guest. Dinnertime was a case in point. We learned to abandon delicious meals in favour of the bland. My wife thrived almost exclusively on tomato soup, crackers and potato chips. Tomato soup with crushed crackers had a consistency that she found comforting. Just the feel of it helped, she said, even if she could not taste or smell it. She said the dish took her back to her mother's kitchen, where tomato soup was just the thing to cure the cold day doldrums, a bit of warm sunshine in a bowl. She craved potato chips because she could taste just a bit of the salt and so each crunch came with the hope that her taste buds would revive soon. She was slurping and crunching her way back to health.

The long haul of recovery has taught me to appreciate the what is, rather than the what should be. I have come to appreciate life in its small increments. Two weeks ago, I was at the kitchen window. The recent snow had mostly melted, leaving small white patches in our yard that sparkled in the early sun. Tree branches wiggled their fingers, some with the smallest of buds at their tips. A blue jay landed on one of those branches and then another landed, both squawking as a cardinal crooned in the distance. Still no deer, but no matter. Beauty abounded.

My wife stirred up in the bedroom, coughed a few times and then came into the kitchen. She slumped in her chair and then straightened herself. She took a deep breath and didn't cough. This was progress in centimetres.

I wanted to kiss the top of her head to celebrate, but it was too early in the day for her. Instead, I poured myself a cup of coffee, answered a text on my phone and returned to the window. Two deer stood at the pile of corn, bent over, gathering mouthfuls. One of the does raised her head and looked up at me as she crunched, eyes content, ears relaxed.

'They're back,' I whispered as though saying it too loud would scare them away.

'Who?'

'The deer. They're back.'

My wife offered a fingernail of a smile. 'Well, good for you,' she smirked and stuck out her tongue just a little. The spice was returning.

I felt a knot growing in my throat. I stifled a sob and put my fingertips on the window, just low enough and soft enough not to startle the deer.

My Mom
Jackie Amable

Beatrice Grace (Beliveau) Gendron was born in Swift Current, Saskatchewan on November 15, 1914. She was the third daughter of four born to Frank and Victoria Beliveau. The family homesteaded in Shell River, Saskatchewan across from the Ahtahkakoop First Nation, formerly known as the Sandy Lake Reserve.

I grew up with my mother recounting tales of her childhood and teen years. Her oldest sister Patricia eventually went off to attend teachers' college, the second oldest, Madge, was sickly and unable to work and eventually had to be admitted to a tuberculosis sanatorium in Northern Ontario, and the youngest, Rose, was still a baby leaving my mother to help out with the 'chores' as she always called work. Chores consisted not only of cleaning the home, cooking, and baking but the usual barn tasks as well. One of her favourites was to get the cattle that had migrated to the back of the long farm and into the bush on her horse, a 'paint' called Old Joe, and bring them up to the barn at night. He had a white blazed face with a crazy black eyebrow painted over one eye, which gave him the roguish look that said everything you needed to know about his personality. My mother would recount with pride how she could turn a herd of cattle with her bullwhip by hitting, not the cow in front of her, but the cow in front of that one on the nose. Her face would soften as she would recount how Old Joe was dropped off by drovers taking a herd of cattle to market. He had been born on the trail and they were tired of having to stop to let him feed and then catch up with the herd and carry him on their saddles when they were moving. At first, Joe was raised in the kitchen, in front of the fireplace. Eventually, when he got too big, he would join them for breakfast by poking his head in the window over the sink to check if they were all up and ready to start the day.

The Great Depression had hit and there was no work; nothing to allow a young woman to earn money and begin her life. The Prairies were a dustbowl, not able to sustain a blade of grass. Madge had married and moved to Sudbury, Ontario. Her husband, a qualified machinist, had found work at Inco Mines. Aunt Madge kept urging my mother to come out and look for work in Sudbury as there were possibilities here. At the same time her husband was urging his best friend he had grown up with to come out as well and get work in the mines. Like a good sister, my Aunt Madge would invite her husband's friend over for suppers and eventually my mother married my father, Alford Gendron and had two boys and myself, a girl.

My mother would tell how after my father worked his shift underground at Inco he would jog six to eight miles to the boxing ring, and fight his fight. My mother would take my two brothers who were approximately six and four years of age by bus to the fight hall and watch the fight. There was no such thing as getting a babysitter; money was tight, this was depression time and you didn't trust your children to people you did not know extremely well. Sitting at ringside, they cheered their father on. I asked my brothers once 'Were you not afraid Dad would get beaten up badly, hurt or lose his fight?' They said, at that age, they knew their father was invincible and when he did lose a fight, they knew he would come back stronger. After the fight was over my father would hoist Frank on his shoulders and my mother would hoist Keith on hers and they would walk/jog the five miles home.

Many of the miners in those days would enter sports like boxing or wrestling to earn extra money and represent the mine they worked for. They didn't get extra pay for representing their employer, it was simply a source of pride or bragging rights for both the employer and employee. The mines would sponsor those who were in a professional sport like boxing or wrestling by paying their entry fees, and a little extra money was earned for the family with the winnings. This continued until shortly after my father won Northern Ontario's Heavy Weight Championship.

The day came when the unheard-of happened to my father, who had the reputation of never being knocked out cold and rarely even having an opponent connect with his head. He was knocked out cold and dropped to the mat like a stone. Under normal circumstances, when a fighter wins by a knockout, the gloves would be taken off in the ring to show that it was a fair fight and that there was nothing in the gloves like a weight of some kind. My father's opponent instead took off for his dressing room with his seconds in tow. My mother jumped up and ran after him carrying Keith, holding on to Frank's hand and with one of my father's seconds chasing after her. My mother was five feet tall and 120 pounds but she pushed past the guy standing at the door of this fighter's dressing room and broke through the door just in time to see the fighter's seconds cutting black tape from his hands. He had cheated. Black tape on a fighter's hands inside a glove with the sweat ends up hard. When he connected with my father's jaw it was like being hit with a rock. After that, my father quit boxing. He felt when you had to worry about opponents cheating to win, then it was time to hang up the gloves. Boxing was a means to earn extra money, not to end up dead or injured for life and leave a young family to struggle on.

Years later when I was a teenager and we were living in Port Credit, my father happened to meet a man who had fought the same circuit with him. They recognized each other walking down the street and of course old stories came out and they did a bit of catching up. They said their goodbyes and wished each other well. I remember my father saying of his old friend, that could have been me. The guy had a cauliflower ear and you could tell he had been hit in the head too many times. He slurred his speech and at times forgot what he was saying in mid-sentence. My father was very quiet the rest of the evening and you could tell he was thinking what might have happened had he not quit boxing when he did. This friend was a good boxer and was champion material, though he never did get a Championship under his belt.

Besides being hard and dirty work, mining was a life for gypsies back then. A man would be promised at least 10 years' work. But the mine would fill up its work quota, and before the year was out, it would close and everyone had to scramble to find work in other mines and move their families, eating up any savings in the meantime. The peculiar thing was that my mother always knew before anyone else did that they were moving. She would suddenly get this inexplicable urge to clean house from top to bottom, throwing out anything no longer needed and repacking whatever should be packed. At some point, my father would come home with this look on his face and my mother would simply say, we are half packed, you go ahead of us, find a job, let us know where and we will join you.

In 1950 they decided to move to Niagara Falls, Ontario where my father, by then a blaster by trade, was hired to blast the tunnels that tourists now go through under the Falls. As the Horseshoe Falls would erode, they would go underneath to rebuild them and the tunnels were needed for the men working on the Falls. My mother worked as a waitress at one of the local restaurants and would recount how William (Red) Hill Jr had gone over the Horseshoe Falls on August 5, 1951 to his death in one of his daredevil stunts. He had come in to her restaurant the night before and drank all night, playing 'Danny Boy' over and over on the jukebox... until the restaurant closed for the night.

My brothers had grown tall and flourished with the Niagara air and fruit, something that was not easily had in the North. My mother, being from solid French-Canadian heritage, canned just about every fruit and vegetable imaginable and not just a basket of peaches here and there. Bushels of whatever: grapes, peaches, pears, plums, tomatoes corn. She made every relish there was a recipe for. She baked her own bread from scratch as she considered eating bought bread was a sin that carried a punishment close to going to Hell on a bobsled. For entertainment she quilted. I cannot recall my mother ever buying a bedspread, a bottle of jam, or a loaf of bread until I was in my late teens. But as she got older and the grocery store was literally across the street, somehow Hell had frozen over and she bought jams, jellies and loaves of bread.

After I was born in 1953, with 15 years' difference between me and my brothers, my family moved back to Northern Ontario... back to the mines where the money was. However, they made a stop at my Aunt Madge's farm in King, Ontario. We were to wait there until my father found work at a mine and sent for us. Everything we owned—stove, fridge, furniture—had been packed and tarped down on the back of a half-ton Ford pickup and then got unpacked into the loft of the barn. My mother, always needing to keep busy, helped with the 'chores' around the farm, of which there was no shortage.

That year, the Summer was hot, humid, and stifling. A few months in, the inevitable happened. Tempers got short and flared, and my mother decided to leave. She got my brothers together and with their help loaded everything back on to the back of the pick-up and started shifting gears. With the boys beside her in the cab and me lying on their knees, she headed up the long hill out of my aunt's farm and north to join my father. A storm had come in with strong winds and heavy rain. With nowhere to stop to wait it out, she kept rolling through, with wipers on high, wheels rolling and me blissfully sleeping away. The tarp had become loose, so when an overpass finally came up my mother drove under it, pulled over and got out to tie the tarp down. She often said the wind screamed like a banshee overhead and she had to hang on to the side of the truck to keep from being blown away as the wind was funneled in like a wind tunnel. We all sat there for a while until the storm died down and we were able to continue on our way. Later Mom found out the storm was actually Hurricane Hazel, which had caused a path of destruction through a good part of the country. As a result of the rain, the hill on the farm was so badly damaged that they were stuck for three weeks waiting for things to dry out enough to be able to get their cars out.

Life continued with my father working in various mines in Northern Ontario. My mother kept the family fed and clothed. She sewed my dresses and slacks and even Winter coats and knitted our mitts and socks. When my father was injured in the mines and unable to work, she worked as a waitress. Through all of this she learned the stock market; penny mining stocks. Everything was familiar, the names of the mines, the producers, the ore... The *Northern Miner* and *Good Housekeeping* magazine were staples in our home, and I grew up with the stock market being discussed over breakfast.

We lived at the mine site, an hour from the nearest town hospital. While other women 'coffee-klatched,' my mother was heading to town to the broker's to see what the markets were doing. After spending the day at the broker's, she would pick up a few groceries and head back home in time to make supper. My mother was a patient, kind and thoughtful person, but like most short women—she was only five feet tall—she compensated for her lack of size with a temper and piercing blue eyes that could drill right through you. When she'd had enough of whatever unfairness was happening, she had a way of slapping back everyone involved. At the same time, she also had a sense of humour that would have you rolling on the floor in tears. Her blue eyes would sparkle as she would come out with an apt one-liner for the moment, always hitting you when you least expected it.

Since my mother had been raised with only girls and my father with three sisters and one brother on a farm in northern Saskatchewan, they were used to women doing whatever work was needed. They didn't have a 'that's women's work or men's work' attitude, which was unusual in those days. Often my mother worked shoulder-to-shoulder with my father loading furniture, repairing the car, etc. My mother would wonder how the other families managed when most women left everything up to their men, including driving. Often men would have to come off a shift underground, shower and jump in the car to drive one- or one-and-a-half hours to town so their wives could grocery shop.

One incident from those days remains firmly planted in my mind. It was a daily thing for the older boys, whose fathers were usually 'management' at the mines, to physically fight the kids of the miners. After one of these altercations, my mother didn't send me to school the next day. We got in the car after breakfast and she drove to Sudbury, about two-and-a-half hours from our home, to a shoe store and ordered Oxford shoes with steel toes. I can still remember her face when they came in three weeks later. She was strapping them onto my feet as she looked up at me with that fierce look and slowly said:

'Now you fight, you kick, you do whatever you have to, but you fight, because if you come home one more time crying because of those goons, I will whale the tar out of you. You decide who you are more afraid of, them or me!'

Well, I fought and have never stopped. I can safely say my mother taught me how to fight back.

When my father was getting older and had had enough of mining, we settled in a suburb of Toronto. Now closer to her sisters, my mother did the usual family get-togethers, seeing me through high school, while my brothers started small businesses or worked at different jobs. Suddenly, in one day my mother aged beyond her 55 years when police informed her that her son Keith had been killed in a car accident on his way to work. Although none of us had been raised with our grandparents due to distance, Keith was a constant reminder of my mother's father. He had his mannerisms, his temper —slow and then explosive—his patience and his sense of humour. If you'd taken pictures of my grandfather and Keith at the same age, you would have sworn they were the same man. My mother slowed down after that, no longer the fireball of activity she had been. When Keith was alive, he and my mother would get up in the morning before the rest of us, and the two would talk about anything; future plans, buying a farm, the stock market, news in the family. Now that was gone.

In her older years, unable to walk because of a fall and her hip not mending properly, my mother entered a long-term care home (LTC). At the age of 99 she still had fewer wrinkles on her than most 50-year-olds and her mind was still sharp, as evidenced by the fact that I had to bring her up to date on the news and its effects on the stock market. She could recall the penny mining stocks she had bought in her 40s, how many shares, what price, what company had issued the stock and whether or not she took a loss or profit. Her television was always on one of just two channels: CP24 News on channel 24, where she could see the stock market run, or Channel 4 where she could watch the only soap opera she liked, *The Young and the Restless*. She would chide the PSWs who attended to her, asking, 'Is this what you want to do for the rest of your life? You're bright enough, go back to school and do something. Get a career where you don't have to jump to some boss's whims.' Others would chat away with her recounting their families 'back home;' what life was like in Africa, the Philippines or Spain. And then there were the ones she was teaching about the stock market, how it worked and how to buy and sell.

The day came when Prime Minister Justin Trudeau addressed Canada about COVID. I showed up on Saturday afternoon for my daily visit to my mother at her nursing home, only to be met at the door by one of the PSWs dressed in a gown, latex gloves and mask and advised that the province had just shut down all LTC to visitors due to the virus and in order to protect the elderly. I, along with the rest of the province, saw Premier Doug Ford unequivocally and forcefully state that the elderly in LTC would be a priority and everything would be done to protect them. His famous cry was 'We will have a ring of iron surrounding the nursing homes.' My mother's roommate had her son pick her up, which left mother alone in the room. Since she was bed-bound, she would have no contact with the rest of the elderly there. As only staff would go in and out of her room, she should be safe.

On May 3, 2020 she passed away from COVID-19. I remember when I was informed by staff at the home that she had tested positive. At that point there had been 29 infected and five deaths due to COVID. I had three face-time meetings with my mother. She was in pain and angry and cursing me for leaving her in the home. She kept telling the social worker who was dressed in full PPE that she looked ridiculous and should go home and put on some decent clothes. The day came when the nursing home phoned that she had already passed away. I had been scheduled to facetime with her the next day. Due to COVID restrictions, I could not bury her until Saturday, May 9.

My boarder, a 38-year-old Palestinian/Syrian here under refugee status, came with me to the funeral home. Having no one who would be able to carry her casket to her grave from the hearse, I was going to have to pay extra for the home to provide four men to do this. Without saying a word, my boarder arranged with five of his friends to carry the casket for me instead. It was a windy, cold day with snow in the forecast. We arrived at the graveyard, and as they were pulling her casket out of the hearse, the snow started to come down lightly. It was not your usual snow. It was in small slivers of curls, like small feathers, and had no moisture to it. As they pulled out her casket, the snow became heavier. As I watched the men carry her casket a thought suddenly came to mind that here was my Christian mother being carried by six tall Muslim men and I could hear her voice saying, 'Just like Cleopatra...'

By the time we got to the grave the snow was coming down heavily. My daughter said quietly, 'Well, somebody is not happy!' as I tried to say a few words and thank the casket bearers for taking the time out of their day to help us. The strong wind was whirling the snow around us, and the air had become freezing. I said to everyone, 'Let's just go; this is going to get worse.' We climbed into our cars, and as our front tires came off the driveway of the cemetery and into the road, the snow and wind stopped as if someone had switched off a light.

My mother would have been disgusted at having had this pandemic get her when she had survived so much. My oldest brother, Frank, had passed away from natural causes three years before her. I am grateful they both went early and did not have to withstand the conditions that the LTC homes are under right now. I watched Premier Ford blubber his way on television at the death rate in LTC, promising that improvements were going to be made, new staff would be hired, existing care workers would receive COVID pay... the list of promises was endless and always included Ford's eternal 'ring of iron.' Doctors and retired nurses through their associations volunteered to go into the LTC homes and assist the already overworked staff. They didn't receive even an acknowledgment of their offer to volunteer. Premier Ford's office was contacted by these associations, but they never received a reply back.

As it turned out, Premier Ford and his ministers responsible for the LTC elderly did nothing. They didn't stop the healthcare workers from working in multiple homes, therefore spreading the contagion from home to home to vulnerable elderly. At the rate this virus traveled through the LTCs, Ontario had the highest death rate of elderly in the world. The famous 'ring of iron' turned out to be nothing more than a 'ring of smoke.' Ontario was given over $12 billion in COVID relief money by the federal government to be put toward the elderly in LTC, and a 'safe return to school' for children according to Peter Weltman, Ontario's Financial Accountability Officer. As of January 2021, none of that money had been used for the elderly or anyone else. Ontario went through the second wave and third wave and still nothing was done about the LTC situation. Residents in some LTC had no air conditioning. The only thing Premier Ford did was announce he was studying the problem. One thing we do know, the Ford government continued to negotiate with the owners of the private LTC homes on turning over the non-profit government-owned LTC to them. It is no surprise that our former Conservative Premier Mike Harris, notorious for the deaths resulting from the Walkerton water tragedy among other things, was now Chair of the Board of Directors of one of the largest private care LTCs. It is also no surprise that this home run by Harris, whose wife reportedly also owns an LTC, has had among the highest COVID infection and death rates in Ontario. In one of his last acts as Premier, Harris allowed private care LTC in Ontario. He was also instrumental in having Doug Ford eliminate all regulations regarding LTC, including yearly inspections. Complaints from residents' families were now resolved via a phone call instead of by a personal visit of an inspector.

At the end of April 2020, Premier Ford asked the Federal Government to provide military help in combating COVID in LTC homes. What the military found was a horror show of abuse in many of the LTCs. But while Ford could not help the elderly, he could and did enact legislation that protected the LTC owners and the province of Ontario from any lawsuits from families whose loved ones had died from COVID in LTC. Fortunately, this legislation was subsequently struck down by the Ontario Court of Appeal.

When a new government is elected in Ontario there should be a public inquiry with a view to implementing criminal charges against all ministers responsible for protecting the elderly in the Ford Conservative Government and Doug Ford himself for the deliberate negligence leading to the death of the elderly in LTC during their term of government.

COVID-19, Death and Dying
Jeanette Grant

COVID-19 would get most votes worldwide in 2020 for being the greatest villain of the twentieth-first century with all age groups. Only a scattering of the extremely agéd live with memories of the 'Spanish' flu at the end of World War I, that took more lives than that war. Faces gouged with scars from smallpox had mainly disappeared by the mid-twentieth century. Few people under 40 would remember SARS, that killed patients and front-line workers alike at the end of the twentieth century. Those under 20 have been spared the scourges of measles, diphtheria, chicken pox, and mumps due to these diseases' near eradication by vaccines. Terror around polio outbreaks is no more.

Polio! Children of the 1940s sure remember that word. We were made to hide from it every Summer as images of iron lungs haunted many of us. Don't go near the water; stay away from crowds! It crawled through both urban streets and rural farms as a slinking rat would, leaving the maimed and dead behind.

Yes, as my 79th birthday looms, I have experienced most of these calamities and have heard stories of the others. Scientists warned long before 2020 that another pandemic would come; it was not 'if' but 'when.' Still, in December of 2019 my worries were few as life was good: family members and friends had nothing major threatening, and life in small town Arnprior was sweet.

My friend noted that my speech sounded slurred. The diagnosis was Amyotrophic Lateral Sclerosis (ALS), a disease that destroys neurons that take messages from the brain to muscle. The disease has no cure. Normally, its progression is slow, but the rate of progression is different for every person who has it. Mine was most pronounced in my upper body, so I would probably lose my speech and swallowing ability first. Horror of horrors had hit me! I was afraid to eat for fear of choking. I was afraid of falling every time I ventured out. Living in ignorance of how this disease would progress was paralyzing.

When I didn't choke to death, my much thinner body and I decided after a few weeks that it was best to live one day at a time with no worrying about what might come. Generally, this had been my pattern in life before ALS, but then had come diagnosis and panic.

By January I was coping quite well, as the month had passed without much difference in my condition. Then came the news of a new virus in China that could be a big threat. I took notice. By February COVID was spreading and March saw the first attempts to slow it with shutdowns. This resembled what had been foreseen: *Pandemic!*

My husband David, my friend Bonnie, her husband Graeme and I met in the park or on the porch to eat or chat as we limited our bubble numbers. Patio tea for two or three was the norm. Masks were a constant. ALS had stripped from me the pleasure of eating in a restaurant, so not doing this because of COVID was nothing new. To stay away from crowds had become my norm before March because my voice was weakening so, once again, my behaviour was not dictated by COVID alone.

July brought another scare; my David had prostate cancer. November was taken over by radiation treatments. December was dedicated to Christmas preparation, having a procedure to insert a feeding tube into my stomach, and learning to use machines to help me cough and breathe as muscles had more trouble due to damaged neurons. COVID was out there causing death and grief and I was busy at home.

Oh, how I missed my volunteering and friends, but I had little time to visit or help others when I was needing so much assistance with my own life. Bonnie and Graeme brought me flowers while wearing masks, and we chatted from the porch. The next week *she* nearly died from a stroke.

As February unfolds, my dreams focus on tulips blooming in my garden where I planted them last Fall. Even though the present COVID shutdown is lifting, I won't be rushing out to restaurants, as my meals are almost entirely liquid and anything I swallow takes ages to chew. No table talk flows because chewing, swallowing and writing notes usually do not work together. Drooling also eliminates pleasant conversation as frequent mopping-up is a new norm. Opening of other stores will not be of much interest because my gait has changed and I need a cane even when, and if, my energy level is high enough to shop.

'Gloomy Gus' may be how you might label me, but I am not. This disease that I have has taken over my body this past year, but there is life in me yet. I can still laugh. Bonnie is improving. In some ways, 2020 was a pretty good year for me because my body held up better than it might have. Even with ALS it would have been better without COVID, as I would have paddled and hugged my friends, but COVID did not change my life-with-ALS as much as it has changed other lives. I know that the pandemic-induced isolation will end, if not when it will end. I've lived through rough times before with disease threatening outside the door. I can't say the same for my illness within; it would end my life even if COVID disappeared tomorrow, even if this predicted pandemic had not yet occurred.

Having a Stroke During COVID-19
Ian Johnson

On April 27, 2020, I had an ischemic stroke affecting my left inferior frontal lobe. The type of stroke I had is better known as a TIA (transient ischemic attack or 'mini-stroke'). I had not been aware of any immediate signs warning that this event was coming. At the same time, I *had* been warned earlier about having atrial fibrillation (irregular heart-beat, or AFib, in abbreviated form) when I received an Apple watch from my younger son, Adam for Christmas in December 2019. I'd had a history of high blood pressure, and for many years I had been on medication to help control it. In addition, I had been diagnosed with sleep apnea in 2012, and had been using a CPAP machine since then. Unfortunately, I was not aware that all these preconditions placed me in a higher risk category for having a stroke.

On April 27, I was trying to take a shower but was unable to properly complete it. My wife, Olga, found me in the shower looking dazed and unable to speak. She recognized that I had suffered a stroke, and needed to get to our local hospital as soon as possible. At the time, I felt I was in a 'cloud.' With Olga's help, I finished my shower and got dressed, after which we left for the hospital.

At the hospital, emergency department staff recognized that I had had a stroke, and started to treat me immediately. I was in the emergency department for a few hours, and was then moved to the stroke unit. As I moved to the unit, I realized that I was leaving Olga. This marked the start of my 'separation anxiety.'

During my first few days in the stroke unit, the specialists had determined what treatment was necessary to facilitate my recovery. I shared a room with three other stroke survivors. As far as I can recall, I was the only person in that group who was mobile and able to walk. I don't remember much of what happened during my first couple of days, except that I still had my cellphone and charger. One of the more memorable moments of those early days was the phone call I made to Olga on the third day, to see how she was doing. The call shocked her, because I was now able to speak and understand what she was saying. Two days earlier, I had been in a daze and unable to speak. We both treasured this moment and were grateful that I had made such an amazing recovery so quickly.

After four days, I was moved to a room on the seventh floor of the Nova Scotia Rehabilitation and Arthritis Centre. Olga was asked to send along some books and clothing for me to use during the rest of my six-week stay at the Centre. Once again, I was able to share a room with three other people, separated only by curtains around our beds, a desk, and a chest of drawers.

After moving to the Rehab Centre, I was able to catch my breath and start my life again. But I felt cut off from Olga, my sister Meg, her husband Danny, my older son James, my younger son Adam, my stepdaughter Natasha, and my friends. Because we were in the midst of COVID-19, as a patient, I was not allowed to visit with anyone from outside the Centre, nor could I leave the Centre on my own. Under normal circumstances, I would have been able to spend weekends at home as part of my recovery process. Being confined to the Centre twenty-four-seven and separated from family and friends had a profound impact on my mental and emotional wellbeing, as I struggled to fight depression and anxiety.

One early memory I had had after moving to the Rehab Centre was how I reacted when I took my first shower after the stroke. An RN took the time to assist me with the shower. I recall how much I enjoyed it, and how pleasant it was. After the shower, she put me back to bed in clean pyjamas. As a result, I felt much better and was able to sleep very well.

I had met earlier that first afternoon at the Rehab Centre with the head of my health care team; a physiotherapist. She explained how the therapy sessions would work and how busy I would be. I then arranged for some initial appointments with the providers of my team. I had four therapy appointments each weekday, including physiotherapy, occupational therapy, speech and language therapy, and recreational therapy. My other big-time commitment was to take two hours of rest at some point during each day. At first, I didn't realize how important this was, but daily naps have continued to be a part of my life, even at home.

Family support was another important aspect of each day. I talked with Olga several times a day; this was absolutely vital to my recovery. I also spoke regularly with Meg and Danny, James, Adam, and Natasha, all of whom provided support crucial to my wellbeing.

Even before my stroke, we'd been having a family Zoom chat each Sunday. After my stroke, this link was especially important to me. One crucial event was a combined staff and family Zoom call during my third week at the Centre. This call helped me to get reoriented, and to start to think about leaving the Centre.

Towards the end of my stay, the recreation therapist, in conjunction with Meg and Olga, arranged a special concert just for me. It took place at the Rehab Centre, with Meg at her keyboard and Mark, one of Meg's music group members, on his trombone. The duo played outside in front of a large window on the ground floor, while I stood inside watching, listening and enjoying the music. It really helped me feel comfortable about getting ready to leave. It was so great to see Olga and Meg, who I had greatly missed seeing in person. It was also very soothing to hear many of my favourite jazz pieces such as 'Sweet Georgia Brown' by Django Reinhardt and Stephane Grapelli,

'Take Five' by Dave Brubeck, and 'So What' by Miles Davis.

In addition to my regular therapy sessions, I was invited by the Head of Recreation Therapy to assist with the gardening program on the sixth floor. I helped with watering the vegetables and flowering plants, and was later able to help move them all outside when the weather became warmer. With my earlier gardening experience, I was able to orient other patients to the sights and sounds of gardening. This proved a great way to meet other patients and help everyone feel better. I really appreciated the opportunity.

I have learned that each person's stroke recovery is different. Each person recovers in their own way at their own speed. Due to the nature of my stroke, I have unfortunately lost some of my intellectual faculties, such as what is termed 'executive functioning,' (that is, I have reduced ability to think abstractly and to hold on to information), but fortunately have suffered no loss of mobility. I am able to walk and have no paralysis. In this connection, I would like to say how much I have benefitted from my fellow stroke survivors, who were very supportive while we lived together at the Rehab.

I would also be remiss if I didn't point out how much each staff person gave each day to us as patients. They did everything they could to help us feel better. Many thanks to the staff and students who assisted us each day.

I left the Rehab Centre on June 12. It was a triumphant day, and I really appreciated seeing and holding Olga again. My wife and family welcomed me home with a special dinner. This welcome made a big difference as I started on my external recovery.

I was soon referred to the six-month Acquired Brain Injury Outreach Program. The therapists in that program have been amazing! They have had a profound impact on me and my family. I feel incredibly grateful for their expertise and compassion, as I continue to make progress in my stroke recovery.

By the time I left the Centre, I was already well on my way toward a full return to normal life. I was able to resume living jointly with Olga, and to do many of the things I had done previously, such as reading, gardening, and playing the trombone. At the same time, I felt more relaxed and less stressed than I had prior to my stroke. I was so pleased to return home!

Ma mère, centenaire de la COVID
Jany Lavoie

Le 12 mars 2020 était une journée comme les autres au bureau, jusqu'au moment où on nous a dit : « Apportez votre portable à la maison ; vous aurez possiblement à travailler de chez vous pendant quelque temps ». Presqu'un an plus tard, le gros des troupes se trouve encore en télétravail. Ce changement en était un parmi tant d'autres qui allaient chambouler nos vies dans les mois à venir.

Ce qui a causé le plus de soucis à ma famille et moi, c'est le fait que notre mère quasi centenaire se retrouvait cloîtrée dans sa résidence pour personnes âgées. Les mesures prises pour protéger les résidents avaient leur raison d'être mais isolaient dangereusement ces personnes de leurs proches et de leurs familles.

Nous pouvions apporter de la nourriture et des achats à la porte d'entrée à l'intention de notre mère. On la voyait alors un court moment, avec pour témoin un préposé qui tenait la porte entrouverte… Le cœur me serrait à chaque fois que j'y allais ; c'était comme visiter quelqu'un en prison. Elle faisait sa vaillante, mais on sentait, lors de ces brèves rencontres ou encore au téléphone, qu'elle perdait de son aplomb et de son courage habituels. Au moins, il n'y avait toujours pas d'éclosion du virus dans les murs.

Un jour, pour la voir et lui parler en direct, on a eu la bonne idée de faire un « Roméo et Juliette ». On se rendait au bas de son édifice, on l'appelait avec le cellulaire et elle sortait sur son petit balcon, son sans-fil à la main. Nous pouvions converser pendant un bon moment.

Je vais toujours garder cette image : bientôt centenaire, toute frêle sur son balcon au 4ème étage, le cheveu longuet rebroussé par le vent, ma mère tient son petit téléphone rouge à l'oreille. Elle me regarde et me parle avec intensité, comme si sa journée tenait à ce moment de présence, de vraie présence d'une de ses enfants, en bas dans le stationnement.

Que ces mois ont paru longs ! On a eu la chance que son lieu de vie soit épargné de la COVID, mais la crainte nous tiraillait chaque jour. La première rencontre en personne a eu lieu dehors, à l'occasion de la fête des mères, après trois mois d'isolement. Je me souviens que ma mère semblait un peu absente, comme s'il lui fallait se réhabituer à l'éclat du soleil et à l'intensité de vraies présences. Mais rapidement, dans les semaines qui ont suivi, elle a retrouvé son allant, son appétit de vivre.

En juillet, on a fêté ses 100 ans. Le party était plus petit que celui qu'on aurait préparé en temps normal, et assujetti aux consignes de santé publique, mais en fin de compte mieux ajusté à ses besoins : en famille, partager un bon repas tout en jasant, en riant et en se remémorant de bons souvenirs.

En vous quittant, chère lectrice, cher lecteur qui avez aussi vécu cette aventure de la pandémie, voici la chanson écrite pour les 100 ans d'Yvonne : Sérénade à la Moum (sur l'air de Sérénade à Madame, de Guy Béart) :

Chère Moum, chère Moum,
quelques mots pour toi,
qui as traversé le siècle d'un bon pas…
De ta tendre enfance, petit bébé surprise
à l'an 2020, centenaire de la COVID,
tu as vu passer bien des gens bien des choses,
de quoi rendre quelqu'un un peu morose!
Mais toi tu as toujours dans l'œil quand tu souris
L'amour immense de la vie
L'amour immense de la vie.

À l'automne 2020 nous avons connu une deuxième vague de COVID. Alors qu'à l'été nous pensions être revenus à une vie plus normale, un nouveau confinement a été mis en place. Heureusement, cette fois, et jusqu'à ce jour où j'écris ces lignes, ma mère a pu accueillir, une à la fois, une personne proche venue à la rencontre de sa lumineuse longévité.

Gatineau
Le 1er mars 2021

Aging Lament
Ann McMillan

Bills, bills, bills, bills,
Pills, pills, pills, pills,
Ills, ills, ills, ills,
What is new today?

Wrinkles, wrinkles, wrinkles,
Crinkles, crinkles, crinkles,
Keratosis, keratosis, keratosis,
Halitosis, halitosis, halitosis,
What is new today?

Arthritis, arthritis,
Cystitis, cystitis,
Phlebitis, phlebitis,
Spondylitis, spondylitis,
Diverticulosis,
diverticulosis,
Tuberculosis, tuberculosis
And cancer and gout are also about,
What is new today?

Pneumonia, influenza,
Psoriasis, gonorrhea,
Bursitis, chlamydia,
And, finally, COVID.

Watching Mom Deteriorate Through a Nursing Home Window:
Diary of a caregiver in the midst of a pandemic
Susan Mills

I am an essential caregiver to my mom.

Mom, or as others know her, Barbara Mills, is a resident of a 61-bed long-term-care (LTC) facility near Ottawa.

At 85, she has weathered this pandemic's brutal toll on the elderly. But not lightly, and not without the help of family.

Mom grew up in Toronto as an only and lonely child and so, after marrying Dad, she had six children, followed by 11 grandchildren and two great-grand-children. We lived in Arnprior, Ontario, and she worked part-time assessing tax returns until she retired and began volunteering in the very LTC home where she now resides. For 15 years, she accompanied residents to medical appointments and helped them with their afternoon bingo.

In 2012, Mom had a ministroke and in 2016 she was assessed with dementia. Two years later, she moved into a one-bedroom apartment in a senior's building where she received home care twice a week.

On a very cold day in February 2019, she left the apartment and was later found outside on a bench not knowing where she was or where she lived. The police were called and she was taken to hospital.

A month later, Mom was in long-term care. She was mobile and participated in crafts, music and, of course, bingo. I felt it was the safest place for her. Her physical needs were being taken care of and she had some daily stimulation. Visits from me and the rest of the family meant she still had a good quality of life.

Even after she broke her hip and ended up in a wheelchair in September 2019, she worked with me and her physiotherapist to use a walker so that we could still take short outings.

As her caregiver, I was there every evening over supper because she tended to eat quickly, so it was better to slow her down. My siblings also visited, and if I could not make it in the evening, I arranged for a family member to go. I also went to see Mom on weekends when I would do her hair, and we would reminisce and read the newspaper together while enjoying tea and a treat. Or we'd go to my place for lunch, do exercises or attend activities at the LTC home.

As a caregiver, you ensure a continuity of care: I know my mom and her history and I can tell if something is off.

Fast forward to March 14 of this year: I received a call from Mom's LTC that visitors would be locked out because of this new virus. We weren't totally surprised as we had already heard about deaths in senior's homes overseas and in British Columbia.

Within days, I'd worked out a plan to do window visits. Staff and I agreed that 10:30 a.m. was the best time: Mom was generally awake and staff would be able to bring her to her ground-floor bedroom window then. I was working from home due to COVID-19, so I could arrange to take my break then, too.

The night before our first regular visit, I taped a sign on her window: 'Susan will be here at 10:30.'

For nearly six months, I was there every morning.

At the beginning, Mom was good and seemed to understand why we were not able to come in. She was able to hold her phone, and communicate well. During the window visit, I would have her do exercises and, when her tea came, we would just talk.

I sang 'You are my Sunshine' to her every day and asked her not to give up.

As time went on, I noticed changes in her. She could no longer hold the phone so we put the phone on speaker; she soon needed a straw and lid for her tea; she could not understand directions to lift her legs or arms; and conversation became more difficult. Often her response was simply, 'Yep.'

I was watching her deteriorate before my eyes.

With activities inside the LTC substantially reduced, she was left without meaningful engagement. Through the window, I could see what the lack of stimulation and isolation was doing to her.

I became an advocate. I wrote a letter to our local paper and e-mailed my local MPP and the Ministry of Health and Long-Term Care. I started tweeting and speaking to the media about the harm being caused to our seniors by not allowing family caregivers into the homes.

Then in June, Mom choked at breakfast. She needed CPR. I received a phone call and was granted an exemption to visit for one hour on compassionate grounds. When she noticed I was there, she gave me a huge smile. She knew she was not alone and she rallied.

The next day, I was back to window visits.

When visitor guidelines were revised in July to allow indoor and outdoor visits, distanced and masked, I tried, but with Mom's declining eyesight and her poor hearing, it was not a positive experience. In fact, during the inside visits Mom didn't know who I was and just went to sleep. It was better for Mom to be able to see a full face through a window.

Each day brought further cognitive, mental and physical decline. More and more times she failed to recognize us; more and more times there was just silence.

On August 14, five months to the day after we were locked out of the LTC, Mom told staff she wanted to give up.

That day, my sisters and I sat outside her window for hours. When Mom reached for our hands, we could only touch glass.

A few days later, her doctor called and she was taken off all non-essential medication. I was allowed a one-hour compassionate visit.

Then in September, caregivers were allowed back into LTCs.

These days, my sister and I are Mom's designated caregivers. We are only allowed in one at a time, so we rotate with one going in the morning and one in the evening. In the morning we are restricted to her room and we do her hair, because if you look good you feel better.

Generally, we play games, work on the whiteboard, read stories, feed her pudding and talk to her while she has her tea. In the evening we are allowed to take her to the dining room and feed her, and then bring her back to her room and get her ready for bed.

Her quality of life, while not ideal, is better than it was in the Spring. And she is happy to have my sister and me there.

But with this second wave of COVID washing over us, we might not be there for long. I will continue to use my voice to fight for access to my mom: family caregivers should be considered partners in the care team, and they can be, with proper PPE, screening and testing.

All residents need to be treated with humanity, dignity and respect. And for now, that involves me and my sister being there for Mom and making sure she can visit with the rest of the family... through the window.

Life Support
Teresa Patterson

I sit at the table in my dining room with my iPad open, ready to talk with the nurse in the COVID Unit.

The woman in the bed has sparkling eyes which are closed now and might well remain that way. She has a beautiful face. There are IV bags hung on poles, plus a feeding tube. A catheter is in place, and in the next few moments a ventilator will be added.

This dear woman was brought here from a nursing home following a COVID outbreak. The most vulnerable of the population have been hit very hard and there is not much that can be done. The scientists and politicians continue to advise everyone to wear masks, wash their hands often and practice safe distancing. The whole world is affected and millions of people are infected with this virus, yet there is still a certain percentage of the population who complain and indeed protest that their rights are being violated. If any one of those individuals had to trade places with me right now, they would surely reconsider.

The nurse is now taking me through what is going to happen. The tube will be inserted and the machines will take over the breathing. The woman I see in the bed will likely only live a few more days, so I must say goodbye now, over a computer screen.

Through tears that fall gently and silently down my cheeks I have resigned myself to the inevitable.

The saddest part of this is that I am 72 years old and the woman in the bed is 46. It breaks my heart that I am losing my daughter to a disease that ran rampant through her workplace; her workplace where she devoted all of her working life to looking after the older generation, making them comfortable, bathing them, dressing them, holding their hands when they needed it. And now she will die with the same compassionate nursing care, but without any family by her side. Nursing staff must deal with this every day, and I'm certain it is harder and harder every time.

The nurse on duty with my beautiful daughter has put her on life support. The nurse will stay on line with me for a while, then call me again, maybe a few more times until it is all over.

Life for all of us has taken a new course. I'm not sure I will ever recover from these changes.

Thank you for listening. Stay safe.

A Mother

COVID and Mental Health:
A Personal Perspective
Jon Peirce

Let me begin by saying that I came into the COVID-19 pandemic as one of the most fortunate and privileged of Canadians. As a retiree and pensioner, I didn't have to worry about going to work and getting exposed to the disease, whether at the workplace or traveling to and from work. And it wasn't necessary for me to make elaborate, cumbersome work-from-home arrangements. Nor—unlike many younger people of both sexes, but especially women—did I have to worry about homeschooling my kids, keeping them amused, or balancing my responsibilities looking after them with work responsibilities. While I worry about my kids for other reasons, they've long since reached the age of majority and left home. I neither have to support them financially nor look after them twenty-four-seven.

Most of all, I came into the pandemic economically privileged. Not that I'm by any stretch rich, but my four small-to-medium-sized pensions among them provide me with enough to live on, and a bit to spare. All four have continued through the pandemic. And that 'bit to spare' grew somewhat bigger, quite simply because there was nowhere near as much to spend it on. Travel, a big expense for me in most years, with annual trips to Maine to visit my sister and twice- or thrice-yearly trips between Halifax and Ottawa, became a virtual impossibility. Restaurants, at which I would normally eat once or twice a week, yielded significant savings by virtue of their being closed, first from mid-March to early June in Nova Scotia, and then from early October through late February in Quebec. And I spent a good deal less on gas because there was really hardly anywhere to go, particularly during the pandemic's first wave. I was even spending less on things like dry-cleaning because I had little, if any, occasion to wear the kind of clothes that require dry-cleaning. Taken together, this resulted in an average saving of $150.00 to $200.00 per month, some of which I immediately donated to various good causes. The rest would come in extremely handy to help pay for, first my move from Nova Scotia to Quebec, and then, later, my hernia surgery in Ontario. But I digress.

I was also privileged in that Nova Scotia, where I spent the first wave of the COVID pandemic as well as most of the mid-cycle 'thaw' period, was about as safe a place as any I could have chosen in which to spend the pandemic. It had among the lowest case rates in the country, both in absolute numbers and per capita, and, by late Spring, among the highest recovery rates.[1] It was among the first provinces, along with others in the Atlantic region, to be able to say it had actually wrestled the disease to the ground. By early Summer, there were frequently periods of a week or longer in which no new cases at all were reported.

At the same time, Nova Scotia is about the *worst* province to be in for anyone experiencing any sort of mental illness. Even before the pandemic, its mental health system was in tatters, as I can attest from firsthand experience, as one who has long suffered from anxiety disorder and occasional fits of depression, and who has in recent years had a number of increasingly unsatisfactory encounters with that system. The worst of those encounters came in the Spring of 2019, when I found myself in the grips of a depressive fit more serious than any I'd known for a decade. Having phoned my old counsellor, only to discover that he'd given up general practice entirely in order to specialize in adolescent psychiatry, I went to my GP to ask for a referral to a psychiatrist. Now, I certainly wasn't expecting any sort of miracle. A province which makes people with crippling arthritis wait 19 months for hip replacement surgery, as I had had to do four years previously, isn't likely to have a large stable of psychiatrists at the ready to help people with mental health issues. But as cynical as I'd become about the health care system, and as prepared for bad news as I was, I wasn't prepared for what my GP—a fine man, I must add—told me. Which in a nutshell was: unless I was on the verge of inflicting outright mayhem on myself or someone else, the healthcare system couldn't help me. I would have to locate a therapist or counsellor myself… and pay for it myself. 'You do have an insurance plan, don't you?' he added, in an attempt to soften the blow. I did; one which, if memory serves, offered about $600.00 over a year for mental health services. Something like enough for three, or possibly four sessions with a psychologist or clinical session worker. Something like offering a man with a gangrenous wound a bottle of hydrogen peroxide. In my nearly 50 years in Canada, I'd never had a health are experience even remotely comparable to this one. To all intents and purposes, mental health had been removed from the list of services provided by the Nova Scotia healthcare system, through the back door.

After a single, spectacularly unsuccessful session with a psychologist of the gestalt persuasion, which was followed by various equally unsuccessful attempts to locate a therapist at a price I could afford on my pensioner's income, I pretty much gave up, essentially resigning myself to remaining more or less depressed so long as I remained in Nova Scotia. And over the Summer, with the help of much deep breathing, better weather, long swims at the Lido pool at the Waegwoltic Club, and some travel to Ottawa and Maine, my depressive fit lifted somewhat, though it would not disappear completely until I left the province the following year.[2]

While I felt *physically* safer in Nova Scotia than I would have almost anywhere else in Canada, that sense of security came at a high cost, namely that of near-complete isolation from other people. Even before the pandemic, the lack of a supportive family and close friends nearby had made me feel quite isolated, though I'd long done my best to keep myself involved in the world through activities as varied as Seniors' College teaching, community theatre acting, choral singing, and participation on a number of volunteer boards. Once the pandemic hit, all these things that had, to a degree, helped preserve my sanity and emotional equilibrium came to an abrupt halt. Now I was forced to go days and even weeks without physical contact with others, or even live, in-person conversations.

At first, I had my cleaning woman Colette for company once every two weeks. This certainly helped. After she had finished cleaning my apartment, we would enjoy take-out Chinese together, and then go for a walk around the neighbourhood. While she was able to continue coming, I retained some sense of being able to communicate with another adult. But before long— well before the end of March—she was forced to stop coming. Most of her clients had asked her not to come once the pandemic started; it would no longer have been possible for her to earn a living cleaning. In order to be able to access the CERB program, she was forced to give up any remaining clients. This left me completely alone. Not until May, when things loosened up enough that I was able to have one person in my house, which allowed Colette to return, would I experience any in-person conversation with anyone, beyond the incidental sort of talk I had with clerks at the grocery, liquor, and drug stores and fellow walkers on the streets of Dartmouth.

As one need not be a genius to discern, with the start of the pandemic and the end of hugs, all other direct physical contact, and in-person conversation of any kind, not to mention theatre and singing, my already significant mental health issues quickly worsened. Within two weeks of the lockdown's start, my heart was often racing and I was having trouble sleeping. After I bought some cannabis oil at the provincial weed store and started using it at bedtime, things improved a little, but not enough. I began to fear that if things kept on as they were, I would soon become really sick from stress and lack of sleep. So it was that, with considerable regret—going off the drug three years earlier had been a major achievement for me—I got a new prescription for the anti-anxiety drug Paxil, which I immediately began using on a daily basis, first 10 mg. per day, and then, before long, 15. Once I went back on the Paxil, I was again able to sleep at night—most of the time. But by mid-April, after a month of lockdown, even it was not enough. A Friday night in mid-April saw me experience one of the most severe and terrifying anxiety attacks I'd known in my 60 years dealing with anxiety disorder.

I have no idea what led me to experience such a severe attack at that particular time. Granted, I was always rather anxious throughout that first wave of the pandemic, when no one knew or understood what was happening or what was going to happen, or how long we were going to have endure being in lockdown. But I can't remember any particular thing, or things, that would have led to a severe attack happening at that time. Very likely it resulted from a more or less constant state of higher stress than I was used to over a long period of time (in this case, five weeks).

The thing actually began on Thursday as a minor stomach disorder. Around noon that day, I first had cramps, then a soft stool. On Friday morning, I had diarrhea. At about the same time, I experienced the racing heart and agitated kidneys, with the constant urge to run to the bathroom and the feeling of the bladder's never being totally emptied, that had characterized most of my previous attacks. Despite all of this, I was able, perhaps due at least in part to a comforting telephone conversation with my girlfriend, Ann, in Ottawa, to have a pretty decent night's sleep on Thursday night, with only two bathroom breaks. And through most of Friday, I actually felt fairly normal. By noon, my stomach seemed to be on the mend. I was able to do my writing and take my 45-minute walk as usual, though I noticed I was walking more slowly than usual and feeling some stiffness in my back. I even got in a one-hour nap on Friday afternoon, something I often did when getting up fairly early. That night, I ate a normal dinner and then watched some sports, a retro baseball game and part of a retro hockey game. All part of my typical agenda at that time.

It was when I tried to get to sleep, starting a bit before midnight, that I realized something was quite seriously wrong. Though I normally get to sleep quite easily—if anything I tend to have trouble *staying* asleep—that was not the case on this particular Friday night. First. I couldn't get to sleep for an hour, an hour that became two. At that point, I took an extra hit of cannabis oil. I did not take Clonazepam at this time, as I feared it would not react well with the cannabis. Perhaps this was a mistake, but the Internet literature I'd read suggested that the combination might not mix well.

I wasn't sure whether this was a kidney infection or a massive anxiety attack. The occasional pains in my flanks, along with the racing, hyperactive kidneys, suggested that it could be either one. In any case, I couldn't sleep and couldn't sleep, and it was driving me crazy. So, I got up around 1:45 and sent a whole bunch of e-mails to close friends and my daughter Lauren. Then I tried to sleep again around 2:30. Still no luck. So, I got up a little after 3:30 and did what many women of my acquaintance might have done, but no other man I'm aware of: started a frenetic general housecleaning. First, I put the dishes in to soak. Then I started a load of laundry, the first of three I would do that night. After the dishes were done, I started sweeping and mopping various floors. By the time the last load of laundry was done, around 6:00, I had cleaned most of the house; a couple of rooms including bedroom and office were still left to go. They needed the vacuum cleaner, which I didn't want to run in the middle of the night. By this time, I was sweaty and a bit stiff from all my unwonted exertions. Until three weeks earlier, my beloved cleaning lady, Colette, had been doing all my housecleaning for me. Before that, in Ottawa, I'd had another cleaning lady. I hadn't done this kind of serious housecleaning for myself for at least 15 years.

Exhausted, I showered and dressed for the day. Around 7:00, I lay down on my bed, fully dressed, and managed to get about an hour and a quarter of sleep. This had been my first all-nighter since the birth of my daughter, Lauren, at which I assisted, in 1982. Even then I had managed to get bits and pieces of sleep lying on a cot in the delivery room next to my wife Pat. Between them, those bits and pieces had added up to a more than an hour and a quarter.

By the time I was up and had had a bite to eat, it was time to call the Woodlawn Medical Clinic to see if I could get an appointment with the duty doctor. The receptionist, who was quite concerned at my having stayed up all night, agreed to have him call me around 9:40. Just after 10:00, the call came. The duty doctor asked me a few questions about my symptoms, including whether or not I had a fever. On hearing the symptoms, he suggested I come in so he could probe my belly to see if it was in any way distended. Fortunately, I had a mask that a kind friend from the local Caregiving Group had given me a month or so earlier. Had I not had a mask, I wouldn't have been able to enter the clinic. (This was several months before masks would become *de rigueur* in any indoor public setting; at this point, only doctor's and dentist's offices were requiring them).

There was so little traffic on the roads that I was able to make the five-kilometer drive to the clinic in seven minutes instead of the usual 10 to 12. It felt weird to wear a mask, but eventually, after taking off my glasses, which kept rubbing up against the mask, I got the hang of it. Luckily the mask was big enough. After waiting another half hour, during which I deposited a urine sample into a vial, I finally got to see the duty doctor, a pleasant enough older chap. After probing my belly, he determined there was no distention. He seemed to think that some sort of urine blockage was going on. I did not dispute him—my flow had indeed been iffy of late—but I also didn't think this was the main source of the problem. Truth to tell, my urine flow had been iffy for some years, both before and after my 2011 brachytherapy treatment for prostate cancer. To me, an iffy urine flow was just part of everyday life.

At this point, we seemed to be at cross-purposes, he insisting on the blockage and I insisting there was something else going on. Finally, he phoned in a prescription for Flo-Max to the drugstore directly below the clinic, and wrote me a requisition for a blood test, which I was fortunately able to obtain on the spot, the blood clinic next door not being very busy. He told me I should phone my regular doctor on Monday morning to discuss the test results.

Unfortunately, there was a two-hour wait to get the Flo-Max prescription filled. I was irritated at having to drive all the way home and then back again, but accepted the situation as there appeared to be no alternative. I used much of the time cooking and then eating a big brunch of fruit, cranberry juice, scrambled eggs, toast and coffee. Finally, after a further wait at the drugstore, I got my prescription around 2:00 p.m. and drove home. The rest of the day was pretty much of a write-off. I couldn't focus on anything, and felt tired, really tired, but still wasn't able to sleep. I wound up frittering the day away on the Internet and watching sports reruns. The only constructive thing I was able to do was to take down the daily plague data, so I could write the journal entry later. In the evening, not really hungry but wanting to put something in my belly to prevent serious ketosis, which seemed liable to result from overworked kidneys and an empty stomach, I ate a big bowl of oatmeal, which I washed down with some more cranberry juice and followed with a piece of coffee cake. I sent some more e-mails to Ann and other close friends. Then I took a Clonazepam and tried to sleep. No luck. Half an hour later, I took another Clonazepam and tried again. Still no luck. By this time, it was getting on for 10:30. I knew I *had* to have my sleep that night, or I would get really sick. So, a little against my better judgement, I took a third Clonazepam, the first time in my life I'd ever taken three of those pills in one evening. To my immense relief, it was third time lucky; within a few minutes after taking the third pill, I was asleep.

I would wake up for one bathroom break in the middle of the night, and then a second time around 7:00. Seeing no reason to get up at 7:00, I went back to bed and was quickly asleep, waking up 'for good' at 10:10, just in time for our St Margaret's virtual church service. The service was beautiful and moving, as Charles Bull's services always were, with amazing music contributed by our music director, Emanuel Serra. As for me, thanks to my long sleep, I felt about as close to 'normal' as it was possible to feel in those times, with no sign of either stomach trouble or anxiety. For the briefest of moments, I actually felt as if I could relax a bit. But all too soon, these feelings of pleasant relaxation would be completely overshadowed and overpowered by feelings of dread coming out of Portapique, a tiny Nova Scotia town not far from Truro, where I'd just taught a Seniors' College course. It was in and around Portapique that the deranged serial killer Gabriel Wortman had murdered an as-yet undetermined number of people; the eventual death toll would turn out to be 22.

In retrospect, I may have been fortunate to have had my anxiety attack when I did. If I hadn't already had it, the serial murders, about which the news media kept publishing stories and pictures for days after the horrific crimes, would almost certainly have induced an even worse one than the one I suffered, literally on the eve of Wortman's shooting spree. Still exhausted from my sleepless night, and more than a little zombified by the biggest dose of Clonazepam I'd ever taken, I sat numb, in shocked horror, as more and more details about Wortman's horrific shooting spree emerged, although much of that numbness would change to anger as it became apparent that the spree might well have been averted by more proactive police measures, such as paying closer attention to complaints from victims of Wortman's numerous previous attacks on women, and from people who had witnessed those attacks.

As could easily have been predicted, the event generated widescale anxiety and panic reactions, post-traumatic stress disorder, and a host of other mental illnesses in its wake, particularly in places like Truro, near the scene of most of the crimes, and where Wortman's car had actually been observed on the streets.[3] The already severely overtaxed and understaffed mental health system was clearly in no position to deal with such a massive collective trauma as this. The fact that the shootings occurred during the pandemic, when physical contact was discouraged and, in many cases forbidden, only made matters that much worse. Having to deal with such a tragedy on top of the huge economic and emotional stresses already inflicted by the pandemic seemed—and still seems—almost more than people should be expected to bear.

Interviewed in December, eight months after the tragedy, provincial bereavement, grief and wellness coordinator Serena Lewis said healing might take months, or even years.[4] It may have helped that the mourning for the 22 shooting victims became a very public event, with a moving three-hour virtual vigil live-streamed free to all on April 24, six days after the shootings.[5] But while the vigil may have brought a certain measure of closure to some, it could not undo all of the emotional damage caused by the shooting. Many, said Lewis, were continuing to struggle with PTSD well into December. For some, seemingly routine sights such as an RCMP car were enough to trigger horrific memories of the rampage. Others, such as Portapique resident Leon Joudry, who lost 13 of his neighbours in the rampage, would feel compelled to put their houses up for sale and move away from the area to try to escape the nightmarish memories associated with those houses.

While I wasn't as severely affected by the mass shootings as were those who lost relatives and friends, or who lived closer to the scenes of the crimes,[6] the rampage certainly did not improve my mental state. Through the rest of April and into early May, I would suffer frequent bouts of low-level depression. Having already medicated myself, with Paxil and occasional Clonazepam, as much as I thought safe, I could do no better at this point than take to my bed, hoping to escape the depressive fits by sleeping more than usual. Though this strategy didn't end the depressive fits, it did make them less severe, and shorter, and was arguably as effective as anything else I could have done at the time.

Things would start to improve in May, when the province opened up a bit and I began to be able to have real in-person conversations again. They would improve even more in June, with a return to live church services, the reopening of restaurants, and the reopening of the Waegwoltic Tennis Club and its wonderful salt water pool, the Lido. But although these welcome developments made my daily life pleasanter, they still did not address my fundamental mental health issue, which was my essential isolation from other people, resulting at least in part from my being a complete misfit as well as a 'come from away,' and hence a second-class citizen, despite my decade-long residence in Nova Scotia.

Maslow's 'hierarchy of needs' described my situation to a 'T.' I was striking out completely on the 'connectedness' level of that hierarchy. Only moving out of the province, which I finally decided on at the end of May and actually did at the end of August, would address this issue.[7] Despite the superficial barriers posed by the language issue, in my new home of Gatineau, Quebec, close to my two grown children, my new girlfriend, and many old friends from work and the literary community, I quickly came to feel the sense of connection with others that I had never felt in Nova Scotia, try though I had to reach out throughout my time there. Even during the severe lockdown we endured in January and early February of this year, I felt far less isolated in Gatineau than I'd felt in Nova Scotia years before anyone had ever heard of COVID.

What are some possible conclusions to be drawn from the mental health issues I experienced during the COVID pandemic? While there are many such possible conclusions, for the present I'll confine myself to two. The first is that the mental health system can't be separated from the healthcare system as a whole. There is no firewall between people's mental wellbeing and their physical wellbeing. Who knows but that with a stronger and more proactive mental health system in Nova Scotia, Gabriel Wortman's serious mental health issues might have been detected in time to avert the tragedy of April 18, 2020? At the very least, a stronger and more proactive mental health system would have left the province in a better position to help the friends and relatives of Wortman's victims, and others profoundly affected by the tragedy.

The second conclusion is the need for provincial health authorities to take mental health effects into account in designing and enforcing lockdowns and other restrictions aimed at combatting COVID. During the first wave, from March through early June of 2020, this was generally not done, with the result that those living alone were almost completely isolated from other people, a situation as likely to breed mental health issues as a stagnant swamp is to breed mosquitoes. By the time of the second wave, in the Fall of 2020, this issue *was* being addressed in the new round of restrictions. In virtually all Canadian jurisdictions, including those like Quebec, which instituted strict lockdown measures in general, those living alone have been able to have close contact with one other household. While this hasn't by any means completely eliminated the sense of isolation and loneliness resulting from strict lockdown measures, it has certainly made lockdown periods more bearable. Once the pandemic's third wave is over, and politicians, public health authorities, and policy-makers are able to step back and take a broader look at COVID restrictions with an eye to seeing how they might deal with future pandemics, it would be worthwhile for them to explore possible measures to mitigate mental health issues for members of other particularly vulnerable groups, such as single mothers or two-person households consisting of elders, one of whom is caring for the other and the other is suffering from a disabling disease such as Parkinson's, Alzheimer's, or ALS.

In the meantime, I can thank my lucky stars that, as a near-lifelong sufferer from anxiety disease, I've managed to come through this seriously anxiety-producing pandemic as well as I have. I also hope that everyone reading this piece has been fortunate to come through the pandemic as well as I have. Hopefully, none of us will ever again experience such an event.

Gatineau, Quebec
March, 2021

Notes

[1] For the purposes of this essay, 'recovery rate' is defined as the number of recoveries divided by the total number of non-fatal cases in any given jurisdiction. It is normally expressed as a percentage.

[2] My departure from Nova Scotia and move to West Quebec is explored much more fully in my essay 'Farewell to Nova Scotia,' which appears in the 'Milestones' section of this almanac.

[3] This I heard from my former Truro writing student and fellow almanac contributor Dianna Davison-Veber, who lives in Truro and says that at one point she herself saw Wortman's car.

[4] For more detail, see Brennan Leffler and Ross Lord, 'Emotional Aftermath: Families of Victims in Nova Scotia Shooting,' *Global News*, December 12, 2020. Except as otherwise noted, material for this and the previous paragraph has been drawn from Leffler and Lord's article.

[5] Jackie Vandinther, 'Victims of Nova Scotia Rampage to be Mourned at Virtual Vigil.' *CTV News*, April 21, 2020.

[6] I say 'scenes' rather than 'scene' because the killings took place in 16 different locations.

[7] For more detail, see 'Farewell to Nova Scotia,' work cited in Note 2 above.

Drinking During the Pandemic
Jim Petrie

The first wave of the Pandemic began with this news from my doctor: 'Jim, you need to start an exercise routine.'

I said, 'Okay. I've been involved in exercise all my life. It's only been the last few years that I let myself go. I've been a runner for a long time, I've been to hundreds of aerobic classes over the years, I do Yoga and I was a champion black belt in Tae Kwon Do. All I have to do is reintroduce exercise to my body.'

Then she said, 'You're also going to have to lose five percent of your Body Mass Index (BMI).

I said, 'Well, that's only 10 to 11 pounds. No problem. That'll come off with exercise. What else, doctor?'

'You need to quit drinking,' she said!

'Well, two out of three ain't bad,' I sighed.

The diagnosis was 'a fatty liver.' Even though they weren't sure what caused a 'fatty liver,' I naturally assumed it was the pint of whiskey I was consuming most nights that was the culprit!

Becoming sober was something I'd wanted to do forever.

I remember as a rebellious teenager, my dear mother saying to me, 'Jimmy, I see where you've been drinking with your friends a lot lately. The odd beer I'll tolerate but don't you be drinking that hard liquor. You'd be better off not drinking any alcohol at all. Do you hear me, Jimmy?'

'Yeah ma, I hear ya,' I said. But all I really heard was, 'The odd beer I'll tolerate.' Who would be supplying this 'odd' beer, I wondered?

Ma gave lots of good advice. She raised six siblings before me, four of whom were boys. Her advice stayed with me over the years although I didn't always abide by it.

The first wave of the pandemic in Nova Scotia had everyone scared, but most people listened and conformed to the new world of lockdowns and regulations from our Chief Medical Examiner, Dr Robert Strang, and the Nova Scotia Health Authority. My bus driver job was temporarily suspended and Cheryl, my wife, took a temporary leave of absence from her Tim Horton's cashier job. I went on the Canadian Employment Relief Benefit (CERB), and the Canadian Government generously supplied me with $2,000.00 a month for the next five months. God Bless Canada and Justin Trudeau! My kids were grown up and on their own now, and my expenses were few. It reminded me of the Summer after my father died, which I will discuss later.

97

Cheryl and I thought that the lockdown would be a good time to catch up on that 'honey do' list. Cleaning usually involved loud rock and roll music and a big box of beer but doctor's orders changed that for me. Cheryl liked to drink beer and after a couple of weeks on the wagon I was back drinking again with gusto. I said to myself, 'I'll start another Dry Spell on Monday.' But Monday never came. I felt like a failure and I don't like failing. I thought about going to Alcoholics Anonymous and admitting to this dependency once and for all but, at the same time, I didn't want to do that. Admitting to something and failing weren't in my personal constitution. Continuing to drink against my doctor's orders was, apparently!

As a young man, I did drink a lot, but did I have a drinking problem? Not only did I, but there were some early signs that a concerned sibling or caring parent would have picked up on in a regular family environment. Mine was not like that. There were many dysfunctional families in the coal mining towns in Eastern Cape Breton, and after years of abuse, never physical, my mother left my father in the Summer of 1977, just before the start of my graduating year from high school.

'Bo,' as my father liked to be called, went into a deep depression aggravated by his many other ailments. He held on just long enough for me to finish grade 12 and another year in community college. A week or two after I graduated, he passed away. He had no will to live and no life to look forward to. It was a sad commentary for a young man of 66 in an old coal miner's body. A friend came over that night with a box of beer and offered his condolences.

I was now 20 years old, alone, in a house that was paid for. It was Summer-time in Dominion, Cape Breton. I'd just started a new job (my first) that Summer with very few expenses. I was Kid Rock, all Summer long in '78. I was caught somewhere between a boy and a man.

Drinking was the name of the game and it continued through the 80s and 90s. There were many times when I would quit drinking but never with any real intention to stop permanently. I'm reminded of this quote by Swami Sivananda:

> Put your heart and mind and soul into even the smallest tasks. This
> is the secret to success.

I didn't do that. My Dry Spells were plentiful, thankfully, but they were short... A dry birthday, a dry long weekend, a dry week or a dry month... which all elicited hearty praise from friends. I appreciated their kind words but always felt I could do better.

What I did do in the late 90s was take a piece of advice from my mother and stay away from the hard liquor for a good number of years: seven. Then the Newfies moved in next door! I never met a Newfie I didn't like and this 'nest' was more generous than most. They introduced me to Gibson's Finest whiskey. One said, 'There's not enough 'Os' in smooth,' to describe this taste.

I was back in the saddle barking and chasing parked cars again.

Damn Newfies!

They moved out about 10 years later and I started another, rather successful Dry Spell. I started before the holidays in 2012 and when Christmas started, I had a week or so under my belt for motivation. I sailed through the holidays and January for an all-time record of 37 days sober. Then Day 38 was like I'd never missed a day. I continued to drink almost every day for years until one day, again before the holidays, I put together a dry run that took me into February for a personal record of 47 days. Again, there was more praise from friends, but day 48 and beyond were the usual.

In the Fall, the second wave of the pandemic started and the Nova Scotia Health Authority issued some new regulations once again. After six months off work, I was glad to get my job back. I was one of the lucky ones. It was early Fall, October 25, 2020, when I decided to get a head start on the holiday Dry Spell figuring that breaking my 47-day record would bring me into mid-December when I would normally be just starting a Dry Spell, and with some previous experience I might not only break the old record, but become the person I'd always wanted to be: a sober one.

This time it worked. I succeeded by setting small goals. First, from October 25 to the end of the month I didn't drink. Then the full month of November would give me 37 days. That also worked. Then, I'd only have to go till December 11 to have a new personal sobriety record and pick up on my past experiences from there. Now I was in record territory. As I was sailing through January, the 100-day marker was February 2, which was enough to keep me from settling for the holiday/January scenario. As my feet hit the floor on that 100th day, I began to realize how easy this actually was. The short-term goal was to complete one full season (Winter). As I write this, it is March 20, 2021, the first day of Spring and almost five complete months without a drink. My most recent liver tests showed no increase in numbers on one of them and a decline in numbers on another. That's good news in these crazy times.

I never again want to experience the disappointment, the morning after, of drinking to feel good the night before, because the joy of being sober every morning is a much better feeling. Now, the pandemic's third wave is rolling through our country and our variant cases are rising dramatically. Yesterday, I registered for my vaccine appointment. We are making progress against this COVID-19 virus and its variants.

I am proud of this country of Canada and all its front-line workers and first responders. They are real-life heroes in this pandemic. I am especially proud of Canada's Ocean Playground and Nova Scotians like Dr Robert Strang who have guided us through this disaster so far, by keeping ahead of the curve with the help of our border, the Atlantic Ocean.

I'm sure there's a wise woman, looking down from the heavens, who would be proud of her youngest son on seeing that he had finally listened to her sage advice.

SECTION 4

Humour

The only thing that's harder to do than to create humour is to explain or analyze it. I don't even propose to try. What I can say is that our inventive authors have come up with all sorts of ways to help us laugh at one or more aspects of the pandemic. Su Mardelli's short story, 'It's Not My Fault,' portrays the plight of an entrepreneur who carries recycling just a touch too far during the pandemic. What's not to love about a guy who's willing to auction off recycled celebrity face masks? Gavin Murphy invokes the language of the tennis court in describing his COVID vaccination experience. Jim Pellegrin (aka Dr Q.) offers all manner of COVID-related advice in the 'Spring Planting' edition of his COVID bulletin. And David Shaw turns everyday events like shopping for toilet paper and getting one's house cleaned into little gems of humour. The section closes with a short 'Speech before St COVID-Vaccine,' by one William Shakesneedle. And then I invite our readers to come up with things about COVID and the pandemic that they have found funny.

It's Not My Fault
Su Mardelli

December 17, 2020

To: The Honorable Maurice Mendel, Governor of the
State of █████

Dear Sir,

My name is Felix Wright and I am writing to
request your official pardon for my criminal
conviction. I am currently serving a five-year
sentence for grand larceny and causing wrongful
death. But I assure you, it's not my fault. I am
humbly confident that once you read my entire letter,
you will come to the conclusion that the events that
transpired were random and not of my doing.

I am an entrepreneur. I started an auction
website www.halfeatencelebritysandwiches.com, over
ten years ago after stumbling upon this untapped
sector of the consumer market.

It all started with Jason Totemblake, the
famous quarterback. In a way he was the inspiration
for my unique business model. I had read an article
many years ago about how Mr. Totemblake's half-eaten
French toast was successfully auctioned off for one
thousand dollars. For years, this nugget stuck in my
head until one day a metaphorical pick-axe came
hurling through the air and dislodged it.

I was working as a bartender in a respectable
establishment in Brooklyn. One quiet evening a very
handsome man walked in with a beautiful brunette. I
realized once they approached the bar that I was
about to serve the famous Shakespearean actor Sir
Gerald Rooney and his gorgeous wife. They ordered
drinks but he received a call which caused them to
leave quickly. Too quickly in fact— Sir Gerald's
whisky cocktail still sat there on the bar untouched.

---- 1 ----

102

I immediately remembered Mr. Totemblake's unfinished sandwich all those years ago, and wondered if this was a gumptious opportunity beating at my brow. I carefully wrapped the glass with the untouched drink in Clingfilm and took it home.

After a sleepless night churning the idea over in my head, I decided to test the waters on eBay. I started the auction for 'Sir Gerald Rooney's untouched Old Fashioned cocktail' at $198. Almost instantly I received a bid. I was incredulous! Then within minutes there was a competing bid for twenty dollars more. Then more bids. It became a bidding frenzy until the time expired and the thespian's cocktail was purchased for $3,589 by an ecstatic buyer. I followed up with that buyer, a true Shakespearean fan, and received prompt payment.

The next day I scoured the tabloids for celebrity sightings. I saw a paparazzi photo of Mariah Swift, the famous reality actress, outside her apartment building—a building that I recognized. With the help of our mutual friend Ben Franklin and his twin brothers, it was easy to befriend the doorman Alberto to alert me the next time she ordered take-out. Alberto called the same evening to let me know that Ms. Swift's pizza would be delivered within the hour. All I wanted was the box it came in.

The next day I picked it up. To my great delight 'M. Swift, Pepperoni' was written on it. I posted it on eBay as 'Mariah Swift's Pizza Box', starting the bid at forty-nine dollars. By the time the auction ended, the empty pizza box with her initials scribbled on the front had sold for $1,045. While I make a mean Old-Fashioned, I'm sure you agree that my bartending days were over for good. This untapped opportunity needed to be exploited and I knew I could do it well and satiate this growing demand to the devoted celeb-foodie fan base. So I quit my job, started my website and spent the next decade growing my business and my network.

My network was critical. It consisted of paparazzi, doormen, maids, waiters, and similar

---- 2 ----

working folk who lived in the shadows of the rich and
famous — with full access to their world. They were
the ones who lovingly wrapped the semi-masticated
sandwiches and other half-eaten comestibles, and sent
them to me to auction off. It was a cash-rich
business and I gladly paid a finder's fee to all the
people that played a part in it. In fact, I was
creating thousands of jobs for the gig economy.

I hired my best friend Joey, whom I've known
since we were eight, to be my bookkeeper. He too was
a gastronomic aficionado of the humble bread grub. He
was also quirky with a few odd habits, like his
passion for escalators and elevators, but he had a
incredible eidetic memory and meticulous record-
keeping skills. He remembered every auction and every
bidder--which was better than keeping box files. We
made a great team and we became known as the bona
fide site for authentic celebrity posh-nosh. I
wonder, your Honor, if you have heard of us?

Our Top 3 sellers were always toasted cheese
sandwiches, PB &Js, and chicken shawarmas. These
usually sold for over a thousand dollars, even from a
B-list celebrity. Weird vegan and sprout sandwiches
from famous supermodels also received surprising
traction, in fact a couple of these tasteless rolls
sold for over eight hundred dollars. Sometimes a
gourmet sandwich would garner attention for its
audaciousness, like the 'Bullion Burger' with gold
leaf and beluga caviar. That fancy patty's starting
bid was seven hundred dollars and it sold for $4780.
Our best days were always July 5 and 6, right after
Independence Day. Celebrities would patriotically
munch through fare that our ambitious sellers
passionately pilfered. Several times the site would
crash from the visitor traffic as hundreds of
celebrities' burgers, hot dogs and other delicacies
found their way to the auction block.

Eventually, even Has-been celebrities strapped
for cash would contact me to sell items. My site
became the income lifeline for many defunct stars. We
started to diversify, adding underwear, toilet seats,

---- 3 ----

104

hair brushes, water bottles, and all sorts of knick-knacks. Here are a few:

The dying-breath-in-a-bottle of the murdered pop star Tinkerbell, sold for $1500. The bubblegum chewed during the trial of the famous serial killer, Shirley Spears was sold for $360. Air from Wavesmith's last live concert was ferociously fought over and closed at four thousand dollars to a lucky fan. A slice of the birthday cake of Lilo, the famous porn star, was our biggest winner, selling for $8600.

In 2019, we had over three million visits a day to the site, two hundred auctions a month, three full-time employees, and over one thousand gig employees all across the country. I was proud of the jobs we'd created. The future looked so bright. Then it all screeched to a halt in February 2020. Everyone was in COVID-19 Lockdown. Against the protests of my devoted buyers, I was forced to temporarily close down the auction site. We struggled for months looking for opportunities to reopen— the situation was bleak.

Finally in June we heard some great news. The mayor announced that despite COVID-19 restrictions, Fourth of July celebrations would go on, 'one way or another'. Encouraged by the news, I heard that '*COVID be damned!*', a rich heiress was throwing a swanky July 4th party at her rooftop penthouse, promising a spectacular view of the glorious fireworks. There would be hundreds of guests attending— a smidge of New York's rich and famous. All this intel came from our sassy ex-marketing executive Mizzy, who had joined a face mask company after we had to close down.

There was so much secrecy around this party it was like a speakeasy. You couldn't talk about it to anyone, but everyone who *was anyone* signalled they would attend. It was anyone's guess what the final number would be but whatever it was, it was a lot! Joey and I were so excited at the promising haul of bid-worthy morsels that we volunteered to work the party as bus boys, much to the party planner's relief.

---- 4 ----

Disaster struck on the night of the party when we found out that all the food and drink we cleared had to be *trashed immediately* because of COVID. Joey and I were so upset, we ditched the bussing duties and decided to leave. We stopped by Mizzy, who was working at the party check-in desk handing out the face masks to the arriving guests. She had come up with the brilliant idea to get them to write their names on the front of the mask with these gold and silver markers. The smell was so toxic that some celebrities just autographed a mask, refused to wear it, and asked for a plain one. The face mask company had given strict instructions to Mizzy that any used face mask was to be discarded, and she was dutifully tossing them into black garbage bags.

Joey and I stood next to her watching these garbage bags fill up with hundreds of *autographed face masks*. It's no wonder that we got the same idea at the same time: we were willing to bet that our fan-fierce buyers would pounce on these 'Pre-loved Celebrity Masks'. We couldn't let this celebrity memorabilia go to the garbage dumpster; there was a fortune waiting to be made! So Joey and I went dumpster-diving.

Am I right, your Honor, in thinking it was a necessary pivot for our business?

We left, each carrying two big garbage bags full of signed face masks. We couldn't wait to get started. Once we were back in my home office, we got to work immediately mass mailing buyers, prepping the masks and so on. Hours later, Joey left to get sandwiches and I swear to you, your Honor, that that was the last time I saw him. In fact, I had no knowledge of the deadly fate of my bookkeeper until the detectives showed up a couple of days later with the awful news. Believe me, I was frantically searching for him, because I desperately needed help. The auction had gone live that morning and just as we had anticipated, our loyal users were rabid for their celebrity fix—the first seventeen face masks had already sold for over six thousand dollars! At this

---- 5 ----

rate, we were on track to bag an easy quarter
million dollars from our dumpster treasure dive. That
meant we were set to net almost one hundred thousand
dollars *each*. What a haul! It was a genius stroke to
shift the core product to face masks. Everyone was
having speakeasy parties—we just had to find them.
Best of all, there were plenty of Ben Franklins to go
around; enough for me, Joey and all our partners.
Right, Governor?

So why would I kill him?

Like I explained to the detectives, I was in my
office alone for three days straight— the auction was
so hectic I was lucky to sneak in five minutes for a
bathroom break. Each bid had a stampede of bidders,
and I had to multi-task just to keep up. Without
Joey, I was doing all the photography, uploads, and
chat, not to mention bookkeeping as well. Thank
goodness I had a fridge stocked with bread, cheese,
strawberry jam and other goodies, otherwise I would
have starved. And like I also had to explain to the
detectives, the little pro-photo studio set-up in
with the camera, backdrop, and lights was to
photograph the face masks. What other reason would
there have been?

I was in the middle of the auction when the
detectives came knocking on my door. At first I
thought it was Joey, and my initial instinct was to
hug him and then yell at him to get to work. I was
surprised to see the two detectives instead, and
shocked at the tragic news they delivered. But they
had caught me neck-deep in the many demands of a live
auction so I may have seemed distracted and
unconcerned. Believe me, I was torn up at the loss of
my best friend. But the show had to go on.
Unfortunately, the detectives deduced that my
reaction was suspicious. It fit nicely into their
theory that after we stole the masks, Joey and I had
had a fight and I pushed him down the escalators to
his death. My criminal conviction is based on that
ridiculous theory. I'll admit I'm no saint and maybe
I've committed a few faux-pas in my life, but believe

---- 6 ----

me when I say this was a freak accident. It was not
my fault.

Because I knew Joey well, I feel I can offer
the best explanation. I do admit that Joey and I had
had an argument (as the neighbours told the
detectives). The evening was stressful and we had
quarrelled over opening bid prices. He went for a
walk to cool off, eat falafel sandwiches and joy-ride
on an escalator. See Joey loved escalators— they
calmed him. Ever since we were kids, he'd loved
horsing around, riding the escalators backwards; down
the Up and up the Down. We would race against each
other and he usually won. He must have been letting
off some steam, reliving his derby days running up
the Down escalator. But Joey was also two hundred
pounds heavier than in our childhood days. No doubt
when he finally reached the top he must have been out
of breath and woozy from the fried patties bobbing in
his stomach. He'd probably lost his balance and
tumbled backward over the middle rail, all the way
back down exactly to where the security guards found
him, crumpled at the bottom of the Up escalator with
a broken neck. RIP Joey.

See, your Honor, poor Joey's death was a
tragedy which had nothing to do with me.
I wholeheartedly hope that you will consider
pardoning me. I aim to start a new website www.pre-
lovedcelebritymasks.com and create much-needed jobs
for our economy.

Thank you for your time and consideration.
Your servant.

Felix Wright
CEO & Founder
www.half-eatencelebritysandwiches.com
Inmate #49841, B— Penitentiary
P.S. I hear there will be an inauguration in a few
weeks for the new President. I hope everyone wears a
mask.

---- 7 ----

108

Office of the State Governor

████████

December 31, 2020

Dear Mr. Wright,

    I was deeply moved by your letter. In these challenging times the State must support prolific entrepreneurs like yourself who are able to create jobs.

    Thus I have granted you a full pardon for your transgressions and you will be freed immediately. We wish you the best of luck in all your future endeavours. Please do not hesitate to reach out should you need help in your new venture. As a small token of appreciation for your job-creation efforts, kindly find enclosed two tickets to the Inauguration. Many A-list celebrities will be attending. Note it is a black tie event and face masks will be mandatory.

    I look forward to seeing you there.

Yours truly,

M. Mandel

Maurice Mendel
Governor of the State of ████████

P.S. I have always wondered what LiLo's birthday cake tasted like.

January 17, 2020

To: The Honorable Maurice Mendel, Governor of the
State of ███████

    Thanks Maurice. Coincidentally, it's LiLo's
birthday the day after the Inauguration. Let me know
if you're still curious about her cake.
    See you there.
    Sincerely Yours,

Felix Wright

Felix Wright
CEO & Founder
www.pre-lovedcelebrityfacemasks.com

COVID-19 Vaccination and Tennis:
Is the Doctor's Son a Man or a Mouse?
Gavin Murphy

Are you a man or a mouse? That question ran through my mind as Sally drove me to Ottawa City Hall on 6 April 2021 for my first COVID jab. It was also the start of the outdoor tennis season the following day, so it looked like a possible early season victory in more ways than one. I would get my vaccination and have a tennis knock the next day. COVID would be sidelined with elimination not far behind. But wait! Things were not all that rosy. Tennis is my drug of choice and I was worried that the jab in the arm might affect my game.

Things along the vaccine road started out swimmingly. I managed to book my first jab and follow-up appointment online with little difficulty. I have to admit it would have been tough getting up at the crack of dawn—which in my semi-retired world is 8:00 a.m.—to book. Mercifully I was already up at that ungodly hour, as contractors were building a new front porch on my 105-year-old heritage house and I wanted to remind them, as always, to be gentle with my garden as crocuses and daffodils were starting to bloom.

With my booking in hand, and rather chuffed with my computer skills, I thought things were unfolding the way they should. Then it sunk in deeper and hit me like a Roger Federer serve. Weren't some of the medical and scientific boffins out there warning about vaccine side effects? Yes. Nevertheless, I figured it was worth a gamble. Who wants to die of COVID, anyway? As well, I could hit the tennis courts knowing my COVID vaccinations were rolling along like an on-serve tennis set. Not a bad tactic when you realize the alternatives are decidedly grim and definitely final. As is the case with a desperation lob in tennis when the opponent moves to the net, there is really no other option.

All seemed in order except for the potential lingering effects from the jab. Rational thinking won me the first set, except now I had another problem. The sight of needles freaks me out. As I was mulling over this dilemma, I received a call on my cell phone. I seldom use my cell for phone calls so I thought it must have been a scammer masquerading with the Canada Revenue Agency to tell me I was in big trouble and would be arrested forthwith unless I followed their guidance. It was early April and the height of the tax preparation season, so I thought I would smoke out this charade. Or maybe it was an offer for duct cleaning, which is hardly relevant as my home is hot water heated. Don't these operators ever give up, I thought to myself as I picked up the phone. Though I greeted him with a rather surly tone to my voice, the calm and relaxed man on the other end of the line asked for me by name. Ah ha, I was right, a deceptive and dodgy scammer working the phone directory.

I was about to give the caller a piece of my mind, until he identified himself as calling from Ottawa Public Health. He advised me the vaccination team were running ahead of schedule and wanted to know if I could come in earlier than the 9:10 p.m. appointment. Thankfully, I had not blown my top. I welcomed the revised game plan to get the jab two hours earlier than originally expected. Same court, just a new start time. I was about to finish off the COVID curse. I considered that a straight sets victory.

Cometh the hour, cometh the man, and now the hour of reckoning was nearly here. I needed to get into the zone and it was time to man up. When I arrived at City Hall and registered, I asked the slightly harried woman signing me in if the jab would affect my tennis game. She looked up incredulously as if she couldn't believe her ears. She had probably been asked all kinds of ridiculous questions during the registration process, and perhaps this one might have taken the cake. She wisely said she didn't know, and suggested I speak to the nurse who would give the jab. This made good sense, along the lines of a tennis smash shot to the corner at a critical time.

So, onto the next stage of the vaccination process and a little more waiting. The intensity was building up like the fifth set of a Wimbledon finals match. Then my name was called. The time had arrived at long last for a convincing victory over COVID. 'Game, set and match!' I thought as I got up from my chair and headed to my vaccination destiny.

As I waltzed over to trainee nurse Alicia and saw her tools of the trade, I almost fainted. Good grief, should I carry on or resign myself to something like a tennis walkover defeat? Maybe the time had cometh but not the man? No, I was going to deliver a winner. Alicia was engaging as we exchanged pleasantries. I thought it would be good to put her at ease. I didn't want her to miss the sweet spot. That would be a non-starter, like a ball hit out of bounds. Of course, she was actually calming down a scaredy cat senior citizen. Alicia told me I would receive the Moderna vaccine and there was nothing to it, really water off a duck's back. Easy for her to say as it wasn't her arm. And she wasn't a tennis player, as I learned from asking her.

I convinced myself to alter my game strategy, so I said something like 'OK, let's get on with it.' I had come this far and there was no turning back. In for a penny, in for a pound is one way of looking at it. Then that penny dropped and reality crept in. What would the others think if I defaulted? They would probably brand me as a rookie. I decided I wasn't going to bail now and forfeit. Remember to man up my man, I said over and over to myself as I watched Alicia prepare the vaccine. Nobody wants to play tennis with an unvaccinated opponent. It was an obvious call, comparable to a tennis passing shot.

As Alicia flicked the nasty-looking needle and vaccine with her fingers I considered there might still be time to pull out and concede. No, I said to myself, I just need to dig a little deeper and adjust. I sheepishly asked her if the jab in my arm would affect my tennis game. After all, it is a little hard to serve if your arm hurts. After rolling her eyes in disbelief at such a bizarre question, Alicia said probably not. Out of an abundance of caution she also suggested that I get the needle in my left arm. I considered this a bad strategy, approximating a return tennis shot into the net. So, I piped up and told her I was a southpaw. She then pointed out I could get the vaccination in my right arm. That was a good coach's call. As she readied herself and I rolled up my shirt sleeve, the woman at the registration desk rushed over and asked about my tennis and jab conundrum. Alicia gave her helpful guidance and I chimed in that I remained undefeated this season. I hadn't lost a game yet. Mind you, I also hadn't won any.

All was now in place for the jab. I finally revealed to Alicia that I hated needles and would have to look away. Barely disguising her laugh, she said OK. With that confession off my chest, I was now ready. A few seconds went by and I asked when she would begin. Another laugh and a roll of the eyes told me she was finished. Truth is the jab was done and dusted in a flash. I hadn't felt a thing. A tempest in a tea cup, really. Alicia had hit an ace serve.

I was required to remain on site for 15 minutes after the vaccination to make sure there were no immediate complications. As mine was the last arm of the day for Alicia to jab, I could see her packing up; no doubt she was thrilled to knock off and head home two hours early. After the short wait, I collected my COVID vaccine documents and walked out into a chilly Ottawa early Spring night. I was halfway there in the two-step vaccination process and with no side effects, in fact no double faults. And I was good to go with tennis, a super tie break victory for me.

On the way home, I realized my COVID performance had been a tad over the top. I promised myself I would act more like a man and not a mouse for the reprise when I got the second jab. After all, I was in the safe hands of Ottawa Public Health, and they knew how to serve up vaccinations.

How did the season's first tennis match go the next day? True to form, I lost. The season was only starting and I just needed to work a little more on the backboards. Practice makes perfect in vaccination hesitancy, tennis, and manning up. So, I consider the COVID experience a three-set Grand Slam victory.

Dr Q's Pandemic Bulletin:
Spring Planting Edition
Jim Pellegrin

Tired of seeing your same weary face on Zoom? Your skin turning an odd, pale colour and sprouting crazy ghost roots like an old potato forgotten in the dark? Sick of your baggy COVID outfits?

Well, Dr Q is here to tell you that hope is on the way. Don't throw away those snappy clothes you used to have fun in! Dust off the old credit card! Practice talking to yourself in the mirror, so you are ready to talk to other people when you're face to face with them. Adios, Zoom!

Already you see maskless old people beaming as they walk down the street, falling on friends and babies with hugs and kisses. Of course, these folks are double-immunized and safe, to themselves and to others, but still they should refrain from understandable gloating and wear masks in public and socially distance themselves, if only to be good examples. And non-immunized young people should not envy old double-shotters. Who is likely to live longer, after all, shots or no shots?

So, honor the COVID dead, and protect the living. Get immunized, somehow, and stay safe, and we will kill the COVID by Fall. Adios, COVID, you murdering son-of-a-bitch!

Dr Q's COVID Vaccine Hotline

Q: Will taking the vaccine make me a genetically modified organism (GMO)? I would rather die than be a GMO!

A: No, you would not turn into a GMO and be shunned by your squirrely friends. You can still wear your 'Non-GMO' baseball hat, if you must. And you might consider why you are willing to die for a food fad.

Q: Is it true that the COVID vaccine will mess up my DNA, so then me and my girlfriend will make weird babies?

A: No. The vaccine will not mess up your DNA. Judging from your question, you were likely a weird baby yourself, and your mother still loved you, or at least kept you alive.

Q: If we are fully immunized, I know that we can safely visit with family and friends. Does that mean that we have to?

A: No. You can still avoid people you don't want to be around. Just tell them you want to be extra safe and hold off for another 10 years in case of new viral mutations.

Q: Is gluten used in the manufacture of COVID vaccines?

A: No. COVID vaccines are gluten-free, as if it mattered. Please, only one question per caller.

Q: What about peanuts and tree nuts?

A: Oh, for God's sake, try to think about somebody besides yourself!

Q: All right, then, what about my service dog? He's an essential worker, isn't he? Can I donate my vaccine dose to him?

A: No! And beware of dogs. Dogs love the pandemic, and want it to go on and on. The last thing they want is for everybody to go back to work or school, so of course they will do whatever they can to keep you from getting the vaccine. Do not be tricked out of your vaccine by your pets!

More COVID Time-Killer Tips

Try to daydream more. Why limit yourself to night-time dreams that you can't remember anyway? Imagine you are a bird, for example. If you were a bird, you could fly anywhere, anytime, right? You'd be free. Imagine you could fly to Costa Rica and hang out with the rainbow macaws and the lazy, happy monkeys napping in the treetops. Better yet, dream you are a happy, lazy monkey napping in the treetops.

So go ahead, daydream your head off; no one will know. You'll get good at it in no time, but remember, do not drive and daydream you are in Tahiti at the same time.

Next, open up your pirate chest full of old photos, and dive into the past. Linger over snapshots of tow-headed toddlers and beautiful young people with radiant smiles. Think about it; those Greek gods and goddesses were *you*! Do some time travelling and enjoy the old vacation photos. Look at you, zooming from place to place in private jets: Baja, Paris, Nice, Peru! How good it all was, how exotic and colorful and rich!

Looking for more projects? Start by making a list of everything you've lost in the past months or years, then turn the house upside down looking for them, all the while cursing demons and plumbers and bad children for stealing them. You'd be surprised what might turn up if you keep searching; earrings, socks, car keys, even skeletons of lost pets and forgotten old flames.

COVID Color

Time to liven up your drab, grey COVID-mind with some bright Spring color. Order a bunch of seed catalogues and read them over and over, murmuring the wonderful names of the vegetables to yourself: Beauregard and Georgia Jet sweet potatoes, Honey and Pearl sweet corn, Detroit Red beets, Stonehead cabbage, Rattlesnake watermelons. Don't miss the adorable babies propped up on gargantuan pumpkins, the smiling little girls holding baskets of flowers. And all the useless kitchen gadgets; apple peelers and corn strippers and chopomatics and cherry pitters. Go ahead, order the silliest of the lot, and have it mailed to a friend.

And just when all seems lost and overwhelmed by the COVID darkness, turn to the flower section and give your eyes a dose of red and white roses, orange poppies, sky blue lilacs, and crazy zinnias, cheerful and colorful as a box of kids' crayons.

COVID Mastery

Now that you have ample (or more accurately, too much) time on your hands, think of two activities you've always wanted to excel at, but didn't get the chance to. Let's say you pick a musical instrument (for God's sake avoid the trumpet and the accordion) and poetry. Now just start from the bottom, and master them. Do not be discouraged by failures earlier in life; don't forget, you used to have other things to do. Also, remember that you can't fail if your standards are low enough.

Now you must play one song every day on your old violin, no matter how badly, and write one poem every day, no matter how awful. Soon you will be scratching away at 'Baa, baa black sheep' as well as any third-grader, and you will be churning out reams of doggerel poetry that will make your highbrow friends wince and run for cover with hands over their ears. Be braced for this kind of audience attrition. Think of it, if you can, as an opportunity for more practice in private.

Exclusive interview with Dr Anthony Fauci, Saviour of the Republic

Dr Q: So good to see you smiling, Tony. What can Americans do to get going again?

Dr F: Good to see you, too, Rudolfo. You might consider a fresh Zoom shirt once in a while. Anyway, we must agree on what matters: kissing in public places, bacon sandwiches, disagreement, cutting-edge fashion, literature, generosity, water, a more equitable distribution of the world's resources, movies, music, freedom of thought, beauty, love.

Dr Q: Whoa, Tony, what a romantic outburst. So unlike you! Did you really say that just now?

Dr F: Well, actually, Salman Rushdie said it a long time ago. Still, you can't blame me for feeling a little giddy. It's Spring, we have a vaccine, the end is in sight. Who wouldn't be joyful?

Dr Q: I see we're almost out of time, Tony. Do you have a final message for the American people?

Dr F: Rudolfo, the message is simple. Honour the dead, protect the living. Get vaccinated, be safe, be happy.

Dr Q: Thank you, Tony. You're just so cute! If we weren't Zooming, I'd kiss you.

Dr F: Maybe next time, Rudolfo. God speed!

Dr Q's Poetry Corner

> Today I tasted life. It was a vast morsel.
> A Circus passed the house—still I feel the red
> in my mind though the drums are out. The Lawn is full of
> south and the odors tangle, and I hear today for the first
> time the river in the tree.
>
> Emily Dickinson

Whoa, I guess Emily is feeling her oats, too.

    I'm afraid that will be all for today's Bulletin. If you come up with some better COVID vaccine questions, call your private doctor and don't expect a call back. Otherwise, my staff and I will be happy to help you navigate the stormy sea of COVID misinformation and political idiocy. Until then, in the words of the great Dr Anthony Fauci,[1] 'Get vaccinated, stay safe, be happy.'

Dr Rudolfo Quackinthebush,
M.D., PhD., LSMFT, SOS,
Knight of the Round Table,
your one-stop source for free COVID advice

---

[1] Go to our website for great deals on Fauciwirerims and white coats.

The Toilet Paper Apocalypse
David Shaw

The grocery stores in North Toronto were rapidly running out of toilet paper. Not sure why, but obviously people had started to hoard it. Stores weren't yet off limits, so Candace sent me out to start our own hoard. But wherever I went, the shelves were empty. I was ready to give up when Candace heard from a neighbour that the Metro store at Bayview and Eglinton had just received a fresh supply of vanishing paper product. So, I went there anticipating bad parking (since the store was in the midst of some ongoing construction) and maybe ravenous crowds.

In my earlier search I had come across a woman who had snagged the very last 12-pack... I suspected that had our roles been reversed that a battle might have ensued. So, I rushed over to the Metro in question and sure enough there was a goodly supply of several name brands and not that many people trying to purchase them. So, I snapped up three 12-packs and headed for the checkout. When I got home, Candace was not impressed.'

You should have bought it *all!* she growled. 'We're going back!'

So, back we went and Candace took a large cart while I took a small cart to get some things for that night's dinner. When I caught up with her, she had ten 12-packs in the cart and wanted me to push it. Anyway, we paid (didn't get too many nasty stares; none that I noticed) and then stuffed them into the car. Got them home where Trevor and Holly took them to the third floor and added them to the burgeoning store of Armageddon supplies. Since then, we haven't been to a store or much else...

Pandemic Fragment: Eden III
David Shaw

In which Alzira our Portuguese cleaning lady returns from the abyss. Coming on public transit, no less. Candace met with her at a distance of almost 12 feet to discuss what needed doing. Then Candace, Sophie and I went to the studio at the end of the garden to attempt to work until such time as Alzira was ready to attend to said studio. At that time, it was only safe to move to the Finns' side of the house (where Alzira had not been). Alzira is Sophie's favourite person so this was not easy and included whining, barking and some door scratching. Eventually at around 6:00 p.m. we were able to return and prepare our dinner. There are other things like the home schooling of our granddaughters but I won't get into that right now. The Alzira Experience now happens once every two weeks… we're in the midst of one right now as I write this in the Finns' part of the house. And the discombobulated nature of it all resulted in missing Sophie's outing so she did all her numbers indoors plus the charger for my computer got marooned in the studio with Alzira and my computer ran out of juice. Groundhog Day in a fortnight.

The Speech Before St COVID-Vaccine
William Shakesneedle[1]

This day is called the Feast of St COVID-Vaccine. He that outlives this day and comes safe home, will stand a tiptoe when this day is named and rouse him at the name of COVID. He that shall see this day, and live old age, will yearly on the vigil feast his neighbours and say 'Tomorrow is COVID-Vaccine.' Then will he strip his sleeve and show his jab and say 'This jab I had on COVID-Vaccine.' Old men forget; yet all shall be forgot, but he'll remember, with advantages, what feats he did that day. Then shall those names, familiar in our mouths as household words—Pfizer-Biontec and Astra-Zeneca, Johnson & Johnson, Moderna and Janssen—be in their flowing cups freshly remember'd. This story shall the good man teach his son; and the day of St COVID-Vaccine shall ne'er go by, from this day to the ending of the world, but we in it shall be remembered—we many, we happy many, we band of masked comrades; for those today that roll their sleeves with me shall be my comrade; be they ne'er so vial, this day shall gentle their condition; and people in Ottawa now-a-bed shall think themselves accursed they were not here, and hold their masks and physical distance cheap whiles any speaks that jabbed with us upon Saint COVID-Vaccine.

Podium finish in the Misappropriation Olympics
With apologies to The Bard

---

[1] AKA Bob Barclay

A Wee Humour Contest

What, exactly, did *you* find funny about the COVID pandemic? Come on, there must have been something, even if it was the sight of the no-longer youthful man or woman struggling under the weight of four 60-roll packs of toilet paper just as the Scott's delivery truck was pulling up beside the grocery store. Grocery stores, drug stores, liquor stores, the line-ups for all of these stores: all could provide good material to the skilled observer.

As for me, the funniest thing I saw was not in any store or store line-up but on Highway #417, better known locally as the Queensway, and not normally a place one associates with humour. And, no, the humour was not in any way intentional, but that didn't make it any the less real. I refer to an illuminated sign, flashing in bold, fully capitalized letters the stern warning: 'COVID-19. Stay 2 metres apart.'

'I'll try to do that!' I said to myself, as I started thinking about how best to extricate myself from the maelstrom of over-aggressive car and truck drivers and mindless motorcyclists making up the Queensway's traffic flow.

Dear readers, we're interested in hearing about *your* funniest COVID moments. Send your humourous items to Ann or me. Once the almanac is published, we'll gather them all together for you to vote on. The contributor of the item you all find funniest will win a copy of the almanac, autographed by yours truly.

Ready to go? Are we having fun yet?

Stay cool and stay safe.

Jon Peirce
jonpeirce@hotmail.com

SECTION 5

COVID
and Me

*T*he pieces in this section focus on people's personal experience with COVID, with an emphasis on how the pandemic has affected their everyday lives. As I reread the pieces while assembling the section, I found myself impressed, and in some cases, quite amazed by the ingenuity shown by the authors in adapting to the pandemic.

While missing her usual dragon boating, Deb Bertrand had little trouble filling the time that would normally have been spent on the water with gardening and nature walks with her daughter and granddaughter, during which all enjoyed taking pictures of the mushrooms they found and then trying to identify them. Brent Coates, in his philosophical essay, views the pandemic as an event which, like the apocalyptic or prophetic writings of old, is designed to 'pull back the veil and reveal the underbelly of reality.' And Dianna Davison-Veber found 2020 'a time for clear reflection, super Spring cleaning, organizing, resting, reading, gardening, thinking—and lots of time to do it in,' even as she missed her usual get-togethers with family and friends. Sasha Dominique's performance poem 'COVID et le Temps' hammers home the huge changes wrought by the pandemic in almost every area of daily life, from eating to hand-washing.

In his amusing memoir, 'What's a Pandemic?' Bill Horne offers some perspective on the current pandemic by describing some of his experiences working for the Department of Foreign Affairs and International Trade (DFAIT) during the previous H1N1 pandemic. Meanwhile, despite the unpromising sound of the title of his memoir, 'Damn COVID!', Neven Humphrey describes what turns out to have been a reasonably successful adaptation process.

Georgia Johnson's brief essay is almost heartbreaking in its portrayal of the pandemic's effect on the life of a widow living almost entirely for her family and her church. Short story writer Su Mardelli, not without humour of her own, paints a vivid picture of the pandemic's effect on an older man left on his own without enough to do while his wife visits a new grandchild.

The section ends on a quietly positive note, with Elizabeth Zimmer's piece, 'COVID's Small Mercies.' While still hating to eat alone, Zimmer says she has come to treasure the hours of solitude this new circumstance allows her. 'I no longer feel it necessary to contribute an opinion to every discussion,' says Zimmer. 'The plague has left me time to think, to remember, and to formulate a sane way forward.'

How COVID Changed
My Outlook on Life
Deb Bertrand

On January 1, 2020, I woke up with a bad cold. Stuffed up, dry cough resulting with a fever. Thinking back, I now wonder if it was the COVID virus. It was hard to shake, but after about 10 days I was back to normal.

February proved very normal. My excitement was mounting because I was joining some friends for a vacation in their Cape Coral, Florida rental home the first week of March. I was busy buying new swimsuits, ensuring that my medication supply was sufficient, and packing my bags. Since my friends were already down there, I flew for the first time by myself. Everything went smoothly. It was a gorgeous home with a salt water pool and hot tub. It had everything you could want in a vacation home, and we enjoyed perfect weather.

While we were down there, the news was full of talk about a virus that had broken out in China back in January and that was rapidly spreading throughout China and neighbouring countries. It was very disturbing to hear, so we stocked up on hand wipes and sanitizing liquid for our return home to Canada. On March 7, we returned on a late flight. At that time, we were not really concerned about contacting the virus, but we nonetheless sanitized our hands and everything we touched at the airports and on the plane.

A week later, WHO announced that the virus had turned into a worldwide pandemic. A lockdown came into effect and everything closed with the exception of grocery stores and drug stores.

I am not going to bore you with the details of how COVID unfolded in Canada. You know all about that. This story is about how I made the best of my circumstances during this crazy year. I did not contract the virus on my flight home, and since my husband had conditions that could compromise his health, I was the main errand runner to get groceries and prescriptions, going out only when necessary.

Of course, I am not the type of person to be happy sitting around and doing nothing day in and day out. I love to read and do research on topics of interest. During this lockdown period I took on-line courses on herbal remedies and teas, and even learned how to embroider and started sewing again. I also did video yoga and muscle building (for seniors) and took long daily walks through the Galilee woodlot and trails. Keeping my distance from negative and fearful people was at the top of my list. It was important to keep my mind, body, and spirit in the best of health and to keep my routine as normal as possible.

When the month of May came around, I was ecstatic. Although the weather was cool, I was in my garden cleaning it up, turning over the soil, and planning what I would plant. Sadly, the dragon boat team would not be able to have a season that Summer, so I had to find other ways to maintain my physical health. I therefore worked on my garden, continued with my walks, and discovered different trails to explore with my daughter and granddaughter. To our delight, there was an abundance of fungi/mushrooms on the trails. We had fun taking pictures and trying to identify the various mushrooms.

I truly feel sorry for people who are not able to get out into Nature a few hours a day. During all this time I stayed away from news media and negative people. Twenty years ago, I went through breast cancer, considering it an interruption in my life. And I learned a multitude of lessons at that time, making changes to the way I think, eat, and care for my physical body. Dealing with COVID was just another interruption, which would provide more lessons to be learned.

People were forced out of employment or had to work out of their homes, small businesses were closing down, and daycares were closed; a series of unfortunate events. There was an increase in COVID cases, especially among the seniors in homes. At this point, the federal government kicked in and started to dish out money left and right for almost anyone who applied. Most people these days are totally dependent on the Government to bail them out and provide a living for them when times get tough. I was lucky because I was retired and living on pensions that didn't change. But all this got me thinking about going back to the basics and becoming self-sufficient.

I was already gardening and growing more types of herbs because I was interested in making my own medicinal teas and tinctures, but that wasn't enough. In order to be more self-sufficient, I needed to source more locally-grown vegetables, fruit, and herbs and learn about foraging and drying and preserving.

Being retired and living in an apartment in town, I am limited in what I can do to become self-sufficient. But along with growing, preserving, and drying food, I can take up sewing and knitting again, and learn new crafts. Small local market garden organizations are always looking for volunteers to help out, in exchange for free foraging. It was win, win when I got to collect rosehips and red clover in October.

In the Fall there was again a wave of panic leading to shortages of food and supplies for the Winter, so I decided to create a 'bugout' bag. Keeping in mind what a crazy year it was, I wanted to be prepared for food and supply shortages, power outages, and even for a short-term evacuation. Call me crazy, but it doesn't hurt to be prepared. Besides drying and preparing my herbs for storage, I also signed up for an on-line course, Ontario Master Naturalist Program. It is an eight-week course out of Lakehead University in Orillia. It is the only such course in Ontario, and they decided back in the

Spring to offer it on-line four times a year. Lucky me, I got into the Winter program and I am loving it. It is helping me deal with lockdown and exercising my aging brain. Spring can't come soon enough, because I have so many ecosystems to check out. Even though it is Winter, we still have an outdoor assignment every week.

Especially during lockdown, it is very important to stay connected to family and friends, and to meet new friends through FaceTime and Zoom. From July to January my son was based overseas. Thank God for FaceTime so we could stay in touch. The rest of the family stayed in touch with one another through Zoom. Holidays and celebrations were very different but we stayed connected. The Prior Chest Nuts, my dragon boat team, are staying connected through Zoom meetings, fun nights, and exercise classes. I also joined a few organizations of interest and met new people. The MacNamara Field Naturalists Club is right in Arnprior, and I also joined the Ottawa Herb Society because of my love of herbs, as well as the Ottawa Valley Weavers & Spinners Guild. My friend Louise and I are taking on a special project in the Spring: to grow our own flax and process it into linen. The Ottawa Guild will provide a wealth of information on this particular process.

Just to be clear, I did have some down times over this past year. With no dragon boat season, I felt quite disconnected. I missed the camaraderie and full body workout we get while paddling in the boat. The thought of not being able to travel or even make plans to travel really threw me for a loop. And it was so sad not being able to visit my mother in the nursing home.

Still, something positive is coming out of this pandemic. It is providing everyone some time to sit back and look at life as it is. It is teaching us to enjoy the time spent with family and to allow children to have fun times and to be taught skills by their parents. It is sad to realize that we are so dependent on the government, and that we have lost the ability to be self-sufficient. I am full of gratitude for good health and will continue with my new adventures. I fully anticipate that this pandemic shall pass and that we can get back to semi-normal with renewed wisdom and experience.

Through My Lens
Brent P.D. Coates

You don't have a life, you are life
Eckhart Tolle
We understand death for the first time
when the hand is placed upon someone we love
Madame De Stael, 1766-1817

What the ancient apocalyptic, revelation or prophetical writing delivered was a story that pulls back the veil to reveal the underbelly of reality. It uses hyperbolic images, unusual celestial arrangements, floods, and mysterious lunar activity. Contemporary science fiction would be today's version; suddenly you're placed in an utterly different world, where what you used to call normal doesn't apply anymore. This seems to describe our present situation with the COVID-19 pandemic.

It is meant to shock: this is an apocalypse happening to us in our lifetime that's leaving us utterly out of control. We're grasping to retake control, but we now know in a new way that we can't totally take control. Wars and earthquakes etc., can be viewed as the beginning of the birth pangs of some-thing new. Is the world really falling apart? Is the idea of progress obsolete? Apocalypse is for the sake of birth, not death. Yet most of us hear this as a threat. Anything that upsets our normalcy is a threat to the ego, but in the Big Picture, it really isn't. Falling apart is for the sake of renewal. In other words, is there a lesson that this has to offer? It points to everything that we take for granted and says: Don't take anything for granted! An apocalyptic event sets the stage to reframe reality in a radical way by flipping our imagination. It's not meant to strike fear in us as much as to launch us onto a radical rearrangement. It's not the end of the world. It's the end of worlds— our worlds that we have created. It's what it takes to wake people up to the real, to the lasting, to what matters. Our best response is to end our fight with reality-as-it-was. Resist being trapped in the past. A cultural and emotional evolution shifts our perspective and rearranges our molecules, first at the individual and then the community level.

The new perspective could continue to move us further into a world that works for everyone. What perspective do we need to hold to be able to embrace and integrate an apparent disaster and then have the ability to examine and create a different future. Is this not the essence of the human spirit?

In a way it is like changing the lens in a camera or actually the lens in our eye. When the cataract is removed, there are several things we see differently, or more clearly: we notice things we didn't see before. When a critical number of individuals shift their perspectives the community shifts. In the aftermath, a new image may not present itself clearly all at once. Bits and pieces get tried and formulated and a new normal gets put in place; the process may take a while. We humans are designed to evolve in an increasingly positive cooperative form, towards increasing diversification and towards integration of greater complexity. Human beings, like every other living organism on this planet, are *cybernetic systems,* that is, where the outcomes of actions are taken as inputs for further action.

With the death of a dear one, a piece of my life has been taken away. I've been left with time to retrieve memories, but I must come to terms with the obvious: I too will die. Death is an ongoing thing; the decay and renewal of our bodily cells is an ongoing process. There is no such thing as life *and* death; they are not two separate activities but one activity taking place simultaneously. Like the front and back of your hand, they are one. Two parts of the same, yin and yang: at some point one process overtakes the other. Mortality is the fundamental reality of our existence... we are mortal 'beings' on this earth. It's said to be a manifestation of divine consciousness.

Everything has a cycle, is in motion, each with its own timepiece is passing away. If we don't hold this counterpoint in mind, we do one of two things: we take this world too seriously, or we try to hold on to everything. We think it's all going to last, but it isn't. The 21st century, the United States of America, Canada, capitalism, our churches and our political parties, and all the rest are evolving and in their own time moving along and passing away. To recall the Buddhist heart sutra 'Gone, gone, entirely gone,' some people may live on in old movies—but even celebrities and stars do die. We can take this as a morbid lesson, or we can receive it as the truth ahead of time, so we're not surprised, disappointed, and angry when it happens to us. Using James Lovelock's 1970 term 'Gaia,' which has become part of our lexicon, we are now more conscious and fully aware of our mutual belonging in the all-connected web of life, of all life on the planet. We are a part of the whole of it—part of a large living organism. And not necessarily as an essential, critical part. We go forward with a wider sense of identity as a unique and integral part of the living body of the planet and there's more to 'you' than your physical being. We get our earthly existence from the planet and we give it back to the planet. The contemporary philosopher Ken Wilber explains it as a holon. Everything is a holon, a part that replicates a piece of the bigger whole.

The spiritual message is really simple, though it may be hard for anyone who only exists in the sensual world to accept. It is saying that nothing is permanent. Apocalyptic literature tells us to be prepared for that, so we won't be shocked or scandalized when someone dies, or something is destroyed.

You might learn this truth the moment after you hear of the death of one of your parents, when the rug is pulled out from beneath you. Or during that moment when you go to the doctor and get a fatal diagnosis and are told you have three months left to live. Or when your house is destroyed by a tornado or flood. Again, the message is not meant to be heard as a threat, but as a truth: nothing lasts forever. Our great hope is that there will be something we can grasp onto, something that's eternal. We want the absoluteness of our life, eternity, and we can't fully find it here.

We exist in an indifferent universe that has no inherent meaning, in a world of passing things where everything changes and nothing remains the same. And yet, we want to find some sort of purpose for our own individual existence in the short time of our physical presence here. The only thing that doesn't change is change itself. It's a hard lesson to learn, but it helps us appreciate that everything is a gift; we didn't create it. We don't deserve it. It will not last, but while we breathe, we can enjoy it, and know that it is another moment of life. People who take this moment seriously take every moment seriously, and those are the people who are ready for death—departure from our earthly existence. The contemporary Franciscan monk, Richard Rohr, blogs that if our spiritual journey is not leading us into an eternal now, an eternal moment, an always-true moment, then we have not lived the moment at all.

I am a piece of creation and the source of creation is throbbing within me—here to explore and experience the highs, the lows, the pains, the sorrows and all the experiences of the gift of life. When time becomes history, will the generations for whom we are the ancestors see us as enlightened beings aware of our unique and integral part of the living body of earth, aware of our cosmic presence as Conscious, Cosmic beings?

> *You are not a troubled guest on this earth,*
> *you are not an accident amidst other accidents, you were invited*
> 'What to Remember when Awakening'
> David Whyte

COVID
Dianna Davison-Veber

I am alone.

2020 and COVID are here.

2020 *used* to represent hindsight and good eye vision. It's here now. I lived during the time of polio, measles and various other epidemics, so I'm fully aware of quarantines and appropriate procedures; however, this one is different.

In Nova Scotia, COVID first hit early in 2020. Our Premier asked us to 'Stay the blazes home!' For 10 weeks, I did just that. I'm a country girl who plans ahead, so I arranged for three months of advance medications—before the drugstores started limiting us to one month at a time. My wonderful neighbour picked up any groceries I needed. I took care of everything else to be done outside the home prior to the lockdown—then the vacation began. 10 *weeks!*

I have never been so totally alone—and aware of it—in my whole life! Not seeing family or friends, not going to classes, not going to band practices. *Home!* I do have a telephone and a TV, and I know how to record.

2020. A time for clear reflection, super Spring cleaning, organizing, resting, reading, gardening, thinking—and lots of time to do it in. Never before.

Telephone conversations with family and friends began in earnest. Everyone was having difficulty with the impact on our freedom and movement. Things we did, we don't do even now. 'Let's go for coffee, meals, shopping.' You would think before you went anywhere.

My first venture out happened after 10 weeks. I phoned my local market to find the best time to go there: 10:00 to 11:30. I was the only customer. Perfect thing! I did this with the grocery store, the pharmacy, etc., etc. It *worked!* But I was terribly anxious the first time. Still, I passed the information along to friends. It worked for them as well.

I was starting to adjust; then killer Gabriel struck!

One Saturday at 10 a.m., my Dartmouth sister phoned to tell me, 'There's a killer gunman in your area. Lock your doors to everyone!' I telephoned all my neighbours and friends, who in their turn telephoned others, warning them. I got my 'Thank-yous' later because they hadn't known. Most would have been outdoors when killer Gabriel drove by—within 100 feet of my house—killing people at random.

Numerous friends later told me about killer Gabriel's near-misses; they'd seen bullet scars. RCMP Officer Heidi's children live near one of my friends, and every time information about the crime hits the media, it makes it difficult for them. Horrible!

I saw the aviation Snowbirds perform in the sky over Truro—then there was the deadly crash in British Columbia.

Later, my neighbour's husband was on *HMCS Fredericton* when the ship's helicopter crashed… and the crew saw it.

Then there were the fishing boat fatalities. All these tragedies on top of COVID.

COVID and me. I still stay home as much as possible, but I talk on the phone a *lot!* When in public, I mask, socially distance and wash my hands frequently. I do have a people bubble, and now, once a week, we go to a restaurant for lunch, *early*, following all protocols. It's nice to see a face besides my own.

I discuss many everyday things with my phone buddies: venting, expressing frustration, and how they're adjusting. But people are learning to communicate again, bringing relationships closer. Kindness. Re-establishing old connections. The similarities are amazing! We don't know the future, only the past, hence the irony of 2020 (hindsight).

Medical? Doctor phone visits are good.

Death and dying? Extra sad! Not being able to make hospital visits, to travel to visit the sick and dying, share the grief, or even say good-bye is *extremely* sad. Virtual visits just aren't the same as in-person ones.

Humour? It's critical! It lifts the spirits, and for a few moments, you feel a bit better. Examples:

1) Why is there no COVID at the North Pole? Because the elves San-ta-tized everything there!

2) When I go to the hospital or doctor's office and I'm in the COVID checkup lineup, I tell them they forgot the two most important questions: a) Have you kissed anyone; and b) Are you pregnant?

Conclusion? We only have today.

Today is the present.
A present is a gift.
Use it wisely.

COVID et le Temps
Sasha Dominique

Le Temps
Souvent maître du monde
Maître de notre vie
Dont on se plaint
Trop souvent
Qu'il nous manque;
On court après lui
On l'attend
On l'espère
Et tout à coup
POUF!
En une journée
Le 13 mars 2020
Il devient omniprésent
Prend trop de place
On ne sait plus
Quoi en faire
Comment l'occuper
Comment l'apprécier
Comment l'apprivoiser
Et le redécouvrir
Lui faire une place de choix
Dans notre quotidien
S'en faire un allié
Il nous surprend
Car on est si peu habitué
À sa présence
Et du fait qu'il ait
Tout son temps
Maintenant
En ce moment
Pour nous
Pour chacun de nous
À travers le monde;
C'est incroyable!
On s'en réjouit
À tâtons

Car on ne sait pas
On ne sait rien
Sur sa présence
Ou son absence
Future
Dans quelques jours
Dans quelques mois
Personne ne sait
Ne peut prédire
Sa durée
Mais pour l'instant
Il est là
Et bien LÀ;
Il faut lui tendre la main
Le serrer dans nos bras
Lui faire savoir
Qu'il est le bienvenu
Et qu'il sera mis à profit
Pour de nombreuses tâches
Que l'on remet toujours
À plus tard
En disant que ceci se fera
Lorsque nous aurons
Du TEMPS
Eh bien, le voici
Ce fameux Temps
Offert
Sur un plateau d'argent
Il nous fait signe
De s'occuper de lui
De profiter de lui, même
Quelle générosité!
Une fois la surprise passée
On s'active
On lui confie des choses
Ménage
Lavage
Repassage
Cuisine
Rénovation
Il nous conseille
Nous aide à faire le tri
On donne, on vend, on échange

133

On aère notre espace
L'aménage autrement
Le Temps
Supervise le travail
Réorganise notre vie
Nos activités
Rendues très limitées
Dorénavant
On se met à prendre des marches
Au quotidien
Avec les gens de notre bulle
On croise nos voisins
Que l'on ne connaissait pas
On leur jase à distance
On fait des rencontres virtuelles
Avec des collègues
Des amis
La parenté
Même si elle n'est pas éloignée;
On fredonne une ritournelle de 20 secondes
En se lavant les mains
Fréquemment
Très fréquemment
Nos mains n'aurons jamais été
Aussi sollicitées
Pour la désinfection
C'est un droit de passage obligé
Dans les commerces
Les restaurants
Les entreprises
Les endroits publics intérieurs
On n'ose plus ouvrir la bouche
Quand on croise des connaissances
De peur de les contaminer;
La Dame en noir rôde
Puissante
Omnipotente
À travers le monde
Elle ne néglige personne
Nous sommes tous égaux
À ses yeux
Et sous son emprise;
Nos dirigeants

Nous préviennent
Nous suggèrent
Nous recommandent
Nous exhortent
Nous prient
Nous confinent;
Le petit écran
Prend la place du grand
Centralise la culture
La monopolise
Les artistes se réinventent
S'ils le peuvent
S'ils y croient
Les commandes en ligne
Les « pour emporter »
Et les livraisons
Se multiplient
C'est la nouvelle façon
D'aller au restaurant
Tout en restant
Chez soi;
On divise le pays
En zones de couleurs
C'est ça qui nous définit
Qui nous accorde des permissions
Ou non
On se croirait dans un grand jeu
De société
On avance notre pion
De quelques cases
Encouragés
Puis
On doit le reculer
Question de débordement
Dans les hôpitaux
Et de courbe
Non aplatie
On se décourage
On voit défiler
Les jours
Les mois
Les saisons
Les occasions de rassemblement

Qui n'auront pas lieu;
Les mesures se resserrent
C'est pour notre bien
Pour la survie des gens
Je suis en faveur
De ces politiques
Je vois au-delà
De ma petite personne
Je comprends l'importance
De ce qui nous est dicté
Et je respecte tout
Recommandations
Suggestions
Mesures
Interdictions
Permissions, aussi
Car il y en a
Il est encore possible
De se sentir libres
Malgré tout
Il suffit de savoir
Apprécier
Ce que l'on a
Ce qui nous reste
Il suffit de savoir
Regarder
Autour de soi
Et écouter
Saisir l'essentiel
Vivre tout à coup
Le moment présent
Vraiment
Présent
Et en apprécier
Chaque instant
Pendant
Qu'il en est
Encore...

Temps.

What's a Pandemic?
Bill Horne

Er, what's a pandemic?
This might not be exactly related to COVID-19, but if you give it a chance, you will see the connection. And every bit is true.

Just after time began, when I had finished my undergrad and grad studies in Political Science, and was thinking that marriage would be a good idea, and figured a job would also be a good idea, I underwent The Interviews for a Job.

Two offers stood out: Bell Canada as a manager in training, and what was then called DFAIT, now Global Affairs Canada, as a foreign service officer in training.

My fiancée and I carefully analyzed both offers, and while DFAIT surely was appealing, with global travel assured, the money Bell was offering was too good to pass up. I ended up with 30 years at Bell, as a middle manager of many things. Life was very, very good.

Soon after retirement, my phone rang. It was a head-hunter from Nortel. Some of you may recall Nortel, at the time one of the most successful electronics companies ever. They were looking for someone with my Bell experience to take an assignment in Bogotá, Colombia, to figure out why the telephone company they were running there was not making any money. I leapt at the chance, discussed the financial benefits with my wife, and headed off. Learned enough Spanish to function well, and soon discovered why they weren't making any money, fixed that, and was very happy to collect my just rewards. Oh, I also started the Terry Fox Run in Bogotá, but that's another story.

The Nortel contract led to some additional contracts with Nortel back home in Ottawa, and one day a new employee showed up who had been with Foreign Affairs, and wanted a chance in private industry. She opened some doors at DFAIT, and suddenly I was where I had seriously wanted to be some 35 years before. It was like coming home. I'd earlier earned certification as a professional project manager. It was like heaven, working with overseas missions on all kinds of projects.

And then I got word that the new H1N1 pandemic had started ravaging the world. It was not as serious as COVID would be, but still worrisome. For whatever reason, my director general thought I would be the guy to do whatever it took to protect the some-12,000 employees and their families and zillions of locally engaged staff. I'd learned that for whatever reason, DFAIT had earlier dispensed with all their medical staff, and my boss seemed to think

I could replace them. To this day, I still recall saying, 'What's a pandemic?'

My boss told me that I should contact Dr Theresa Tam, who was then the Deputy Chief Public Health Officer. (Yes, the same Dr Theresa Tam as today, of course now the Chief Public Health Officer.) I think she took pity on me, but we became pretty good buddies. I did indeed learn what a pandemic was. We very quickly decided we had to buy enough H1N1 vaccine for all DFAIT employees and families world-wide, plus all our locally-engaged staff at all missions. I hired a summer student to help with all the calculations of how much vaccine and how many locally-engaged nurses and other bodies/equipment, etc., we needed, and soon went to my director general with the request. I was very well-prepared with all the facts and figures, expecting a gruelling session. He listened to my spiel and asked one question: 'How much will this cost?' The simple answer was $684,000.00, a number I think I will recall forever. He said, 'OK, do it.' I was a bit surprised, to say the least. I had assumed it would take forever to get approvals, fill out endless forms, etc. His comment was simple: 'If anyone asks, just send them to me.' To this day I have no idea where the money came from. And nobody ever asked; they just did whatever I requested.

It had also come to my attention that a new shipping container for vaccine had recently been developed. H1N1 vaccine required normal refrigeration, not the super-cold temperatures we now require. We tested a box on the side of an airport runway in Nairobi for 24 hours, and the box passed perfectly.

So, we needed to buy a whole slew of those boxes, figure out how to 'recycle' them back and forth from Ottawa, and on and on in logistics. Dr Tam and her staff were incredibly patient and helpful in all this.

The whole exercise went extremely well. We only had one mild case of H1N1, the High Commissioner to Singapore, who recovered nicely.

I remained around DFAIT for several more years, and had pretty well morphed into the 'go to guy' on medical issues around the world. One day I got a call from an African mission, requesting help with an outbreak of leptospirosis in the country. I actually knew what it was and had a pretty good idea of what to do about it. But I still checked with Dr Tam, just to be sure.

Dr Tam was in attendance at several World Health Organization meetings around the world, representing Canada, and someone had decided it would be good for me, the DFAIT project manager *cum* medical guy to go as well. We went to the United Nations, Vietnam, Egypt and China. On some trips my wife came along and we combined the official trips with some vacation time.

This rather amazing adventure lasted until 2014, when I finally retired, this time for good. One thing I learned for sure was what a pandemic is.

Damn COVID!
or
How I Survived a Pandemic
Neven Humphrey

One: The First Wave

The year 2020 was supposed to be a great year for me. I was going to go to lots of book fairs, and sell plenty of books; I was going to go to Halifax and Anthro East Coast in August; and I was going to do a lot of fursuiting. (For those who don't know, fursuiting means walking around in an animal-like mascot costume.) Thanks to a worldwide pandemic, and people too stupid to protect themselves, all of this just wasn't to be.

The year started out well enough. The Gatineau Anime Winter Festival was on the first weekend in January and I, of course, attended in fursuit. I participated in panels, watched a few sample animes, and even posed with a JPop group. Needless to say, I had a lot of fun there.

Unfortunately, things didn't start out that well in the job category. At the beginning of January, I was hired by DND for a 10-month contract. My new boss (who looked like a bad clone of the late Quebec actor Paul Buissonneau), instantly took a dislike to me, and then constantly berated me and deliberately made my job difficult. A week later, I complained to his superior, and he fired me. Soon after, though, I was hired by Service Canada as an Information Officer; and despite a few glitches and assignment changes, I am still working there, hopefully until my contract ends, in December.

Meanwhile, February brought Winterlude, which was again OK this year. I went a few times, including in fursuit on Opening Night. The shows I attended all involved French hip-hop and its crude language. Except for a few cinema wheels, there weren't any original displays, and the activities were the same as in the years before. Little did I know then that this would be the last big event that I would attend this year. Indeed, something worse than a comet was soon going to impact Earth.

That something was named Novel Coronavirus (or COVID-19), a disease that mysteriously appeared in the Wuhan region of northern China in January and then spread to nearby countries. At that point, people predicted that it was going to be bad. And when it hit Canada, everything was suddenly placed on stand-by. Inevitably, as the case level in this country started to rise, event after event got cancelled, due to fear of COVID spreading even more. Just after St Patrick's Day, the country went into full lockdown. Businesses, except for the most important, closed, forcing thousands of workers to either go on Employment Insurance or work from home. Public places like malls, restaurants and theatres closed. Even churches were forced to shut down. The Ghost of 1918 had returned.

The situation deteriorated further in April and May, with over 1,000 cases and hundreds of deaths per day, but then things slowly started to improve, so that by mid-August, there were only about 400 new cases a day nation-wide, and nearly no deaths. Consequently, public places started to open again, but with everyone inside wearing masks and staying at least two meters away from each other. Unfortunately, the situation was still too risky for cultural events, especially those normally held indoors, thus there were no book sales on the horizon, and nowhere really to fursuit. My Summer was ruined!

Do you think I'm exaggerating? Well, what *can* you do during the Summertime when there are no social and cultural events going on? Sure, the movie theatres had opened again, and restaurants had enacted effective social-distancing plans for their diners, but you can go to the movies or to a restaurant any time of the year. Summer is the season to go outside and have fun; but having fun is very hard to do when you have to keep your distance. Summer is also when you visit museums. In 2020, they would only open in the fall and, even then, you needed to reserve tickets to get in. Finally, Summer is when you walk around and listen to the different accents of visitors. But Canada had long since closed its borders to tourists, and who knew when they would open them again. Thus, your only real options are taking long walks or jogs outside, or staying inside, trying to stay cool, lying in front of your fan or AC unit.

So, what *have* I been doing this Summer? As I said before, I work at Service Canada on the COVID line, so that takes care of weekdays. I also meet fellow members of Toastmasters every two Tuesdays on Zoom; and since the local church reopened, I've started serving as churchwarden again. The rest of the time, I'm on the computer, either watching videos or movies, going on Facebook, or writing my bunny story, which should be finished by the end of the year.

A major consequence of the COVID pandemic for me is that I haven't been able to see my mother, who lives just south of Quebec City, since last Christmas, and I probably won't see her until next Christmas. Normally I see her at least four times a year. I usually go at Easter, at the end of June, on Thanksgiving Weekend, and during the Christmas holidays. The first time was during the worst of the epidemic in Canada, and the second and third are impossible since Greyhound has cancelled service in Quebec for the near future. But while I can't go and see her, I do keep in touch with her every Friday by phone.

Another consequence of the COVID pandemic is my inability to travel. Even when I didn't have much money, I always tried to go on vacation somewhere at least once a year. This year, I was supposed to go to Halifax, but the trip got cancelled for obvious reasons. I hope that I'll be able to go next year, but I'd also like to do another trip, this one to Europe. Which country should I go to? I'd really like to go to the UK, but that's one of the European countries hardest hit by the pandemic. While Slovenia and Croatia are doing fine, there might be a language barrier for me in those countries. Of course, things might change by next Spring; there might be a vaccine. Alternatively, the situation in the U.K. might improve greatly. Anyway, I think I'll wait until October before making my final decision.

Two: The Second Wave

Along with the return to school, September has brought an increase in COVID cases. While there were never as many as 2000 new cases in a day during the Summer, there have never been fewer than that many during the Fall. In fact, there are sometimes as many as 4000. Still, the situation is not without its 'silver linings:'

1. There are relatively fewer deaths and 90% of new cases have already recovered
2. No one's planning a full shutdown yet
3. We're not in Europe, with their tens of thousands of cases in some countries.

Still, the overall situation is quite the bummer. Every club I belong to, except for Toastmasters, has announced that its next season has either been postponed or cancelled; even bowling has been cancelled. How will I occupy my weekends? More important, how will I get my exercise? I'm going to have to figure that out.

And speaking of Europe, Canadians are banned from traveling there. Nevertheless, I have chosen where I'll go next year: Croatia and/or Slovenia if I can travel in May, and Germany if I have to wait until December.

With Winter coming on, will things get worse due to indoor living? And I'm still not sure if I can go home for Christmas—though I hope to do so by train. In addition, (as if the COVID situation weren't bad enough), another scourge will soon be rearing its ugly head: seasonal influenza. I'm definitely getting a flu shot this year! And hopefully a COVID shot next year.

So, in conclusion, 2020 sucks, and I hope 2021 will be better.

To those who refuse to wear a mask, I can refute all your excuses:

*   'It's my freedom of choice.' It's my freedom of choice to walk along Yonge Street completely nude, but that's not going to prevent me from getting arrested. Wearing a mask in public places is a provincial law, a law meant to protect people from the disease of COVID, and to stop it from spreading. So, you can practice your freedom of

choice, but please do it where you won't damage people's right not to catch Coronavirus.

- 'The Coronavirus threat is overblown.' The World Health Organization says at least 50 million people have caught Coronavirus around the world, and at least 1.0 million people have died. (That's as of Fall, 2020, when this section was written.) But hey, what do the leading experts on health and disease know about health and disease?

- 'The mask causes disease.' Only if you dab it with feces and then put it over your face.

- 'I can't breathe!' Calm down, and breathe normally; air does pass through the mask if you don't hyperventilate on purpose.

- 'It's discrimination to force me to wear a mask.' Then you don't know the definition of the word 'discrimination.' Dictionary.com defines discrimination as 'Treatment or consideration of, or making a distinction in favour of or against, a person or thing based on the group, class, or category to which that person or thing belongs rather than on individual merit.' Anti-maskers are not their own group, class, or category; they're just individuals who refuse to wear masks. And discrimination means constant harassment; as soon as the pandemic is over, you will stop being 'discriminated' against.

- 'I tested negative for Coronavirus.' Coronavirus has an incubation period of up to 14 days; so, one day you may not have it, and the next day, you may. And some people may not show symptoms, yet still have Coronavirus, and be able to spread it.

- 'It's not macho.' Spreading a potentially fatal disease is not macho, either.

- 'I can't get the virus.' Oh, lucky you. Unfortunately, we don't believe you.

- 'No one can see my face, or hear me talk.' We can see your face once the pandemic is over. And the mask doesn't muffle your voice that much.

- 'It's a sign of communism.' No, it isn't; non-communists wear masks, too.

- 'The advice on wearing them keeps changing.' Scientists, who know about Coronavirus, have always said to wear a mask. It's the politicians, trying to please their bases, who flip-flop.

Three: Third Wave, April 2021

Can it get any worse? Now, I had expected the pandemic to get really bad, since Health Canada said the numbers were going to get higher, due to people staying mostly indoors during Wintertime. And that's exactly what happened, as new cases went up to 9,000, but then quickly went back down to the levels we saw last October. And since people in Canada started to get vaccinated, everyone thought we would soon see the light at the end of the tunnel. (By the way, I did go stay with my mother for the Christmas holidays. We respected the rules; and so everyone was fine.)

But then came the variants, deadlier and more contagious. And starting in March, the number of new cases rose again, to reach nearly 10,000 a day. The rate of vaccinations also rose week after week, so personally I was starting to wonder what was going to happen first: being vaccinated or being dead. Myself, I'm getting vaccinated in May with Astra-Zeneca, no matter the remote risk of getting blood clots. I'll be getting it not far from where I live, at the family clinic.

Meanwhile, I've discovered the Virtual Reality world. Indeed, in order to get a virtual booth to sell my books at the Virtual Furnal Equinox, I had to install the VRChat app on my computer, and then spend at least 10 hours on the app. Which I did, and after many trials and tribulations, I finally succeeded, and eventually set up a booth at the event, (where I sold seven books).

On the way, I discovered a new way to make friends and keep in touch with them; so, I just might stay on VRChat. No, I don't have a VR helmet, and though that doesn't stop me from going on VRChat, it does limit what I can do there. For example, my avatar, (VR character), has no freedom of movement except by tapping keys on the keyboard, and even that is limited, and quite clumsy. But I might get a helmet, and even have avatars custom-made for me. I don't know how much it'll cost, though.

Four: The Shot, May 2021

On May 5, I had my first injection of Astra-Zeneca. I was surprised that the injection took over five seconds. I mean, they inject you with half a milliliter of vaccine; it should take less time than a flu shot. But I guess that since it's intramuscular instead of intravenous, it might take longer.

After that, there was intense pain at the injection spot, which I'd expected. And the following morning, I started feeling a little nauseous, though not enough to be a concern. Unfortunately, I soon developed a headache so intense that I was bedridden for the whole afternoon. It dissipated slightly during the evening; but during the night, the nausea came back strongly enough that I spent over an hour in the bathroom. The following morning, I still had a bit of a headache, but it disappeared during the day.

My next injection is on August 25. I hope it's not Astra-Zeneca again, but even if it is, the side effects shouldn't be as bad.

Five: The 'Light,' June 2021

During the week of May 17, Canada reached the 50% mark for people who'd received at least one injection. This is good, since things will start opening up again, However, only around 4% are fully immunized, which means masks will be needed at least until next Fall. By now, though, I've gotten used to wearing one, so that's OK.

At this point, new daily infections are below 2,000 again, as in the first wave. With nearly 70% of people having received at least one injection, I think things will soon be nearly back to normal. And I couldn't be happier. At least in Canada, this pandemic will soon be over. And I hope, for future generations, it won't come back for at least 100 years (cue noise-makers).

Alone During COVID
Georgia Johnson

I've been asked to submit my experiences and thoughts relating to the COVID-19 pandemic and the impact it has had on my life. I'll start by introducing myself: I'm a retired nursery school teacher who on January 06, 2016 lost my husband of 53 years after his long battle with cancer. Learning to function on my own with all the changes it has created has been a challenge, but not quite as big a one as living alone during COVID-19.

Before COVID, I generally purchased fresh fruit and vegetables several times a week. With COVID restrictions, it became risky to shop that often. I felt uncomfortable being out in the stores as often as two to three times a week. My solution was to make greater use of frozen foods. I continued with the frozen option for some time. The result: unnecessary calories and high salt consumption. As well, I've gained weight, as I'm sure many of us have.

Most of us have made difficult changes to our lives and many of us are coping with loneliness. I have to explain that, after I lost my husband, I very consciously decided to focus the remainder of my life on church and family. Unfortunately, COVID has made this extremely difficult. You see, one of my grandchildren lives in Atlanta, Georgia, while I live in Halifax, Nova Scotia. Being able to see my grandchildren is everything to me! I love hugging them and teaching them to bake. With the oldest girl here in Halifax, I was able to do just that. I still see her from time to time and we do bake and have sleepovers. With the youngest, that isn't possible. I haven't been able to hug her for over a year, and it will probably be at least another year before I can. How I miss those hugs! It's tough to explain how much this has changed my life!

My second resolution has to do with my church. In order to be able to 'attend' Sunday services, I've learned how to 'Zoom.' But the process hasn't been easy. To say the least, technology is not my friend; at my age, I'm really not interested in learning new software. Nor can Zoom bring back the many parts of church life that have been lost since the start of the pandemic. There are no church dinners, bake sales, or other social functions of the type I would normally be attending. Given that a lot of my social life is in church, the lack of these many social functions has created a void in my life. I manage to keep in touch with my friends from St Margaret's; however, I just can't wait for church life to get back to normal. My church family and my grandchildren are my life.

In closing, I have to say that as a lady of advanced years, I know my time is limited and I am extremely sad at having to put the most important parts of my life on hold. When you're older, you want to fill every day with living.

Peoplephile
Su Mardelli

At some point it would have been a good idea to leave the house, even if it was just for a breath of fresh air. But at no point did this idea ever cross Brian's mind. The quarantine, in his opinion, was the best idea conspiring politicians had concocted to flatten the curve. And though he had yet to uncover the true motive behind this nefarious lockdown, he was as happy as a cuddled kitten to be at home and away from everyone.

He still had to deal with people all the time, which was exhausting. Before his retirement the previous Summer, his favourite evening wind-down routine had been to sip a hot mug of tea next to his wife, while sharing stories of the latest barrage of nincompoops encountered during his workday. He would unleash tirade after tirade, snowballing anecdotes into distorted *facta et figuras* (facts and figures) of human stupidity. These would elicit sympathetic 'Yes dears' from his wife, who had long since learnt not to share her opinions. Sadly, incompetency reigned everywhere—like this virus—infecting the old and the young alike, omnipresent in the genetic code. Now, for example, he was on the phone with a shipping company who had hopelessly lost his package.

'I'm afraid that's just not good enough, Molly,' he said, shaking his head while adjusting his earpiece. He stirred his coffee, noting again how his sugar intake had doubled since lockdown had started in early March. He theorized that this was a scheme cooked up by the greedy coffee cartels who had 'cut' the coffee beans with brown fava beans to ramp up profit. This brilliant scam not only gave the coffee the colour and strength of a Scottish ox, but also made it more bitter, forcing him to add extra sugar to balance his palate. His theory seemed so plausible that he'd started mapping it out on his living room wall, using red string to connect the pinned newspaper cut-outs of commodity trends to cartoon clip arts of coffee beans, farmers and impish Red Devils.

Once he'd included related industries such as the sugar cartels, the diet centers and the gyms, his theory gained momentum and now looked like a cat's cradle gone awry.

He gave up his mapping when the superstore ran out of red yarn and changed its free delivery eligibility to orders above 20 dollars. On principle he objected, complained, then abstained from buying anything from there, an embargo that was still in effect as he reminded his wife every time they spoke. On the plus side, though, his wife was happy, knowing he could only stomach one large cup of coffee a day.

He shook his head again, catching a glimpse of himself in the mirror over the dining room buffet. His reflective twin, Other Brian, grinned back at him. Still devilishly handsome and sharper than a Crusader's arrow, he thought to himself. His slight paunch was hidden under the frame of the mirror, his upper torso pacing within it like the bobbing half of a puppet in a beachside Punch and Judy show. He was wearing the blue sweater with the white chevron pattern, which made his baby blue eyes and white hair seem brighter than usual. He had four more sweaters left in his closet before a washing day was required. A good thing, he thought, thinking back at all the follow-ups he needed to get through in the next couple of days. It's a bloody full-time job, he signalled to Other Brian, who both nodded and rolled his eyes in agree-ment.

'No, no, no, Molly. Please, just put yourself in my shoes.' He let out an exasperated sigh to reinforce to the hapless Molly how frustrated he was getting. 'Now I understand that you're not a very senior or experienced person in this company, but I don't want a refund. I want my item delivered. That's why I ordered it.'

He snorted, looking skywards, his palms held up as if in devotional prayer to the gods of common-sense. Other Brian looked back with unequi-vocal exasperation at the travail of explaining *the obvious* to the very challenged Molly. Faint 'for sures' could be heard through the headset as Molly kept her infinite politesse together.

'Fine, Molly. I will wait for you to check and call me back. I mean look,' he offered in a moment of unfettered magnanimity, 'if you're short-staffed I'm happy to take a gander in your warehouse and search for my package. I'm sure I'll find it quickly.'

He hung up, satisfied that he had imparted essential process improve-ments to the shipping company's protocols.

'I don't know what they pay those people to do, but it sure seems like a waste of money,' he declared to his current audience of two: Other Brian and the perpetually muted TV. His wife had left at the start of the lockdown to be with Betts and her new baby.

'You don't remember, Brian, how difficult those first three months were,' she had said on the steps of the house as she was leaving. She had pinched his cheek affectionately asking one more time, 'You sure?' referring to the car.

'Yeah, yeah,' he had gestured dismissively. His heart was breaking, but he disguised it well by sighing loudly enough to catch the quiver in his voice before it emerged. 'Take the car, I won't be leaving the house anyway. Everything can be delivered.'

Their youngest daughter Bettina had had several miscarriages before baby Serena was finally born, and he was comforted that his wife would be with them during these unprecedented times. It was more important for her to be taking care of them than of him. He would be fine.

What's next? he wondered, dusting imaginary dust off his hands while recalling his extensive To-Do list. His daughter had asked him to check the WHO standards for plastic baby bottles and compare them to the Dr Brown's bottles her neighbour had gifted her. He sat in his executive office chair, prominently placed at the dining table because it gave him a panoramic view of the entire living area, and readjusted the lumbar. He squinted through his glasses as he opened a fresh page browser—a habit more than a trial— and readied himself for a few hours of immersive reading. He had moved his computer, printer and files out of the small home office into the spacious open-concept living area just before his wife left, preferring to hold court in the big space that offered ample pacing paths, a good view of the front yard and street, and the luxury of eating, working and watching all at the same time. His wife had helped with the transfer, even suggesting he nap on the couch when the work fatigued him. Brian had creased his brow and crinkled his nose as if she had just suggested he marry a horse. 'I'll sleep in the bedroom,' he had replied.

'Whoever napped in their office?' he'd muttered to himself.

Through the window he saw a delivery van pull up on his side of the street.

'I wonder what the neighbours are getting today,' he thought.

He had noticed, over the past few weeks, that delivery vans tended to park on the opposite side of the street from the delivery address. The logic was lost on him. Why would anyone want to walk further than they had to? To his surprise, the doorbell rang and out of the corner of his eye he saw a blurry image get smaller through the front door's frosted glass.

'Ah, it's for me. Clever fellow. Let's see what's due today.'

He clicked on his calendar and noted the various coloured horizontal bars that lined across the days. Each represented a potential delivery timeline from his purchases. Today there was only one; a cyan-coloured bar. He clapped his hands in delight.

Finally, the face masks had arrived. He had been waiting for this package with much anticipation. He was looking forward to sending them to all his kids, hearing the gratitude and relief in their voices when they called to thank him, basking in their knowledge that everyone still needed Dad. After all, only Dad would have selected The Best of the Best. And, indeed, this was so! He had researched the subject extensively, listened to experts' endless debates, read research articles about filtration efficacy, modes of trans- mission, and so on and so forth. He had concluded that non-PPE face masks *would* protect his family, but only if they were made of a certain material and were a particular thickness. He had even called up CBC Radio to share this information with the city's Chief Medical Officer. She'd seemed impressed with his knowledge, though she'd raised a good point about availability. He was therefore delighted when he saw the owner of a local face mask company, who was being interviewed on CTV, detail the salient features of her product which matched his specifications. And the price was reasonable too! He had placed an order immediately, pleased with the ease and simplicity of the website's buying process. The only problem was that he had to wait three weeks for the masks to be delivered. But what to do? Good quality took time. And frankly, the three weeks had passed relatively quickly.

He waited until the delivery van had left, then walked briskly to the front door and opened it wide. Sure enough, bulging out of his mailbox was a white plastic parcel with the sun logo of the face mask company prominently displayed. Perfect! Finally, a company that really cared about treating customers well. These people knew what they were doing and kept their promises. He would send them a five-star rating immediately. He grabbed the parcel and eagerly walked back inside. There he picked up the large scissors, conveniently relocated to the kitchen counter and with a practiced hand sliced the package open. Inside was another plastic bag—the blue transparent freezer kind—in which the masks were packed. He pulled the bag out and held it up in his hand, rotating it like he was appraising vintage wine in a glass, counting the masks—one, two, three, four, five, six... But wait a minute!

He frowned. He turned back to his computer, clicking the mouse impatiently to check his order. He was not mistaken:

12 × double-layered assorted coloured face masks $203.40.

He slammed his fist on the table. He most certainly had *not* received the 12 masks he had paid an arm and a leg for! He sat down and started writing an indignant email to the company. He was frustrated that his fingers were not as agile on the keyboard as the words he was dictating. But the pounding of the keystrokes satisfied him. He was not taking this lying down. Enough was enough. These companies pretending to be socially-conscious and community-minded and all that nonsense. What a load of rubbish! He would not be nice about it, either. As his fingers blasted across the keyboard, he caught Other Brian looking at him nodding: *Good idea Other Brian!* He would report them to the police unless immediate action was taken. And this time he wanted a full refund, including compensation for all the time he had wasted waiting for the masks to arrive. He could have bought cheaper masks that would have arrived faster but he hadn't because of the promises—*i.e., lies*—that the face mask company had made in its advertisements. He made sure all this was written in black and white so there could be no confusion to his intentions. They could be shady, but he was as honest as a sunny day.

He hit SEND and reflexively checked the time. It was 10:09 in the morning. I'll give them until tomorrow, he thought, already drafting a one-star review in his head. He looked at Other Brian in the mirror and gave him a knowing nod. These people would learn not to mess with customers. Not everyone was gullible enough to fall for their hoax.

The phone rang. He looked at the display; a number he did not recognize. Probably a telemarketer, a thought that angered him even more.

'Hello!'

'Hi, good morning,' said a woman with a soft voice. 'May I please speak to mister Brian Patterson?'

'Yes speaking. Who is this? Is this a telemarketing call? If it is, I'm giving you 10 seconds to hang up and you'd better not try to sell me anything!'

But it wasn't a telemarketer. It was the face mask company. 'I just saw your e-mail. I'm so sorry for the mix-up Mr Patterson. I can't imagine how it happened. I packed your masks personally and I was so sure that I counted all the twelve masks. I'm so sorry for my mistake. It was really late at night and I must have miscounted. I just had so many orders to pack and I must have been more tired than I thought.'

Brian was—for lack of a better word—dumbfounded.

The woman went on to apologize again and offered to deliver the balance of the masks in the afternoon.

'How many are you missing? I just want to make sure there are no mistakes this time.'

'Um… Six or seven,' he managed to say in a softer tone. 'Let me count again.'

He picked up the blue freezer bag and this time opened it. He pulled out the masks, each neatly folded and stacked perfectly and counted them aloud one-by-one. 'One, two, three, four, five, six, wait a minute… seven, eight, nine, ten, eleven… twelve.'

Brian felt the saliva in the back of his throat freeze like it had been sprayed with liquid nitrogen and drop with the weight of a wrecking ball.

'Oh, my goodness…' he stammered, 'It's… Oh… oh no… I'm so sorry. There are twelve indeed.'

'Oh, thank goodness! I really thought I had made a mistake.'

Brian felt his legs wobble and his head start to spin. How? How could *he* have been mistaken?

He sat down on his executive chair.

'I'm so sorry,' he found himself saying. 'I'm so sorry. You see at first this morning I…' He managed to mangle some words and sentences together, inserting 'I'm sorry' when he didn't know what to say. Somehow, he ended the call then covered his face with his hand. Even Other Brian did not want to look at him. Brian looked up, furrowed his brow, squinted then gritted his teeth. The masks were packed too tightly, he thought, anyone could have made the same mistake. He could hear Other Brian disagreeing: *You should have opened and counted them first.*

They should have packed them individually, he retorted.

And use twelve plastic bags? Think of the environment!

Well, *recycle* anyone?

Other Brian snorted, then held up his palms in fervent worship to the gods of common-sense: *Oh Lord, save me from this nincompoop.* Brian frowned and crossed his arms. He had always prided himself on his stellar pragmatism. Common sense is what our crawling ancestors used to survive, he used to tell to his children when they fumbled during adolescence.

He stood up and scanned the room around him. His research printouts on historical pandemics were stacked neatly on the dining table. Next to them were box files with his tax forms, appliance manuals, and various bills. On the wall of the living room next to the TV was his tangled coffee collage, and on the media unit were two piles of newspapers and magazines organized into READ and JUNK. These were all projects he had tasked himself to complete. But now, looking around, he couldn't shake the feeling that he was in a mausoleum, a preserved tomb of all his soliloquies. He also noticed the week's dishes piled up in the sink. He kept telling himself he would get round to them soon, but really, he'd tried to avoid the chore until all the crockery was used. It was a constant reminder that despite his large family, he was the only one using them.

Another paternal adage popped into his head, causing him to sigh heavily and drop his shoulders. He picked up his phone and pressed the green button. It rang twice.

'Hello?' answered a soft hesitant female voice. 'Mister Patterson?'

'Hi yes, it's me again. I hope you don't mind.' He felt a blush rising up his face like a red sunrise after a stormy night.

'Not at all. How can I help you?'

'I just want to say how sorry I am. My email, my behaviour... was appalling. I'm so embarrassed and you didn't deserve it. Please, please forgive me.'

'Of course, sir, it's water under the bridge. Think nothing of it.'

'Thank you yes, you see, I'm not like that. It's just that well, I really have no excuse, do I?'

There was a slight hesitation, as if the face mask woman were having an internal debate, before she continued. 'I think it's just grand of you to call me again. It's really big of you. It must be hard to do that and these days people seem to be so angry all the time. I think it's the lockdown and being isolated. It's really not healthy to be away from people for so long. I think, anyway. Are you also on your own?'

'Yes,' he answered quickly. 'Yes, I am. My wife is with my daughter, she just had a baby you see, after trying for so many years.'

'Oh congratulations! Is this your first grandchild?'

'Yes, I mean no, I mean for her it is. I have two other kids, grandkids. I have four kids. Now three of them have children.'

'It must make holidays so wonderful. I love the madness and warmth those little people bring to our lives.'

151

Brian did too, he told her. They chatted, exchanging small talk like kids trading sweets after a Halloween haul. When they finally hung up, Brian felt he could have talked for hours. He was excited, he had enjoyed the conversation with the woman from the face mask company and was eager to share it with his wife during their daily call. It would be a welcome change from the anecdotes of baby Serena's diaper deposits and sleeping patterns.

He sighed happily, picking up his coffee and taking a sip. But then he grimaced. It was tepid. He set the mug back down on the table, wondering if maybe there were a local coffee house that roasted its own beans. He wriggled on his seat to continue his baby bottle research but was now too distracted to focus. He glanced at the face masks now fanned out on the table next to him, reflecting on the past hour.

Brian stared at his pasty grey screen with the flashing cursor and made a decision. He stood up and closed the laptop in one smooth movement. He could see himself in the mirror grinning from ear to ear. It was enough for today. He turned off the TV and grabbed one of the masks. A walk would do him good.

COVID's Small Mercies
Elizabeth Zimmer

For close to 50 years, I earned a good chunk of my living going to the theater and writing about what I found there. I've reviewed dance, theater, film, and all sorts of experimental performance, for radio, magazines, and newspapers on both coasts of Canada and the United States. In 1992, I returned to Manhattan, where I was born. While friends and relatives eased into retirement, playing golf and hosting grandchildren, I soldiered on, tracking press releases, making reservations, and working a double shift: writing all day at my computer, with a dinner break and then a stint sitting still and watching other people move, or talk, or commit all sorts of atrocities on the big screen. And taking notes, and heading home to sit some more and meet a deadline. Sometimes I was so tired I'd fall asleep in my chair.

But a year ago everything suddenly froze. Broadway shut down. Dance companies cancelled their seasons. Movie theaters, gyms, restaurants... all shuttered. The senior center where I spent a couple of hours a week lying on the floor, doing the odd combination of exercises and resting that make up the Feldenkrais Method, closed its doors. Doctors cancelled appointments. My trainer, my housekeeper, my massage therapist, even my physical therapist stopped showing up. Many of us who live alone mourned the absence of human contact, of human touch.

For a lot of people, the onset of COVID-19 lockdowns came as a shock, a psychic blow cushioned by generous unemployment benefits. They had cash flow, but no place to go, nowhere to spend their sudden windfall. A stage-manager neighbor pivoted to making masks on his sewing machine and giving them away. College teachers, shut out of their lecture halls, realized they could operate from anywhere; one friend left our Chelsea building for Mayaguez, Puerto Rico, where she's been teaching remotely over Zoom and helping her mother settle into a new house. Another, flummoxed by construction noise in his uptown apartment and lousy WiFi at his husband's country digs, took his laptop to an upstate city where he keeps his newly widowed mother-in-law company, writing his dissertation and teaching from her home and garden.

I, on the other hand, was merely bemused, and startled by how frightened everyone around me seemed. I live in an apartment complex full of senior citizens who'd dart away, terrified, when anyone approached them. People let their newspaper and mail deliveries sit for days before daring to touch them, and swabbed down their groceries. My work as a standardized patient, pretending to be ill so medical students could practice their interpersonal skills, shifted fitfully to Zoom and then quieted down for the Summer. I wrote about dances on video, filmed in quarantine, until my editor and I couldn't stand it anymore.

But I'm an old hand at this kind of isolation. Laid off from a full-time job in 2006, I've spent years working freelance from home. In the past decade I've undergone three orthopedic surgeries. Confined to this apartment for weeks on end, I got used to going nowhere, with only public radio for company. My idea of a vacation is not having to go to the theater! Being forbidden to walk in the street without a mask prevented me from eating the fattening snacks that delight me about urban life—never mind that the bakeries had closed. I immediately lost 10 pounds. A large cohort of Facebook friends replaced the lobby conversations I'd been missing, and were easier to deal with, given the progressive hearing loss that haunts me, compounded by the difficulty of understanding people through their masks.

Will Friedwald, a music writer with a passion for jazz and popular song, put his Clip Joint, a compilation of clips from old films and television variety shows spotlighting his favorite performers, onto Zoom where, thrice weekly, viewers, many of them similarly expert, can kibitz in the chat while the clips play, and wire tips via Venmo and similar services. Alcoholic beverages are optional. The Joint keeps me up late, but I've made new friends there, and can attend in my nightgown.

I help edit Persimmontree.org, an online quarterly magazine of the arts by and for women over 60. We'd just closed our Spring issue when the pandemic began to threaten the United States, and we sprang into action, soliciting responses to COVID from our readership. Contributions poured in: poetry, prose, drawings, clips of music and film. We published five special Corona sections between May and the November election, and another responding to the events of January 6, before the presidential inauguration.

Life goes on, for those of us lucky enough to escape the virus. The Feldenkrais lessons, uniquely suited to the Zoom environment, multiply: I now take 11 classes a week, working on a mat on my living room floor, and slowly getting to know the people, in their little rectangles, in their own homes, who take them alongside me. Dancers and choreographers are making movies, often only five minutes long—the perfect length for our fractured attention spans. My voice instructor, who lives upstairs, also teaches via Zoom, with surprisingly good results. Theaters around the country are producing new shows, and repurposing old ones, for digital transmission. My senior center has been screening first-run films via Zoom; this is the first year in ages that I've actually seen most of the Academy Award contenders.

And Spring has come again; blossoms and bright leaves and birdsong erupt outside my window. I still hate eating alone, but I've come to treasure the hours of solitude this new circumstance allows me. I no longer feel it necessary to contribute an opinion to every discussion. The plague has left me time to think, to remember, and to formulate a sane way forward.

SECTION 6

Politics

*I*t is perhaps inevitable that the COVID pandemic should have become entangled in politics, at least to a certain degree. Given that the fight against the virus entailed, first, the wholesale shuttering of businesses and the placing of severe restrictions on people's personal freedom, and then, later, the establishment of province-wide networks for testing and the distribution of vaccine, it would have been hard for it not to have become politicized to a certain degree. But the degree of politicization—at times approaching outright weaponization of the pandemic for crass political ends—was something I for one had not seen before, and something I wasn't prepared for. As frightening as it is, the story needs to be known and publicized. We make no apologies for the fact that this is a long, meaty, and sometimes difficult section. In many ways, it is the almanac's most important section.

The section begins with Ann McMillan's piece on Grannies and COVID. Having followed gender issues for the last 50 years, she has noticed that women are carrying more than their fair share of extra pandemic-related burdens, such as those related to child care. Her most important finding is that grandmothers seem to be living the perfect storm, being vulnerable to COVID as well as having families that need support during the COVID pandemic. In fact, Grannies are providing society with an unpaid 'buffer' to help with adapting to the new order, without suitable recognition or reward.

My two pieces, 'Politics and COVID I: the U.S.' and 'Politics and COVID II: Canada,' attempt to outline the extent of politicization of the COVID pandemic in the two countries and some of the reasons for it. In the U.S., politicization of the pandemic has often been quite extreme, both in strongly pro-Trump states such as those in the Deep South and Rocky Mountain region and in those, such as Wisconsin and Michigan, closely divided between pro- and anti-Trump forces. My research has found that high COVID rates are quite strongly related to high percentages of support for Trump in the 2020 Presidential election, and also to the presence of Republican state governors. Even more tellingly, the research cited in the Coda to this paper has found high vaccination rates even more strongly related to high percentages of support for Trump's opponent, Joe Biden, in the 2020 election, as well as to the presence of Democratic or 'non-partisan' Republican state governors. ('Non-partisan' Republicans refers to Republican governors, all serving in heavily Democratic states, who to all intents and purposes have handled the pandemic as Democratic governors would have.) Conversely, low vaccination rates are strongly related to high rates of support for Trump and the presence of Republican governors; this is true particularly in the Deep South.

In Canada, the relationship between purely partisan politics and COVID case rates or vaccination rates is not as clear or as obvious. But this doesn't mean that the pandemic has not been politicized. In most of the country, it definitely has, albeit not to quite the same extent as in the U.S. Most notably, case rates have

157

been many times lower in Atlantic Canada, where the pandemic has to all intents and purposes never been politicized, than in the rest of the country. It doesn't seem to matter what party an Atlantic premier belongs to. The approach to the pandemic has been basically the same throughout the region, whether the premier in question was Conservative or Liberal. This has not generally been so in the rest of the country. Hard-right Conservative premiers such as Alberta's Jason Kenney and Ontario's Doug Ford have been more reluctant to impose strict lockdown measures than premiers from provinces east of Ontario. They have also been quicker to lift those measures, and less willing to enforce the measures strictly while they are still in place. The result is that Alberta, the country's most right-wing province, now has the country's highest overall COVID case rates, and Alberta and Ontario have the largest number of variant cases. Of all the possible causes of higher case rates listed above, enforcement would appear to be the most significant, though this is a matter bearing further investigation.

The section concludes with Alan Lennon's powerful essay, 'COVID Social Responsibility and "The Next Times".' Lennon's sobering conclusion is that while the pandemic may have taught some of us our interdependence, and shown some of us our vulnerability, it has also, with the connivance of a relatively small group of individuals, undermined the social responsibilities that we all have. Without those responsibilities, Lennon says, we will either slowly or quickly decline into a Hobbesian state of nature and life will become increasingly 'nasty, brutish and short.' One can only hope that we all awaken to our responsibilities to one another in time to prevent such a horrific result from coming to pass.

Grannies and COVID
Ann McMillan

Introduction

Life has always ensured that I, as a woman in science with my PhD in Mechanical Engineering from the University of Waterloo in 1976, would take gender issues seriously.

I took note as women came to make up more than half of university students, as well as of new doctors. When women slowly joined the ranks of university professors, management, and fields related to emerging information technology, I imagined the changes that would occur as a result. I was proud when I learned of women, such as Katherine Johnson, who participated in the development and adoption of new space technology. I cheered in 1992 when Roberta Bondar took off to become the first neurologist (and the first Canadian woman) in space. I recognized progress when Anna Mae Hays guided the U.S. Army Nurse Corps in the Vietnam War, and became the first female general in American military history.

I applauded when young women stepped forward into leadership roles far beyond their years; when, for example, Malala Yousafzai became the youngest ever Nobel Laureate for fighting to protect girls' education in Afghanistan, and Greta Thunberg took on then U.S. President Trump with her impassioned statements on climate change.

I also cheered whenever the historic achievements of heroic women of the past were finally acknowledged, an example being Maria Anna Mozart who performed on the harpsichord and toured with her brother, and who was called one of the best musicians in Europe at the ripe old age of 12. Or how about Lavinia Fontana and Sofonisba Anguissola, Italian painters of the 16th century who were widely acclaimed and then almost forgotten. Then there was Henrietta Wood, who made history after the American Civil War by pursuing a lawsuit against the man who kidnapped her back into slavery, and winning.[1]

The celebration of outstanding achievement by women is important but, as I age, the sentiment expressed by Bella Abzug in 1977[2] resonates with me: 'Our struggle today is not to have a female Einstein get appointed as an assistant professor. It is for a woman schlemiel to get as quickly promoted as a male schlemiel.' For those of us who are not on the rarefied spectrum of the truly exceptional, some semblance of equality and maybe even equity would be amazing. It is past time.

Beyond my career, I have raised two daughters into assertive, accomplished young ladies and applauded their progress. I have also raised one son

159

who understands that women are people, too, and who offers his partner all his support as she pursues her career, modelling these traits for his son to see.

In general, over my lifetime, I have seen progress for women in the way they are treated and the way they can live their lives, but I continue to be amazed at how slow and how fragile progress is. In the 70s and 80s when Canada began recognizing a need for equality, being an expert on gender issues was just expected of women in the workplace, an 'other duty as required.' As one of only two women on a Management Team of 32 people at Ontario Hydro's Research Division in the 80s, I spent a lot of my time dealing with 'women's issues' on top of my 'real' work.

Now long retired, I sit back and enjoy the sort of 'me' time that I hope I have earned. Just occasionally, something happens which throws me back into the deep end with respect to gender issues. COVID has been such an occurrence. Just when I thought that things were progressing, at a snail's pace to be sure, I couldn't help but notice that COVID has blown us back into the 1950s or before, and the price that women are paying due to the plague is astronomical and rising every day. This means that society is paying a high price as well, although, sadly, many men may not have noticed yet. It is not entirely COVID itself that is having this effect; it is the economic shutdowns that have been slapped in place with a minimum of sober thought about consequences, largely by the men in power. It seems that, in the face of crisis, the world returns to its paternalistic roots and gives women, particularly women of a certain age, a good slap in the face for good measure in spite of their leadership success.[3]

March 2021 is the second Women's History Month of the COVID pandemic. Perhaps just after that is a good time to have a look at how COVID has influenced us and to provide an overview of the current gender situation by the numbers, in the media, and by personal observation. It offers a moment to reflect on the special role of Grannies as the future unfolds. I wonder whether we will learn anything from our COVID time. If so, the next pandemic could possibly be less destructive of women's lives and less destructive of society more generally. I hope we learn our lessons well.

The Figures, the Issues and Some Anecdotal Information

It has been many years since my last foray into women's issues, so I thought I would enlist my good friend Ms Google to assist me in synthesizing a quick update on the impacts of COVID on women. Her help has been extensive, but the exercise of sifting the wheat from the chaff and trying to tell a story based on it has been somewhat challenging. Let me be clear upfront; this is no balanced academic overview. I have simply let my curiosity and my personal tastes guide my line of enquiry and attempted to tell a story based on the result. Deborah Stone, the noted American feminist says, 'No number is innocent.'[4] I have tried to remember that.

This is a *big* topic with lots of interesting and important extensions into gender and race. I have chosen not to go there. Also, North America is the focus for reasons of familiarity and brevity, though I make occasional excursions to the larger world.

Over the past many months of COVID, there have been occasional bursts of numbers providing a snapshot of how women are doing in the workplace, the usual stage for studies of equity. For example, the number of mothers in Canada who worked less than half their usual hours increased by 70% from February to September, 2020.[5] The comparable number was 24% for fathers. In the U.S., 'four times as many women as men dropped out of the labour force in September, roughly 865,000 women compared with 216,000 men.'[6] As well, female participation in the American work force dipped below 57% in April and May, 2020, according to the U.S. Bureau of Labor Statistics.[7] In a report on COVID-19 and gender equity,[8] McKinsey and Company note that 'women's jobs are 1.8 times more vulnerable to this crisis than men's jobs. Women make up 39% of global employment but account for 54% of overall job losses.' COVID-19 is apparently making women leave the work force in droves. Some 1.5 million Canadian women left or lost their jobs in the first two months of the pandemic. The job losers fell mainly in two age groups: those aged 20–24, and those aged 35–39.[9] There are apparently a number of reasons for this, including:

- Women are typically 'front line' workers in jobs where they can't work from home (e.g., nurses, retail, childcare workers and public-school teachers, personal care workers, hospitality and the arts).
- Women are employed in 'hardest hit' occupations (e.g., in accommodation and food services. In October 2020, of 48,000 jobs lost, 80% were by women).[10]
- Women aged 20–24 appear to have gone back to school in large numbers.
- In the age group 35–39, 'women with children under six made up 41% of the labour force in February 2020, but account for two-thirds of the ensuing exit from the work force.'[11]

Thus, while it is apparent that many more women than men are choosing their education or their parenting responsibilities over their careers in these times, many women's jobs have simply disappeared. Pertaining to the disappearance of women's jobs, as could be expected with labour changes of this magnitude, there are economic consequences. McKinsey & Company estimates global GDP growth in 2030 to be U.S. $1 trillion less than it would be 'if women's employment simply tracked that of men in each sector.'[12]

Employment analysis could fill numerous books, but let's just glance at healthcare. In 2006, 93.8% of nurses were women in Canada, while only 35.5% of practicing doctors, dentists and veterinarians were women.[13] These figures may have changed somewhat over the intervening years. In the early days of COVID women's infection rates were often double those of male health care workers. For example, in Spain, by the end of April, 2020, there had been 28,326 health care workers infected with COVID, of whom 21,392 or 75.5% were women and only 6,924 or 24.5% were men.[14] This probably illustrates that the women nurses were the 'front line' with the patient while doctors had less contact and exposure, as well as a combination of lack of understanding about COVID transmission and inadequate training and use of personal protection equipment (PPE) in those early days. This subtly illustrates one inequity that women experience with COVID. Women have been going to work to care for others even while recognizing that the threat to their health and safety is high, which translates into high risk for their families. Making the decision whether to continue at work or go home to family must be heart-wrenching. It is not clear to what extent health care institutions have stepped up to deal with the gender disparity in healthcare work or offered effective PPE and sufficient compensation for women to risk their lives daily to provide front-line care.

COVID has changed many aspects of women's lives and these changes, in turn, have levered other changes depending on the situation of the particular women.[15] The numbers above indicate that there are more women at home, and with 'working from home' and school closures, there are more families at home in general.

As family life changes, so do the lives of mothers and Grannies. Not only have parents not in front line work been laid off due to COVID closures, and sent to 'work from home' in large numbers, but childcare centres, schools, and colleges and universities have also seen changes. Depending on the location and the severity of the COVID outbreak, facilities have closed to in-person participation, have modified their operation to virtual centres, or have shut down entirely. The situation with respect to child care has profound impacts on how women can manage their pandemic response. If the day care is open, the woman may worry excessively about the health of her child. If the day care is shut, it most often falls upon her to arrange for alternate care or to stay home and look after the child herself. In many jurisdictions, the opening and closing decisions have been relatively short-term and unpredictable, heightening the stresses involved in planning for child care.

A small study by the American Centers for Disease Control and Prevention (CDC) concluded that very small children can catch COVID and spread it.[16] Notably, this was an early study from April to July 2020, carried out in three centres in Utah and it is not clear what mitigation strategies were applied; the children did not wear masks. While 12 children were infected from someone else at the daycare centre, most had none to mild symptoms. These children spread COVID-19 to one in four contacts outside the centre (often including mother and siblings).

A serious concern is that childcare centres could contribute to community spread of COVID. In a major study of 57,000 U.S. childcare providers across the U.S., one group from facilities that stayed open and one group from facilities that closed, no differences in COVID-19 outcomes were reported as long as safety measures were taken.[17] The study, done by Yale University researchers, provided evidence that daycare centres can operate without increased risk to the caregivers as long as they 'practice mitigation and prevention strategies which cost money.'[18] This study focused on the caregivers, since the researchers didn't have data about the children's risk. One of the researchers pointed out that since typically the workers had a small group of children to work with, the situation was significantly different from that experienced in kindergarten to Grade 12 schools with large numbers in the same building.

Another study, co-authored by Dr Camille Aupiais from Hôpital Jean-Verdier in Paris, indicated that children in daycare are an unlikely source of COVID infection.[19] The study was small, being based on 347 children between the ages of five months and four years. The levels of antibodies in the blood were assessed and found present in only 4% of the children. Further, these children had been infected by someone in their home and not someone at the daycare. Levels of antibodies in the blood of the staff were similar to those in a control group of adults who were not exposed to children in a day care setting.

Thus, daycare settings are apparently a relatively safe environment. But what about schools?

Public Health Ontario did a rapid review last July, which serves to frame the issues.[20] Schools in Ontario were first closed on March 13, 2020. The review was based on literature covering not only the current COVID-19 pandemic, but also the H1N1 pandemic. The sources for the review were: MEDLINE; Supplemental (i.e., Embase, PsycINFO, CINAHL, Global Health and Scopus); and Pre-Print (i.e., medRxiv and vioRxiv). The overall conclusion was that 'in the majority of modelling studies, school closures… reduced the total or cumulative number of cases.' Interestingly, however, the reduction was not as great as that resulting from some other actions that could be taken (such as closing non-essential businesses and limiting gatherings), according to some modelling studies. And, according to two studies, school closures may have negative consequences for ICU capacity and mortality due to their impacts on healthcare workers who will then require childcare. There were also negative outcomes for children, including 'decreased physical activity, increased screen time and sedentary behavior, poor nutrition, poor mental health and wellbeing, and risk of child abuse and neglect.'

There have been several investigations of COVID-19 outbreaks in schools reported in the literature; they indicate that there is a low risk of transmission from children in schools. However, 'several pre-print modelling studies predict resurgence' of cases unless additional steps are taken such as 'reduced class sizes, testing symptomatic people and contact tracing.'[21]

The situation with respect to schools is considerably more complex than with respect to daycare. In addition to issues within the school itself, there are issues of care before and after school, as well as travel to and from school. The summary of the daycare situation is complex; a detailed discussion of the issues around schools is beyond the scope of this analysis. Suffice it to say that in spite of research that provides comforting results on the risks of daycare and school, it is apparent that in general, women prioritize their family's perceived health and safety before their own need for a career.

What doesn't seem to have been quantified or even widely discussed is the continuing uncertainty with respect to changes in procedures and even the future opening and closing of daycare and schooling programs and facilities. It is enough to drive staff and parents bonkers not to know whether they can depend on their daycare arrangements past this Friday, and it can be profoundly exhausting. How can a woman plan to work if she doesn't know whether her two-year-old or 14-year-old will be home next Monday?

Most families will figure out what works best for them. When the woman is working parttime, or in a job that pays less than her husband's, her choices may seem to be obvious and logical. Less obvious, and often overlooked, is the fact that when the woman gives up her job, society goes back to the '50s with paternalistic social mores and a shifted balance of power with a home-maker/breadwinner divide.

Let us not forget that as in healthcare, women make up the majority of the staff and teachers in the education system. In fact, 'Today 87% of American teachers are female and those numbers continue to increase annually.'[22] Other developed nations show similar numbers.

Teachers have truly been in the front lines, expected to show up and teach as the system opens and closes, in some cases erratically. They may get a double whammy of stress from both their jobs and their family situations. They work on the one hand without clear guidance as to how to deal safely with the students if schools are open, and on the other hand with challenging technology which may be new to them. However, it is still not very clear if teachers in school are at higher risk than people in communities at large, or if so by how much.[23,24] At a time when teachers are needed more than ever, of the 3.5 million teachers in the US, 38% said they are considering leaving the profession.[25] As with nurses, teachers are aging, and this may be a factor. Apparently, 18% of private and public-school teachers in the U.S. are over

55 years of age.[26] Given that COVID is more serious for older people than for younger ones, is there any wonder they worry about being exposed to COVID in the classroom?

There have been attempts to assess the economic impact of learning losses from school closures.[27,28] Some areas in which these will be found are lost individual earnings as well as losses in Gross Domestic Product, and the amounts are staggering, but quite variable depending on the study.

In addition to these situations in healthcare and teaching, women have traditionally done more than their share of 'unpaid' labour. Charlotte Whitton famously said, 'Whatever women do they must do twice as well as men to be thought half as good. Luckily, this is not difficult.'[29] In COVID times, however, it *is* getting difficult. Childcare is just one type of unpaid work that has fallen back on families to do. Many other home-related tasks, such as cleaning, have also become more time-consuming or more difficult in the time of COVID due to the need for increased sanitizing. Before COVID, 'women already spent about three times as many hours on unpaid domestic work and care work than men.'[30] The UN received data from 38 countries that substantiates that both women and men have taken on a greater amount of work since COVID began, but women continue to do more as well as taking on more care work.

One of the most alarming changes that COVID has brought is the increase in violence towards women. According to the *World Health Organization News* (WHO) of March 9, 2021, one in three women will experience violence in their lives. Worse, 27% of women from 15–49 who have been in a relationship experience sexual or other physical violence from their intimate partners. Gender inequity and norms on the use of violence are a root cause of violence against women. They are influenced by a number of factors including, in the case of intimate partners: 'Past history of exposure to violence; marital discord and dissatisfaction; difficulties in communicating between partners; and male controlling behaviors towards their partners.'[31] With many societies experiencing lockdowns, work from home situations and closed schools, as well as the ongoing threat of catching COVID, it is easy to see why the incidence of violence against women is likely to continue to rise.

At the same time, access to services for victims of violence has decreased during the pandemic. In many countries, resources that would normally support such services are now directly involved in dealing with COVID. According to a U.N. Women brochure, *Impact of COVID-19 on violence against women and girls and service provision,* 'The pandemic and subsequent measures to address the pandemic have disrupted the availability and accessibility of services for survivors of violence.'[32] In addition, while there are insufficient data available on trends in violence since the victims often find themselves in situations where it is dangerous to report, there is some evidence. Canada's

Assaulted Women's Helpline fielded 20,334 calls between October 1 and December 31, 2020, compared to 12,352 over the same period the previous year, said Yvonne Harding, manager of resource development at the organization, as reported by the CBC on February 15, 2021. Between April 1 and September 30, the Helpline received 51,299 calls, compared to 24,010 in the same time frame in 2019. It is good news that the Helpline has received additional funding to assist with the increased volume.[33] Along similar lines, Statistics Canada reports that, based on 17 police services, calls related to domestic disturbances increased almost 12% in the period March–June, 2020, compared to a similar period in 2019.[34]

Canada's figures are echoed around the world. U.N. Women, the United Nations entity dedicated to gender equality and the empowerment of women, has called violence against women the 'shadow pandemic' of the COVID-19 crisis. 'Globally, an estimated 736 million women—almost one in three— have been subjected to intimate partner violence, non-partner sexual violence, or both at least once in their life (30% of women aged 15 and older).'[35] While one would have hoped that COVID would provide the impetus for this issue to be seriously considered around the world, President Tayyip Erdogan announced Turkey's withdrawal from the Istanbul Convention on March 20, 2021. The first binding treaty on preventing and combatting violence against women, this Convention, which came in force in 2014, sought to promote accountability of governments in preventing violence and holding perpetrators responsible. World leaders, including U.S. President Joe Biden, issued public statements opposing Erdogan's decision, and Turkish citizens took to the streets in protest, but the Convention is gone.[36]

Gloria Steinem once said, 'The truth will set you free. But first it will piss you off.'[37] Truths emerging from the pandemic are enough to piss anyone off, especially women. Women are clearly not being rewarded adequately for the risks they take in being front-line workers, in working in healthcare or in education, or for the unpaid work they do. Instead of considering how the pandemic could be used as an impetus toward greater equality, governments have had a tendency to take immediate actions such as closing schools and daycares, which have forced women to choose between their careers and their families, then, partially because of the woman's reduced economic power, to trap them in violent situations, meanwhile reducing their lines of support.

Much of this essay has been based on North American perspectives, but during my work with Ms Google, I happened upon a Report of the Committee on Women's Rights and Gender Equity reporting to the European Parliament 'On the gender perspective in the COVID-19 crisis and post-crisis period.' This report acknowledged that:

Whereas a majority of workers delivering essential services in the current crisis are women, including 76% of healthcare workers (doctors, nurses, midwives, staff in residential care homes), 82% of cashiers, 93% of childcare workers and teachers, 95% of domestic cleaners and helpers, and 86% of personal care workers in the EU;... it is thanks to them for whom physical distancing is often not an option and who thus bear the increased burden of possibly spreading the virus to their relatives, that our economic, social and healthcare systems, our public life and our essential activities are maintained. [38]

What Does All This Mean for Grannies?

One of my most cherished current roles is that of grandmother. While I last hugged my grandson last August, in a hurried and head-averted hug, I think about him every day and worry a little. Grandmothers across the globe share the need to nurture their extended families, protect them from harm, and try to prepare them to make the world a better place.

Until about 30,000 years ago, few people lived long enough to be grandparents in today's sense. In fact, studies of Neanderthal grandparents are based on the study of individuals 30 years of age and older, with the expectation that first children were had about age 15. [39] At some point, there was a surge in the numbers of older individuals; the reason for this is still a topic for research. However, having older individuals in society, 'Conveying wisdom and providing social and economic support for the families of their children and larger kin group,'[40] offered advantages then as it does today.

People over 65 number about 703 million in the world today. [41] There are more women elders than men across the world, as men generally die younger than women. Some 57% of people aged 70 and up and 62% of those aged 80 and up are women. [42] That being said, a lot of what is described in the following applies to grandfathers, too. With life expectancy growing, both the proportion of aged people in the population and the length of time of grandparenthood are also increasing.

Different countries and cultures deal with grandparents differently. In western culture today, children typically leave home and set up their own families. But this was not always the case. For example, in the U.S., '57% of adults 65 and older lived in multigenerational households' in 1900. This number had dipped to 12% by 1980[43] but has been increasing again, with a record 16.1% of the population or 49 million Americans living in a family household that contained at least two adult generations in 2008. [44]

When I decided to write this story of Grannies, I expected to be able to access some current research providing numbers on what women who are grandmothers are actually doing in these COVID times. Ms Google and I spent quite a bit of time searching and searching, without much success. And then a thought struck me. Women in the workforce, whether they are nurses, or teachers, or personal care workers, all contribute to the economic picture of the country. Thus, it is important for economists to capture and document how many of them are contributing through work, and what they are doing as a basis for policy development. Once one retires from paid employment, one has no more economic significance and becomes a shadow person perhaps collecting a pension, perhaps requiring healthcare, but no longer productive in the sense of having a job and therefore no longer of economic interest. Powerful policy-makers do not care about Grannies.

Let's start with trying to figure out what Grannies do. Three categories come immediately to mind: the Grannies who are still pursuing a career into old age; the Grannies who are retired or never worked but who are still mentally and physically able to engage with friends and families; and the Grannies who have some significant impairments and therefore live in a long-term care facility (LTC). While this is an oversimplification, it will help in structuring the following discussion.

Thinking of Grannies who are still pursuing a career, it is relevant to the COVID situation that in the U.S., 'between 1993 and 2009, the share of nurse supervisors and registered nurses between the ages of 55-64 grew from 12.8% to 18.5%.'[45] If we assume the trend for nurses to work until older ages has continued, it is likely that a significant number of practicing nurses are Grannies as well. We have already noted that over 18% of teachers in the U.S. are over 55 and we also note that personal care workers in the LTCs are mostly older women. Other Grannies continue to work in frontline jobs as cashiers, hospitality workers, hairdressers, etc. and are experiencing the ups and downs of the COVID economy where businesses are open one day and closed the next. These fully employed Grannies are deciding in droves to retire to avoid the threat of catching COVID-19 or because their jobs have disappeared.

Thus, with natural aging, lengthening life spans, and the coming of COVID—which appears to have led to a large-scale retirement of Grannies from the labour force—there are more Grannies available on the home front, and they are not likely to be sitting around watching soap operas on TV. The situation for women, especially Grannies who are being drafted in large numbers to provide care for their families and schooling for their grand-children, is changing as the pandemic progresses. As more and more of society is shut down, all women have to do more themselves. First, it was the hair-dressing that went, then the pedicures. Many forms of medical care have been reduced to 'on-line' talks with doctors, which are not conducive to good communication with elderly people who may have issues seeing, hearing and understanding. Thus, the well-groomed and closely monitored Grannie of 2019 may look a bit more haggard and hairy than she did then, and may be called upon to not only look after her own complex grooming needs but help out with those of her family as well. What with providing daycare through her Grannie School and doing the shopping and cleaning as her daughter hangs on to her job, Grannie has every right to look a bit haggard.

Of the 83% of U.S. elders 65 and older who say they have grandchildren, two-thirds say they have at least four grandchildren while of the 52% of U.S. elders between 50 and 64, 47% say they have at least four.[46] If a Grannie has lots of grandchildren it makes sense that she will face a greater demand for childcare provision.

In 2015, a Pew Survey 'found that among U.S. grandparents who have helped with child care in the past 12 months, nearly three-in-four (72%) said they did so only occasionally, while about one in five (22%) said they provided child care regularly.'[47] While I could not find more recent numbers, I would suggest that these numbers have probably gone up.

And, anecdotally, Grannies are stepping up. While working-age women without Grannie-support are stepping away from the work force, those who have mothers or mothers-in-law who are healthy and able-bodied have the support to carry on. It is interesting that although I know anecdotally that this is happening, I could find no recent North American numbers to support this view. There is lots of sociological work about the role of Grannies in the family, but the focus is on such aspects as why Grannies contribute their time to their families. (In the case of COVID, this is usually abundantly clear.)[48]

There has been some work done in Britain which looks at the role of grandparent care and workforce participation. Shiren Kanji finds that 'Grandparents' childcare increases the labour force participation of lone and partnered mothers at all levels of educational qualifications but by different degrees. Grandparents' childcare enables mothers to enter the paid work force.' Further, it 'raises the labour force participation of mothers with a child of school entry age on average by twelve percentage points.'[49]

While 'quick assessments' have been done about many aspects of the pandemic and its management, the only recent assessment of the impacts of COVID on Grannies that I could find focussed on the changes in the lives of healthy older women in the U.K. and South Africa.[50] The study highlights the intergenerational support of grandparents no matter what overall changes occur. It should be noted that the two countries are very different in terms of employment, poverty, and multi-generational living arrangements as well as differing in approaches to manage COVID-19.

In the U.K., grandparents are expected to isolate and avoid contact with their grandchildren, which halts the informal care that grandparents could otherwise provide. On the other hand, in South Africa, grandparents are more often part of multigenerational households where they maintain their role as caregivers. In South Africa the grandparents' income through the Old Age Grant (OAG) often is essential for food and household costs.

The outbreak of COVID-19 was met with worldwide lock-downs. The U.K. and South Africa imposed lock-downs almost simultaneously on March

27 and 28, 2020. Working from home for all but essential workers was imposed, and childcare centres and schools were closed. In the U.K., care arrangements remained open for the children of essential workers. In spite of this, a survey of nearly 20,000 working women carried out in July, 2020 revealed that 'since lockdown 60% of those surveyed have struggled with childcare provision' and 67% 'reported that they had been forced to reduce their paid work hours because of a lack of access to childcare.' Pre-COVID, five million of 14 million total grandparents provided some form of childcare according to AGE UK,[51] who estimated that this childcare was worth about 3.9 billion pounds a year to the economy.

In South Africa, no childcare provisions were offered to essential workers during the lockdown. However, about two-thirds of children live in extended families. In contrast to the U.K., childcare for children under five years old is provided by the market or by kin. Three million jobs were lost in the first three months of lockdown, of which two million were held by women. Parents are starting to return to paid work, but many childcare providers are still closed and grandparents are likely to take on additional childcare despite the risks to elderly people who contract COVID, which are worse in South Africa due to the prevalence of diabetes in older women.

In conclusion, the intergenerational support provided by grandparents is significant in both countries although it is taken for granted. 'Older people as a burden and as recipients of care, coupled with a lack of value associated with unpaid caring work, engenders a "double invisibility".'[52] More thoughts on this later.

What of the frail elderly? Let's have a look at the Grannies who find themselves in long-term care (LTC) homes in Canada. According to *Hillnotes* of October 30, 2020 (updated with January 5, 2021 figures), these homes reported 11% of the total cases of COVID in Canada and 73% of the total deaths. While 71% of deaths occurred in people aged 80 and older, 97% occurred in people 60 and older.[53]

According to the 2016 Canadian census, of the 121,140 people over the age of 80 living in LTC, 73% were women. While men are generally more likely to die of COVID than women, 64.5% of the COVID cases in LTC in Ontario were women.[54] The situation in LTC has been horrific. By March 7, 2021, 15,597 LTC residents had died, a figure comprising 70% of Canada's total deaths due to COVID. Not surprisingly, when surveyed, 96% of seniors wanted to avoid living in a LTC facility.[55]

For months the LTC homes were shut down, which meant that family could not spend face-to-face time with their loved ones. Many LTC residents are there because they have some level of dementia and have issues associated with that. Imagine being one of these elderly folk, unable to see your loved ones, and perhaps getting ill with COVID and dying alone.

Can we unpack the situation a bit to examine what is going on that the lives of these women are respected so little that they are being allowed to die in droves? Who actually provides the care in the LTCs? The Royal Society of Canada, in a June 2020, report, noted that 'nurses are the primary regulated healthcare professionals... with physicians rarely on site.' Further, 'up to 90% of actual resident care is provided by unregulated and unlicensed care aides or personal support workers.'[56]

The report goes on to state that almost 90% of LTC care aides are women, of whom 70% are older than 40 years, and thus often Grannies themselves. Further, 60% have English as a second language, especially in urban areas where many are immigrants. Almost one-third of them work more than one job and '65% report having insufficient time to complete care tasks.'[57]

In Canada the situation of having Grannies caring for Grannies has resulted in a 'perfect storm.' Powerless residents who cannot look after themselves are cared for by employees who are pushed to their limits and not provided with adequate protection, remuneration or training. In Ontario, long-term care workers in independent/private long-term care facilities typically make $19:00 per hour, with those going through agencies for employment in facilities making $14:00 per hour.[58] In spite of the extra pay granted during COVID, this is little inducement for front-line employees to risk their lives.

In the past, these employees have often relied on unpaid family caregivers to provide support and care. When that unpaid support is withdrawn, because families are not allowed into the facility, the employees find themselves in an impossible situation and, without sick leave, they must struggle along trying to maintain stability in their own lives with insufficient resources. In some cases, the situation has been so horrific that staff have eventually not reported to work for various reasons including getting sick themselves, and the deaths of residents due to other more preventable causes than COVID, such as dehydration, have been the result.[59]

By May 2020, Canada was in the middle of OECD countries in terms of the number of COVID-19 deaths per million population, but not surprisingly, Canada did not compare well with other OECD countries in terms of COVID deaths in LTC compared with deaths in the community. LTC residents made up 81% of reported COVID deaths in Canada, compared with an average of 38% in other OECD countries.[60] Canada's mortality ratio comparing deaths in LTC to those in the community was 73.7 as compared with the OECD average of 25.5, by Fall 2020.[61]

So far, politicians have been full of nice words and promises but not so forthcoming with actual interventions to change the situation. Not only does Canada rank poorly, but it is apparently without shame or the political will to change.[62] Given the predominance of Grannies in the picture, there may well be some sexist and ageist holdover attitudes responsible for some of this. In any culture there are standards of behaviour that include the population saying 'we don't do this' to some acts. It would be nice if Canadians would adopt 'we don't kill our Grannies,' as a bit of a rallying cry. The latest wrinkle appears to be that with hospitals filled to the breaking point with COVID patients, governments have decided that some of the elderly who are in hospitals will be moved into the LTC facilities, which now, apparently, are less full than they once were. Hmmm.

Summing up, what we see, with the older generation stepping up, is a phenomenon where this generation is acting as a sort of cushion between the world and outright disaster. By contributing significantly to the pool of unpaid work to allow others to continue to adapt to new means of paid work, they allow families to continue to meet their needs. However, so long as they do not receive due economic recognition for their efforts, the true cost of COVID will never be known. Without data on the contribution of Grannies to COVID survival, we will never understand the full societal costs of the pandemic: nor will we have any sense of whether daughters and Grannies will be able to weather a next storm when the next pandemic hits.

COVID May Force Needed Change

We have had pandemics before, some of epic proportions. From the Black Death to smallpox, to polio to H1N1 to SARS, disease has had significant impacts on our species.[63] Strangely, in recent times, once the pandemic is over, the world has tended to forget, and has gone back to a slightly modified normal. In some cases, such as smallpox and polio, vaccines have led to the virtual eradication of the disease. In other cases, such as the plague, we continue to have recurrences, but we understand the disease and can treat it. Once the immediate threat has disappeared, so has society's interest in thinking about it any more. And so too has the political will to plan for the next pandemic, which we now know is inevitable.

There is historical research that argues the opposing view, for example: 'How three prior pandemics triggered massive societal shifts,'[64] argues that the Antonine and Cyprian plagues, which were most likely smallpox and which killed one-quarter to one-third of the population of the Roman Empire between A.D. 165 and 262, also helped the empire to change from pagan to Christian. The Christians who cared for the sick did better than the pagans who either fled or self-isolated. The Christians developed immunity and proselytized to dramatically increase their numbers.

The plague of Justinian killed up to half of the population of the Roman Empire in the two centuries of its recurrence from A.D. 542 to 755. At the time there were two other powers in the region, Sassanid Persia and the Islamic Rashidun Caliphate. The Caliphate, which was relatively unaffected by the outbreak, moved aggressively to conquer Sassanid Persia and strip

Rome of territory, leaving three major power centers: 'An Islamic one in the eastern and southern Mediterranean basin; a Greek one in the northeastern Mediterranean; and a European one between the western Mediterranean and the North Sea.'[65] In this last, so many slaves were killed that the landowners had to grant the remaining slaves plots of land in order to get the land worked, paving the way for feudalism.

In 1347, the Black Plague broke out in Europe, killing almost half of the 80 million population. Again, labour shortages triggered innovation with improvements to farming, and the development of printing and pumps for various applications. The wealthier peasants moved to cities and developed art and culture, demanding luxury goods only available through trade, and eventually becoming the 'middle class,' which in turn laid the foundation for the Renaissance.

With the COVID pandemic, it would be good if we could learn some more lessons, beyond how to Zoom, work remotely and shop online, and could bulletproof some of our systems and make plans against the day the next pandemic comes around. Significant gains could be made and held for equality of women if this were to occur. Grannies' contributions would be better understood, and dare I say, rewarded?

Of course, at this time there are a number of efforts underway locally, regionally, nationally, and globally to both support and encourage women, especially those in the workforce, and to continue to track women's progress. A mere smattering of these can be described here; they serve only as examples illustrating that the situation is not being ignored entirely. Most of these efforts were ongoing before the pandemic, but some have spawned specific lines of inquiry or specific thrusts related to the current situation.

In Canada, in March 2021, the Labour Market Information Council (LMI) issued *LMI Insight Report no. 39, Women in Recessions: What Makes COVID-19 Different?* Evidently, employment among women remains about 5.3% below where it sat in February 2020—just before the first wave of COVID-19—compared to a drop of about 3.7% for men. 'Most of the short-fall is attributable to losses in sectors like food services and accommodations, where workers deal directly with the public and have been hit hard by lockdowns and restrictions.'[66] Employment for women in low-earning occupations is now 14% below pre-crisis levels, while their counterparts in high-earning jobs have fully recovered. Economist Liz Betsis, one of the authors of the report said, 'Low-earning women were the most severely impacted in this recession of any other income group or any other gender, and to this day, they are the furthest away from recovery.'[67] In other words, there is a class dimension as well as the gender dimension to COVID impacts.

Politically, Canada's Liberal Government has publicly supported equality for women. Prime Minister Trudeau said in a media statement delivered

March 8, 2021, 'This crisis has created a she-cession and has threatened to roll back the hard-fought social and economic progress of all women… To build a fairer and more equal Canada, we must ensure a feminist, intersectional recovery from this crisis.' He announced the Formation of a Task Force on Women in the Economy.[68] This Task Force has a mandate:

> To advise the Deputy Prime Minister and Minister of Finance and the Minister of Middle Class Prosperity and Associate Minister of Finance, and Finance Canada ('the Parties') on policy actions to address the unique and dis-proportionate impacts on women caused by the COVID-19 recession. The Panel will also provide broader advice on advancing gender equality over the medium and longer term, consistent with the goals and policy intent of the *Canadian Gender Budgeting Act* and the Government's Gender Results Framework.[69]

The first meeting of the Task Force was held in early March 2021, with up to three follow-up meetings in March and April. Subsequent meetings will be held approximately every two months until the conclusion of the Panel's work in late 2021. As expected, the first outputs of this Task Force found their way into April's Canadian Federal Budget.

Chrystia Freeland, Canada's first woman Finance Minister, delivered that budget—the first Canadian budget in two years—on April 19, 2021. It was, as expected, full of measures to address COVID. There was emphasis both on elders and on childcare. Starting with an apology to seniors for the LTC debacle, the budget allocated $3 billion over five years toward improving the infrastructure of Canadian LTC systems, and announced the development of a National LTC Services Standard. Old Age Security will be increased for seniors over 75 by 10%, and they will also receive a one-time payment of $500.00 in August 2021. An Age Well at Home Initiative was announced to enable low-income Canadians to age in place. In addition, $50 million over five years was targeted to reducing elder abuse. Finally, the budget allocated support to strengthen data infrastructure and collection for health care.[70]

Also announced was a national plan to provide government subsidies to reduce the cost of child care. Childcare costs vary widely in Canada from Quebec, whose subsidized system costs about $181.00 per month, to big cities like Toronto and Vancouver, where the costs are over $1000.00 per month per child. The aim is to share the costs 50/50 between provincial and federal governments and to reduce the price to $10.00 per day by 2026.[71]

Meanwhile, in the U.S., Kamala Harris is the first woman Vice President. Her career has been focused on improving the situation of women in the U.S. In a recent interview with the newspaper *USA Today*, she stated that COVID has exposed the 'failures and fissures in our society.' She went on to point out that healthcare was being delivered with disparities, black mortality for COVID is higher than white, frontline workers especially in childcare and healthcare are not being treated well, and the working poor (mostly women) have to take public transportation, increasing their risks when they have no paid sick leave, and deal with child care issues, all this on about $15,000.00 a year. At the end of the interview, she spoke directly into the camera to women and said she wanted them to remember that, 'You are powerful, your voice is strong, and you are not alone.'[72]

Worldwide there has been increasing recognition of the gendered nature of the COVID pandemic. The United Nations has stepped up and has a number of groups and projects underway. The U.N. has a portfolio of $17.8 billion of sustainable development portfolios across its operation; these will be refocused on COVID, in addition to the Response and Recovery Trust Fund. There is a focus on education and training, and on providing economic support for the recovery as well as protection from violence. The program has support for women built in at every step, but is far too broad to discuss fully here.[73] Every international organization I looked at has a well-developed plan of some sort to address COVID-19 within their sphere of influence. Some of the specifics have been touched on throughout this essay.

What Lessons Can We Learn for the Future?

Looking behind the numbers, what do we see? Women are typically front-line workers dealing with customers or patients face-to-face. This means that they are vulnerable to catching COVID. Without the protection of adequate PPE, their risks are high. If they do catch COVID, they often do not have sick leave and thus have to leave or work while sick. This being said, the media has noticed women's plight and are telling the story. However, we seem to have forgotten Ruth Bader Ginsberg's declaration that 'Women belong in all places where decisions are being made.'

COVID has had a profound effect on women generally. Advances made in terms of equal pay for equal work, reproductive rights and social equality have been rolled back by the demands to keep moving to survive the pandemic. Attention has been focused on getting through the here and now, and not enough thought has been given to the human cost of rolling back the hard-won steps toward equality that women have achieved in the last decades.

The well-known Prussian philosopher Karl Marx has said, 'Anyone who knows anything of history knows that great social changes are impossible without feminine upheaval. Social progress can be measured exactly by the social position of the fair sex, the ugly ones included.'[74] My sense is that women are too tired at the moment to manage upheaval, but it might well be coming. As my rather superficial tour of COVID-19 and Grannies has shown, while we have been immersed in the here and now, there has so far been little synthesis of the available information, and little thought as to what to do next. As I hope I have demonstrated, there are a myriad of topics that emerge that beg for further study and research. Here are a few obvious ones:

- What impacts has COVID-19 had on the status of women in society and how has society coped to maintain advances that have been made (or not)?
- What are the characteristics of women's leadership that have made women-led countries cope with the pandemic better than male-led countries?
- What are the economic impacts of pressuring Grannies to step up to take on careers and childcare as never before?
- How has COVID-19 impacted the health and welfare of Grannies?

There are also a number of questions around LTC, including the need to move to greater professionalism such as registration for long-term care workers, the need for tighter standards of care, the need for a more stringent regulatory system for pandemic management, and on and on.

This short essay has raised the questions but cannot provide answers. One obvious area that needs immediate work is in the planning for future pandemics. Given that the impact of COVID-19 on women is worldwide in its scope, it is good to know that the United Nations has stepped up through a Gender and COVID-19 Working Group and Project, recognizing that the pandemic hits some people harder than others and that effective responses need to be fact-based. As is customary for these projects, the need for better planning before, during and after pandemics is emphasized in their report, *How to Create a Gender Responsive Pandemic Plan* where 'A gender-responsive pandemic plan focuses on the intersectional needs of women, men, and gender minorities, in planning, data collection, response and recovery.'[75] I found it a good start for considering planning for the next pandemic, based on what we have learned from this one.

In summary, the U.N. report emphasizes that after one pandemic and before the next, lessons learned from the pandemic must be integrated into policies and planning. Data needs to be collected, assembled and analyzed and the results fed back into the process. Knowing that violence against women and children will increase, specific plans are needed to ensure that necessary support services are in place to help abused women and their children. The traditional roles of women and their potential negative impacts can be made visible so that responses are considered. If schools close, it is often women who stay home to look after children. Hence, such closures can have a disproportionate effect on women's livelihoods. Communication efforts to highlight equitable distribution of caregiving and household responsibilities may encourage consideration of other options. For instance, employers can be encouraged to adopt measures that encourage gender equity, such as paternity leave.

Response to the arrival of any new pandemic must be flexible, but can be based on the data collected and the pandemic planning that has already been done. Governments with an updated pandemic plan will be able to act on it in a reasonable and effective way, while those lacking one will need to step back to collect the necessary data and do the analyses on which to base their next steps. They will need to know the priorities, risk, capacities and resources available to them. In both cases, ongoing assessments will be required to monitor outcomes and progress. Policies need to be in place to address a range of health-and safety-related issues, such as ensuring an adequate and equitable supply of personal protective equipment (PPE) for healthcare workers. Other issues needing to be addressed, both for healthcare workers and for others, include the need for safe, affordable quality child and elder care services and for increased access to financial support (e.g., unemployment benefits, maternity protection, paid sick leave, access to insurance).

As the pandemic comes under control, it will be necessary to:

> Support return to work programs that purposefully plan for gender equity (i.e., targeted stimulus activities, trainings, credit, etc.) and target displaced workers, as well as historically marginalized women (i.e., indigenous women, sex workers, women with disabilities, etc.) [and that] continue to provide emergency cash transfers to assist those whose livelihoods have been affected by the pandemic, using systems that allow women direct access to the funds.[76]

These measures are mostly straightforward and quite clear. I wonder why they are not in place already. This is not our first pandemic. The impacts of COVID on our society are pervasive and surely everyone is aware of them.

That being said, women have their own perspectives and need to be much more involved with pandemic planning. As previously mentioned, I fear that as the bitter memory of previous pandemics passes away, the impetus to act also fades. As Margaret Thatcher said, 'If you want something said, ask a man; if you want something done, ask a woman.'[77] In the next cycle, given that women will continue to be in the frontlines, it will be important to engage them in planning in a way that has not been done before.

It does occur to me that the Grannies of our society are perhaps providing a function during these times that they have always provided, but which is much more important today. By being old and frail and in need of care, some of them have acted like the 'canaries in the coal mine' and provided us with an indicator of failures in some of our societal systems. Some, not quite so old and frail, have stepped in to cover off unpaid work, which is typically done by women and generally underappreciated by society. While this has had the great benefit of allowing younger women to keep their jobs and children to be well looked after and home schooled, it has tended to push the pandemic's true economic burden under the rug. And as for slightly younger women, who have been called back into the medical profession in droves, whether as nurses in the ICUs or long-term care providers, their contribution has often been what has allowed systems to continue to function. They bear the stress of knowing that if they get sick and cannot work, not only will their families suffer, but the whole healthcare system may begin to crumble. Their mothers at home trying to hold the family together are often the unsung heroines in the whole story.

When the pandemic is over, life will return to what will quite likely be some sort of new normal. From my position as a grandmother myself, I hope that Grannies across the world will, after having their hair done and their nails manicured, have the energy left to stand up and cheer and take a bow for the contributions that they have made. I also hope that they have the energy to make sure that pandemic planning of the future includes the ways and means to respect and reward their contributions and those of their daughters and granddaughters.

Elizabeth Cady Stanton once said, 'I would have girls regard themselves not as adjectives but as nouns.'[78] In general, grandmothers see their daughters, daughters-in-law and grandchildren as 'nouns.' They understand the importance of who they are and what they represent in the continuity of the human species. If I were to be granted one wish, I would wish the men in power would find the energy and inspiration to see more women as 'nouns' and to include grandmothers in their planning for pandemics. It would also be helpful if economists took a more serious and balanced view of the value of unpaid work in the context of recognizing 'nouns.' We would all be better off if they did.

Notes

[1] I was reminded of many of these examples by 'Celebrating Women Leaders' in the *Washington Post* of March 25, 2021, where many examples of outstanding women's success stories were provided.

[2] Goodreads, Accessed May 4, 2021 at:
https://www.goodreads.com/author/quotes/733319.Bella_Abzug

[3] Taub, Amanda, 'Why are Women-Led Nations doing Better with COVID-19?' *New York Times*, May 15, 2020, updated August 13, 2020.

[4] Stone, Deborah, *Policy Paradox: The Art of Political Decision Making*, ISBN: 978-0-393-91272-2, 1988: 130.

[5] Evans, Pete, 'Canada added 378,000 jobs in September, even more than in August,' *CBC News*, October 9, 2020.

[6] Kashen, Julie, Sarah Jane Glynn and Amanda Novello, 'How COVID-19 Sent Women's Workforce Progress Backward', *Center for American Progress*. October 30, 2020.

[7] U.S. Bureau of Labor Statistics, 'Civilian Labor Force Participation Rate', Accessed May 4, 2021 at: https://www.bls.gov/charts/employment-situation/civilian-labor-force-participation-rate.htm

[8] Madgavkar, Anu, Olivia White, Mekala Krishnan, Deepa Mahajan and Xavier Azcue, 'COVID-19 and gender equality: Countering the regressive effects,' *McKinsey & Company*, July 15, 2020.

[9] Desjardins, Dawn and Carrie Freestone, 'Canadian Women Continue to Exit the Workforce,' *RBC Economics*, November 19, 2020.

[10] Desjardins, Dawn *et al,* 2020.

[11] Desjardins, Dawn *et al,* 2020.

[12] Madgavkar, Anu *et al,* 2020.

[13] Armstrong, Pat, Katherine Laxer and Hugh Armstrong, 'Gender and Work Database,' *Conceptual Guide to the Health Care Module*.

[14] 'COVID-19: Emerging gender data and why it matters', *UN Women*, June 26, 2020.

[15] 'UN Secretary-General's Policy Brief: The Impact of COVID-19 on Women', *UN Women*, 2020, 21 pp.

[16] Edwards, Erika, 'Kids at day care spread COVID-19 to parents and teachers, CDC says,' *NBC News*, September 11, 2020.

[17] Breen, Kerry B, 'Child care programs not associated with COVID-19 spread, large study finds,' *Today*, October 14, 2020.

[18] Breen, Kerry B., 2020.

[19] Preidt, Robert, 'Very Low COVID Transmission in Day Care Centers,' *U.S. News*, February 9, 2021.

[20] Public Health Ontario, *Rapid Review, COVID-19 Pandemic School Closure and Reopening Impacts*, July 27, 2020.

[21] Public Health Ontario, 2020.

[22] The World Bank, 'Data.' Accessed May 21, 2021 at: https://data.worldbank.org/indicator/SE.PRM.TCHR.FE.ZS?locations=US

[23] Schraer, Rachel, 'COVID: Teacher's Risk Similar to other Under-65s,' *BBC News*, March 1, 2021.

[24] Barnum, Matt, 'COVID Cases Among Teachers Appear to be Rising. What does that Mean?' *Chalkbeat*, January 12, 2021.

[25] 'E-News: K-12 Employee Job Satisfaction Plummets,' *Centre for State and Local Government Excellence Newsletter*, February 26, 2021.

[26] Bailey, John P. and Jessica Schurz, 'COVID-19 is Creating a School Personnel Crisis,' *American Enterprise Institute*, May, 2020.

[27] Hanushek, Eric A. and Ludger Woessmann, 'The Economic Impacts of Learning Loss,' *OECD*, September, 2020.

[28] 'Simulating the Potential Impacts of the COVID-19 School Closures on Schooling and Learning Outcomes: A Set of Global Estimates,' *The World Bank*, June 18, 2020.

[29] Goodreads, Charlotte Whitton quote. Accessed May 6, 2021 at: https://www.goodreads.com/quotes/434779-whatever-women-do-they-must-do-twice-as-well-as

[30] 'Whose time to care? Unpaid care and domestic work during COVID-19,' *UN Women, Brief: Gender and COVID-19,* November 25, 2020.

[31] *World Health Organization News,* March 9, 2021.

[32] 'Impact of COVID-19 on violence against women and girls,' *UN Brochure.*

[33] Thompson, Nicole, 'Reports of domestic, intimate partner violence continue to rise during pandemic,' *CBC News,* February 15, 2021.

[34] Pablo, Calito, 'Police Agencies report increase in domestic disturbance calls during height of Canada's COVID-19 lockdown,' *The Georgia Straight,* September 1, 2020.

[35] 'The Shadow Pandemic: Violence against women during COVID-19', *UN Women.*

[36] Yalcinalp, Esra, 'Turkey Ergodan: Women rise up over withdrawal from Istanbul Convention', *BBC Turkish,* March 26, 2021.

[37] Lewis, Helen, 'The Pandemic has given Women a New Kind of Rage', *The Atlantic,* March 10, 2021.

[38] Rapporteur: Francis Fitzgerald, 'On the gender perspective in the COVID-19 crisis and post-crisis period,' (2020/2121(INI)), Committee on Women's Rights and Gender Equality.

[39] Caspari, Rachel, 'The Evolution of Grandparents,' *Scientific American,* November 1, 2012.

[40] Caspari, 2012.

[41] United Nations Department of Economic and Social Affairs (DESA), November 16, 2019. Accessed May 27, 2021 at: https://www.facebook.com/joinundesa/posts/703-million-people-in-the-world-today-are-aged-65-or-older-by-2050-or-just-31-ye/2524995167589688/

[42] *Policy Brief: The impact of COVID-19 on women,* April 9, 2020. Accessed May 14, 2021 at: https://www.un.org/sexualviolenceinconflict/wpcontent/uploads/2020/06/report/policy-brief-the-impact-of-covid-19-on-women/policy-brief-the-impact-of-covid-19-on-women-en-1.pdf/

[43] Gidick, Kinsey, 'Grandparents Play Starring Role in Multigenerational Home Life,' *AARP,* July 23, 2020.

[44] Taylor, Paul, Jeffery Passel, Richard Fry, Richard Morin, Wendy Wang, Gabriel Velasco and Daniel Dockerman, 'The return of the multi-generational family household,' Pew Research Center, March 18, 2010.

[45] Armstrong, Pat, 2015.

[46] '5 Facts about American grandparents,' Pew Research Center, *Factank,* 2015.

[47] *op. cit.*

[48] Coall, David A., Sonja Hilbrand, Rebecca Sear and Ralph Hertwig (2018): 'Interdisciplinary perspectives on grandparental investment: a journey towards causality,' *Contemporary Social Science,* DOI: 10.1080/21582041.2018.1433317.

[49] Kanji, S., 'Grandparent Care: A Key Factor in Mothers' Labour Force Participation in the U.K.,' *Journal of Social Policy,* 47 (3): 523-42.

[50] Cantillon, Sara, Elena Moore and NinaTeasdale, 'COVID-19 and the Pivotal role of Grandparents: Childcare and Income Support in the U.K. and South Africa,' *Feminist Economics*, 27:1-2, 188-202, DOI: 10,1080/13545701.2020.1860246.

[51] Mccarron, Emily, 'COVID-19: the impact on the human rights of older people,' *AGE UK*, May, 2020.

[52] Cantillon *et al*, 2020.

[53] Loprespub, 'Long-Term Care Homes in Canada – the Impact of COVID-19,' *Hillnotes*, October 30, 2020.

[54] Loprespub, 2020.

[55] Taylor, Brooke, '"It's a disaster." Trust in long-term care at an all time low.' *CBC News*, March 8, 2021.

[56] Estabrooks, Carol, Colleen M. Flood, and Sharon Straus, 'We must act now to prevent a second wave of long-term care deaths,' *RSC COVID-19 Series, Publication #20*, 2020

[57] *op. cit.*

[58] On, Avtar, 'Ultimate Guide to PSW Salary in Ontario.' Accessed August 3, 2021 at: https://personalsupportworkerhq.com/psw-salary/

[59] Howlett, Karen, 'Patients died from neglect, not COVID-19, in LTC homes military report finds: "All they needed was water and a wipe down",' *The Globe and Mail*, May 11, 2021.

[60] Canadian Institute for Health Information, 'Pandemic Experience in the Long-Term Care Sector: How Does Canada Compare with Other Countries?' Ottawa, ON, CIHI, 2020.

[61] Sepulveda, Edgardo R., Nathan M. Stall and Samir K. Sinha, 'A Comparison of COVID-19 Mortality Rates Among Long-Term Care Residents in 12 OECD Countries,' *J. Am Med Dir Assoc.* 2020 Nov; 21(11): 1572–1574.e3. Published online September 12, 2020.

[62] Hoffman, Elizabeth, Jeanette Grant, and Ann McMillan, 'Lessons from History,' this almanac.

[63] Latham, Andrew, 'How three prior pandemics triggered massive societal shifts,' *PBS News Hour*, October 1, 2020.

[64] 'Women in Recessions: What Makes COVID-19 Different?' *LMI Insight Report no. 39*, March, 2021.

[65] Sepulveda *et al*, 2020.

[66] Alhmidi, Maan, 'Rolling back progress for women should not be COVID-19's legacy: Trudeau,' *Toronto Star*, March 8, 2021.

[67] Canadian Gender Budgeting Act, S.C. 2018. Accessed May 15, 2021 at: https://laws-lois.justice.gc.ca/eng/acts/C-17.2/FullText.

[68] Miller, Audrey, 'Federal Budget 2021 Highlights summarized by National Institute on Aging.'

[69] Tait, Melissa, 'Ottawa promised $10-a-day child care in the 2021federal budget. How would that work? A guide,' *The Globe and Mail*, April 21, 2021.

[70] Hackney, Suzette and Nicole Carolle, '"You are strong." Vice President Kamala Harris has a Message for American Women,' *USA Today*.

[71] 'United Nations COVID-19 Response.' Accessed June 1, 2021 at: https://www.un.org/en/coronavirus/search?query=COVID+response+for+women

[72] 'Powerful Quotes that prove only Women can save our Planet.' Accessed May 17, 2021 at: https://medium.com/project-2030/21-powerful-quotes-that-prove-only-women-can-save-our-planet-2b97d117a0fe

[73] Rosser, E.N., R. Morgan, H. Tan, K. Hawkins, A. Ngunjiri, A. Oyekunle, B. Schall, D. Nacif Pimenta, E. Tamaki, M. Rochaand and C. Wenham. (2021), 'How to Create a Gender-Responsive Pandemic Plan: Addressing the Secondary Effects of COVID-19.' *Gender and COVID-19 Project.*

[74] *op. cit.*

[75] '60 Empowering Feminist Quotes from Inspiring Women,' *Harper's Bazaar*, February 28, 2020.

[76] Jagannathan, Meera, '14 Early Feminist Quotes that still Resonate Today,' RD.com

Politics and COVID I:
Some Thoughts on Interstate Variations
in COVID rates in the U.S.
Jon Peirce

Introduction

Other things equal, one would expect rates of a highly infectious disease such as COVID to be higher in more densely populated jurisdictions. Again, other things being equal, one would expect jurisdictions of higher population density to feature more crowded housing arrangements, including a greater number of multi-generational families living together, which means an increased likelihood of contracting or transmitting the disease even among people strictly complying with all government protocols around COVID. One would also expect such jurisdictions to have more crowded streets, stores, and public facilities, leading to greater difficulty in maintaining adequate social distancing and an increased number of opportunities to contract the disease, even out of doors.

The U.S. experience with COVID to date does not in any way bear out this preliminary hypothesis. As we shall soon see, the relationship between population density and COVID is closer to being one of inverse than of direct correlation. While some of the least densely populated states rank at or near the top in per capita COVID rates, some of the most densely populated states rank at or near the bottom. In what follows, we shall examine the relationship more closely, with an eye to offering some tentative explanations for the seemingly counter-intuitive phenomenon. The paper closes with some suggestions for further research.

The Historical Context

If, one year ago, anyone had suggested that the two Dakotas would have the highest COVID rates of any states in the U.S. in a year's time, or that other 'Top 10' COVID states would include Iowa and Utah, or that the 'Bottom 10' COVID states would include Washington (an early epicentre for the disease), Michigan, Maryland, and the District of Columbia,[1] I suspect that that person's family and friends would have taken them aside and suggested the advisability of immediate psychiatric intervention. Certainly, the data from the pandemic's first wave (from March through June of 2020) suggested nothing of the sort. For a considerable period of time during that first wave,

New York state, driven by exceptionally high case numbers and numbers of deaths in New York City, far outstripped all other states. For example, as of May 1, New York state accounted for about 27.5% of the country's 1.1 million cases and 29% of its 63,000+ COVID fatalities,[2] despite accounting for slightly less than 6% of the country's population. For its part, Massachusetts was accounting for about 5.6% of the nation's cases and 6.6% of its COVID fatalities, despite having just 2.1% of the country's population.[3] While many (including the present writer) were shocked by the exceptionally high case and fatality figures for New York state and New York City, the overall pattern of high case incidence and fatality rates in urban areas and (at the time) far lower case incidence and fatality rates in less-populated rural areas was in line with what one might have expected. Today, as the left-hand column of Table 1 shows, both New York and Massachusetts rank *below* the national average in per capita COVID rates, while the per capita rates in the two Dakotas are roughly half again greater than those in New York and Massachusetts!

What happened between last spring and the present to bring about such dramatic changes in different states' COVID rates? Quite a lot, as it turns out. The pandemic's first wave, during which most U.S. states (and Canadian provinces as well) behaved more or less as predicted with regard to their case rates, generally subsided, to be succeeded early in the fall by a second wave which would be handled quite differently by state governors of varying political stripe and varying degrees of belief in science and its role in controlling the pandemic. There was a bitter Presidential election campaign, in which the incumbent Donald Trump's handling of the pandemic and insistence on holding live, large-scale rallies, in contrast to the primarily virtual rallies held by his Democratic opponent, Joe Biden, would themselves become major issues. The campaign would result in Biden's defeating Trump. Later, after an equally bitter campaign featuring two tense, testy run-off elections in Georgia, the Democrats would regain control of the Senate, giving them control of the White House and both houses of Congress for the first time since 2010. And finally, during the last quarter of the pandemic's first year, a vaccine against COVID-19 was launched and began to be widely distributed before the end of 2020.

An eventful year, indeed. But we are getting a hit ahead of ourselves here. Before we can comment in any detail on these events and their connection to COVID, let's go back to the preliminary hypothesis with which this paper began, with an eye to considering why, despite its commonsense appeal, it has fallen so far short of explaining interstate variations in COVID case rates in the U.S.

COVID Rates and Population Density

Table 1 (next two pages) offers a quick but nonetheless reasonably detailed snapshot of data which could potentially be related to the states' differing COVID performances. In addition to per capita COVID rates themselves (see the table's left-hand column, in which these rates are rank-ordered in descending order), the data include the states' population densities per square mile (see right-hand column), and as political indicators, the percentage of each state's popular vote earned by Donald Trump in the 2020 Presidential election, and the party of the governor in charge of each state as of the beginning of 2021. We shall be explaining the significance of these two latter indicators shortly.

Even a cursory glance at the right-hand (population density) column suffices to tell us that population density does not in any way explain states' differing per capita COVID rates. Of the 10 states with the highest COVID rates, only one (Rhode Island) ranks in the top 10 or even top 20 in population density, while only three (Wisconsin and Tennessee in addition to Rhode Island) rank in the top half (top 25) with regard to this indicator, and only four of the 20 most densely populated states (South Carolina, Indiana, and Georgia in addition to Rhode Island) rank in the top 20 in their COVID rates.

At the same time, three of the 10 states with the highest COVID rates, including the two highest (North and South Dakota), rank in the *bottom* 10 in population density, while seven of the 10 hardest-hit COVID states rank in the bottom 20 in population density. These states include Utah, Arizona, Oklahoma, Iowa, and Arkansas, in addition to the two Dakotas. Similarly, eight of the 10 *least* densely populated states are in the top 20 with regard to their COVID rates, while another (Montana) is in the top 25. The only one of the 10 least densely populated states which does not rank in the top half in its COVID rates is Alaska, which is by far the country's least densely populated state. While this one finding appears to suggest a possible direct relationship between low population density and low COVID rates, even it must be hedged with certain qualifications, as we shall see later on. And at most, Alaska is but one state. Overall, it is beginning to look as if we are closer to an inverse than to a direct correlation between population density and COVID rates.

A similar pattern of apparent inverse relationship emerges from our examination of the states with the country's lowest per capita COVID rates. Of the 10 states[4] with the lowest COVID rates, two, including the country's most densely populated one, D.C., are in the top 10 in population density, while five are in the top 20 with regard to this indicator, and six are in the top 25. This last group of states includes, in addition to D.C., Maryland (#6), Hawaii (#14), Virginia (#15), Michigan (#18), and New Hampshire (#22).

185

When we expand our selection to the 20 states with the lowest COVID rates, we find that six, these being Massachusetts (#4), Connecticut (#5), Maryland (#6), New York (#8), and Pennsylvania (#10), in addition to D.C., rank in the top 10 in population density, while another five, among them Ohio (#11), Hawaii, Virginia, North Carolina (#16), and Michigan, rank in the top 20, and 12 (all of the aforementioned plus New Hampshire) rank in the top 25.

Does this mean that we should simply assume that COVID rates will be highest in the least densely-populated jurisdictions? No—not really. We are not quite ready to stand common sense on its head to that extent. What it does mean is that we need to look for other variables which may help explain the seemingly counterintuitive phenomena we have just observed. This is where the table's political variables come in.

State	COVID Rates as % of population	% of popular vote for Trump (rank)	Governor, by party*	Population density, people/ sq/m (rank)
North Dakota	13.20% (1)	65.11% (4)	R	10.5 (48)
South Dakota	12.88% (2)	61.77% (9)	R	11.1 (47)
Rhode Island	*12.23% (3)*	*38.61% (44)*	*D*	*1017.1 (3)*
Utah	11.74% (4)	58.13% (13)	R	35.3 (42)
Tennessee	11.52% (5)	60.66% (10)	R	157.5 (21)
Arizona	*11.38% (6)*	*49.06% (27)*	*R*	*58.3 (34)*
Oklahoma	10.87% (7)	65.37% (3)	R	56.1 (36)
Iowa	10.81% (8)	53.09% (21)	R	55.3 (37)
Arkansas	10.79% (9)	62.40% (6)	R	56.9 (35)
Wisconsin	*10.70% (10)*	*48.82% (29)*	*D*	*106.0 (25)*
Nebraska	10.53% (11)	58.22% (12)	R	24.3 (44)
South Carolina	10.26% (12)	55.11% (19)	R	138.8 (20)
Alabama	10.23% (13)	62.03% (8)	R	95.4 (28)
Kansas	10.20% (14)	56.21% (18)	D	35.4 (41)
Mississippi	10.03% (15)	57.60% (14)	R	63.7 (33)
Indiana	9.94% (16)	57.02% (15)	R	183.4 (17)
Idaho	9.73% (17)	63.84% (5)	R	19.5 (45)
Georgia	*9.69% (18)*	*49.24% (26)*	*R*	*173.7 (19)*
Nevada	*9.65% (19)*	*47.67% (31)*	*D*	*25.4 (43)*
Wyoming	9.50% (20)	69.94% (1)	R	6.0 (50)
Illinois	*9.49% (21)*	*40.55% (39)*	*D*	*232.0 (13)*
Montana	9.46% (22)	56.92% (16)	R	7.0 (49)
Louisiana	9.37% (23)	58.46% (11)	D	107.1 (24)
Texas	9.29% (24)	52.06% (23)	R	101.2 (27)
New Jersey	*9.26% (25)*	*41.40% (38)*	*D*	*1218.1 (2)*
Kentucky	9.22% (26)	62.09% (7)	D	111.3 (23)
Missouri	9.18% (27)	56.80% (17)	R	87.9 (29)
Delaware	*9.13% (28)*	*39.77% (41)*	*D*	*475.1 (7)*

Table 1, part 1: Population Density and COVID Case Rates by Population vs. Popular Vote Support for Donald Trump, 2020 U.S. Presidential Election, U.S. States and U.S. as a whole, and Governor by Party as of January 1, 2021.

Florida	9.11% (29)	51.22% (24)	R	364.6 (9)
New Mexico	*8.93% (30)*	*43.50% (36)*	*D*	*17.2 (46)*
California	*8.89% (31)*	*34.32% (46)*	*D*	*246.1 (12)*
UNITED STATES	*8.79%*	*46.86%*	*D (President)*	*89.5*
Minnesota	*8.74% (+32)*	*45.28% (33)*	*D*	*68.1 (31)*
New York	*8.74% (-33)*	*37.75% (45)*	*D*	*417.0 (8)*
Massachusetts	*8.64% (34)*	*32.14% (49)*	*R-NP*	*858.0 (4)*
Ohio	8.41% (35)	53.27% (20)	R	283.2 (11)
North Carolina	*8.37% (36)*	*49.93% (25)*	*D*	*202.6 (16)*
Alaska	8.10% (37)	52.83% (22)	R	1.3 (51)
Connecticut	*8.10% (38)*	*39.19% (42)*	*D*	*742.6 (5)*
Colorado	*7.61% (39)*	*41.90% (37)*	*D*	*50.8 (38)*
West Virginia	7.49% (40)	68.62% (2)	R	77.1 (30)
Pennsylvania	*7.47% (41)*	*48.84% (28)*	*D*	*285.5 (10)*
Virginia	*6.91% (42)*	*44.00% (35)*	*D*	*209.2 (15)*
Michigan	*6.63% (43)*	*47.84% (30)*	*D*	*175.0 (18)*
Maryland	*6.44% (44)*	*32.15% (48)*	*R-NP*	*610.8 (6)*
District of Columbia	*5.95% (45)*	*5.40% (51)*	*N/A*	*11,686.0 (1)*
New Hampshire	5.70% (46)	45.36% (32)	R	147.8 (22)
Washington	*4.55% (47)*	*38.77% (43)*	*D*	*104.0 (26)*
Oregon	*3.75% (48)*	*40.37% (40)*	*D*	*40.9 (40)*
Maine	*3.44% (49)*	*44.02% (34)*	*D*	*43.1 (39)*
Vermont	*2.62% (50)*	*30.67% (50)*	*R-NP*	*68.0 (32)*
Hawaii	*1.98% (51)*	*34.27% (47)*	*D*	*218.6 (14)*
UNITED STATES	*8.79%*	*46.86%*	*D (President)*	*89.5*

Table 1, part 2: Population Density and COVID Case Rates by Population vs. Popular Vote Support for Donald Trump, 2020 U.S. Presidential Election, U.S. States and U.S. as a whole, and Governor by Party as of January 1, 2021.

Note
Jurisdictions that voted for Trump are in plain boldface; jurisdictions (including the U.S. as a whole) that voted for Biden are in boldface italics.

Sources
> For population density data, *Wikipedia.*
> For COVID case data, Johns Hopkins University website, data as of March 10, 2021.
> For U.S. Presidential election results, *Wikipedia* article on U.S. Presidential election of 2020.
> For Governors, *Wikipedia,* list of U.S. governors as of January, 2021.

Jon Peirce

Partisan Politics and COVID Rates
Support for Donald Trump

Unlike population density, support for Donald Trump *does* appear to be related to a state's COVID rates. If we look at Table 1's two left columns, we will see that of the states with the top 10 COVID rates, seven of them supported Trump in last Fall's election. Six of those 10 supported Trump by a wide margin (more than 15%), and five of them (Oklahoma, #3, North Dakota, #4, Arkansas, #6, South Dakota, #9, and Tennessee, #10) also ranked among the top 10 in their Trump percentages, all with more than 60% support for the ex-President. Another, Utah, ranked well within the top 20. Of the three top 10 COVID states that supported Biden (Rhode Island, Arizona, and Wisconsin), two (Arizona and Wisconsin) did so by narrow margins; one (Arizona) is an historically Republican state with a Republican governor, whose entry into the Democratic column in November was regarded as something of an upset victory for the Democrats. The only strongly Democratic state in the top 10 COVID states is Rhode Island, the nation's third most densely populated state behind D.C. and New Jersey. Why Rhode Island should have experienced such high COVID rates when neighbouring New England states such as Connecticut and Massachusetts, also densely populated, did not may bear some explanation. Some possible causes have been offered by Dr Megan Ramney, a Brown University professor and an emergency physician at various hospitals in Rhode Island, who was quoted extensively in a December 9, 2020 article in the *Providence Journal*.[5] These include a very high rate of testing, the state's high per capita proportion of college students, relatively lax lockdown provisions including late closure of indoor activities and allowing restaurants to remain open for indoor dining even as the pandemic raged, and the fact that 'We [have] lots of multi-family and multi-generational homes. . . [which] leads to fast spread, simply because people can't distance from each other. [And] we are a very tight-knit state. . . Family is everything.' Two-thirds of RIers never move out of the state. And we know that our much-treasured family gatherings are often superspreader events.'[6]

While many of the above factors, such as the high population density, large numbers of students, and large numbers of multi-family and multi-generational homes might also have applied in comparable states such as Connecticut and Massachusetts, state officials' lax lockdown regulations and allowing restaurants to remain open may not have applied in those other states. This is an issue which bears further examination, though there is not space to provide such an examination here.

In any event, a single state does not make a trend. In this group of top 10 COVID states, Rhode Island is clearly an outlier—and the one state that has behaved as our initial hypothesis might have predicted.

Turning to the top 20 states with the highest COVID rates, we see that 15 of them supported Trump last November. Of the five top 20 states that did not, four supported Biden by narrow margins; indeed, all four (including Georgia and Nevada as well as Wisconsin and Arizona) were among the most hotly contested, drawing numerous heated challenges of the vote count and even attempts to overturn that vote count from the Trump camp. It is also worth noting that two of those four hotly contested states that ultimately went for Biden (Arizona and Georgia) had Republican governors and were historically Republican states. Notably, Rhode Island is the only one of the top 20 COVID states that voted for Biden by a margin of more than 10%. Our group of top 20 COVID states includes seven of the top 10 Trump states, among them Wyoming, whose 69.9% Trump support was highest of any state in the country. Fourteen of the top 20 COVID states ranked among the top 20 states in Trump support, while a fifteenth (Iowa) was 21st. Nor did Trump win these top 20 COVID states by narrow margins. In all 20, his margin was 10% or greater, his weakest showing in this group being in South Carolina, which gave him 55.1% of its vote. The pattern is starting to look increasingly clear.

A similar story emerges when we look at the bottom end of the COVID spectrum, with the results almost a mirror image of those at the top end. If anything, the relationship between COVID rates and support for Trump is almost stronger at this bottom end of the COVID spectrum than at the top. All 10 of the states with the lowest COVID rates supported Biden in the Presidential election, most by wide margins. In only two of those 10 states (Michigan and New Hampshire) was the race relatively close. Five of the 10 (D.C., Vermont, Maryland, Hawaii and Washington) were also in the top five in percentage of Biden support (and thus lowest percentage of Trump support). Expanding our examination to the 20 states with the lowest COVID rates, we see that 16 of the 20 supported Biden; three of the remaining four (Alaska, Ohio, and North Carolina) supported Trump by relatively narrow margins, with North Carolina, at less than 50% Trump support, a real 'cliff-hanger' whose result was not finally determined until some time after the election. Among the bottom 20 COVID states, only West Virginia, whose 68.6% support for Trump was second only to Wyoming, could be said to have been a solidly pro-Trump state.

In the group of low COVID states, West Virginia is an outlier just as Rhode Island is an outlier in the group of high COVID states. The state's strong COVID performance is particularly surprising in view of its population's high average age and numerous co-morbidities, including smoking and work-related lung diseases. The state's average life expectancy is among the lowest in the entire country. But a variety of particular local circumstances, including a close-knit culture and strong advance planning, appear, in the case of COVID, to have been more significant than the poor overall health of the state's citizenry as well as the more macro-level political factors we have been talking about here.[7]

As interesting and inspiring as West Virginia's example is, however, it must be noted that like Rhode Island in the opposite direction, it is just one state—the exception that helps to prove the broader rule. In its advance planning and careful coordination of its COVID response, it did not in any way operate like a state that gave Donald Trump over two-thirds of its vote. In particular, it stands in the starkest contrast to the two Dakotas, strong Trump-supporting states which lead the nation in their COVID rates.[8]

Democratic vs. Republican Governors

The other political variable of interest for our current study is the party of the governors in power in the different states. As will be explained in more detail later, the party of the governor in power is important in any examination of COVID and politics because, in the American federal system, it is the governors rather than the President of the U.S. who are actually responsible for setting and carrying out COVID-related policies in their respective states.

Turning again to Table 1, we see that the second column from the right lists the parties of the governors in power as of the end of 2020. Overall, the relationship between partisan political support and COVID rates appears pretty much the same for governors as it was for President. The states with higher COVID rates generally have Republican governors; those with lower COVID rates typically have Democratic or non-partisan (anti-Trump) Republican governors. Eight of the top 10 COVID states and 16 of the top 20 (all but Rhode Island, Wisconsin, Kansas, and Nevada) had Republican governors as of the end of 2020. We have already spoken of Rhode Island as an outlier in this group of states with high COVID rates. Kansas must also be regarded as something of an outlier. In connection with Kansas, we should note that it is historically a solidly Republican state, which in the 2020 presidential election gave Trump over 56% of its vote. Its Democratic governor, Laura Kelly, was elected in 2018 under most unusual circumstances—circumstances which cannot really be said to indicate a significant overall change in the state's political culture.[9]

Again, if we turn to the states with the lowest COVID rates, the pattern with governors is basically the same as it was in the Presidential election. By and large, the states with the lowest COVID rates are most likely to have Democratic governors. Of the nine of the bottom 10 COVID states that have governors of any political stripe,[10] six have Republican governors, and two (Vermont and Maryland) have what I have described as non-partisan Republican governors who have not supported Trump and have for the most part handled the pandemic in the same way as their Democratic counterparts.

It is worth noting that the two non-partisan governors noted above, Phil Scott of Vermont and Lawrence Hogan of Maryland, as well as the third non-partisan Republican governor, Charlie Baker of Massachusetts, all govern states ranking among the most heavily Democratic in the country in Presidential elections. It is highly unlikely that any pro-Trump Republican could be elected from states such as these, none of which gave Trump as much as one-third of their vote in last Fall's election. Expanding to the bottom 20 COVID states, the pattern of primarily Democratic or non-partisan Republican governors continues. Of the 19 of these states that have governors, 12 are Democrats and three, non-partisan Republicans, leaving only four (Alaska, Ohio, West Virginia, and New Hampshire) with regular Republican governors. And New Hampshire, despite having a Republican governor, voted for the Democratic nominee (Biden) in the presidential election in 2020, as it has in every presidential election since 2004. It cannot by any stretch be considered a solidly Republican state; it would more accurately be characterized as a battleground or swing state.[11] In addition, New Hampshire borders both Maine and Vermont, two of the states with the lowest COVID rates in the country, a fact which may have had something to do with its own relatively low rates of the disease.

Discussion:
How Political Variables Play Out in Practice
1) President
a) Coordinating National Strategy
How would a President's political ideology affect COVID rates, whether at the national or state level? It may be useful to start this discussion by noting that the President has two critical roles to play in the fight against a pandemic disease such as COVID. First, it is the President's job to coordinate overall strategy against the disease. Second, it is the President's job to set a tone which will—as much through his or her example as in any other way—encourage ordinary citizens to follow regulations and otherwise do their part in bringing the disease under control.

Trump's coordination efforts, overall, must be deemed to have been spotty at best. During the pandemic's first months, he was extremely reluctant to invoke the Defense Production Act (DPA), arguably the strongest tool available to a President in such a situation, suggesting that to do so in order to speed up production of desperately-needed personal protective equipment (PPE) such as medical masks would have amounted to 'left-wing overreach.' This despite the fact that the DPA had been more or less routinely used, for many years, both for military purchases and such civilian purposes as speeding up infrastructure repairs following natural disasters.[12] It's true that in late March, 2020, after weeks of criticism over federal inaction and with COVID case numbers soaring, Trump did, reluctantly, invoke the act. But even then, he said he would use it only in a 'worst-case' scenario, a promise he appears to have kept, to the nation's cost.[13]

While Trump's daughter Ivanka, in her speech to the Republican National Convention in 2020, had suggested that her father had 'rapidly mobilized the full force of government PPE and the private sector' in the fight against COVID, evidence from other, more reliable, sources indicates that this was very far indeed from being the case. On only six occasions was the DPA used to accelerate production of medical equipment to address the nation's supply shortages.[14] An analysis by the non-partisan Congressional Research Service described the Trump administration's use of the DPA as 'sporadic and relatively narrow.' And Biden campaign advisor Dr Nicole Lurie, who had been Barack Obama's assistant secretary for preparedness and response in the Department of Health and Human Services, went much further, saying that despite Trump's having created the illusion that he was using the act, by occasionally resorting to it, 'The truth is that the White House is still failing to centrally manage the supply chain.'[15]

The nation's nurses were among the groups most seriously affected by the White House's haphazard coordination of supply management. All too frequently, shortages of such critical PPE as N95 medical masks used to filter out most virus particles had put nurses at risk. In a report released in August, 2020, the American Nurses' Association found that one in three of its members responding to a survey taken earlier that month were short or completely out of those masks. More than two-thirds of the survey respondents said that their employers required them to reuse their masks—an increase since May. Commenting on the findings, association president Ernest Grant said the lack of domestic supplies had left nurses at the mercy of inferior or even outright counterfeit foreign masks. 'We've been urging the administration since mid-March to use the DPA to ensure that everyone has adequate supplies so nurses don't have to worry that each time they put on a mask they are putting themselves, their patients and their families at risk of infection.'[16]

I do not know what the Trump administration's response to this report was. I would only suggest that it is absolutely appalling that such a report could be written—would have to be written—six months into the nation's worst pandemic in over 100 years.

While sins of omission such as those just described, resulting from the Trump administration's doing little or nothing to coordinate a federal response to COVID, were extremely common, Trump was also guilty of a number of sins of *commission*—instances in which his actions were a positive detriment to scientists or lower-level officials seeking to control the disease in their own jurisdictions. His battles with certain governors over PPE and hospital equipment such as ventilators would become legendary. We shall look at these in more detail shortly. They bear significant discussion because they shed light on one of Trump's most deplorable characteristics: his willingness and indeed eagerness to use a pandemic that had inflicted such horrific suffering on an entire country as a political football, with an eye to achieving his own narrow partisan political ends. But perhaps we should begin this part of our study by mentioning his single most destructive action of all throughout the pandemic: his destruction of the National Security Council's (NSC's) special global health and pandemic unit, which had won widespread praise from experts for its handling of an Ebola epidemic five years earlier, under President Obama.[17] This dismantling of the unit charged with planning and preparing for future pandemics took place in 2018, as part of a broader NSC reorganization that saw that organization's professional staff cut by more than half.[18] That it was a matter of when, not if, the next pandemic would hit was a conclusion any reasonable person might have drawn, given that the 15 years preceding the unit's dismantling had seen three global epidemics (SARS and H1N1 influenza as well as Ebola). The unit's first director, Beth Cameron, said she was 'mystified' by Trump's decision to dissolve the pandemic directorate, which left the country significantly less prepared for pandemics like COVID. The purpose of the directorate, she said, was to be the 'smoke alarm' and get ahead of emergencies and sound the warning at the earliest sign of fire, 'all with the goal of avoiding a six-alarm fire.'

In a classic understatement, journalist Deb Riechmann notes, 'Trump's elimination of the office suggested, along with his proposed budget cuts for the CDC (Centre for Disease Control), that he did not see the threat of pandemics in the same way that many experts in the field did.' His total lack of understanding of the issue had already been demonstrated through his response to a question as to whether elimination of the Global Health and Pandemic unit had slowed the country's response to the pandemic. His reply, on that occasion, had been 'This [the pandemic] is something that you can never really think is going to happen.'[19]

There are no words to describe such an appalling lack of prescience or understanding of the nature of infectious disease in the modern world. I would only suggest that Trump's persistent downplaying of the severity of COVID would certainly have been a factor in his administration's lack of an overall 'whole-of-government' response, described by former Obama Home-land Security advisor Lisa Monaco as necessary in combating any pandemic. As journalist Abigail Tracy has noted, the Trump administration's response to the pandemic has been 'ad hoc, shifting day to day with the mood of a president who has refused to accept that the buck stops with him.'[20]

While Trump's attitude toward the disbanded pandemic task force has been perhaps the most dramatic manifestation of his inability or unwillingness to accept responsibility for the actions of his presidency, his refusal to accept that 'the buck stops with him' has also coloured his relations with the state governors largely responsible for carrying out the fight against COVID in their own states. Instead of doing what he could to work in tandem with the governors, or even stepping aside and staying out of their way, he repeatedly sought to blame the governors for his administration's failings. And far from helping states with their procurement efforts, he even allowed his own federal agency (the federal Emergency Management Association, or FEMA) to outbid the states on critical supplies, in the process driving these supplies' prices up and pitting state against state in a process one governor (Andrew Cuomo of New York) has described as something akin to an eBay auction.

'We're not a shipping clerk,' Trump told governors critical of what they saw as inadequate federal efforts to obtain such medical supplies as hospital beds, face masks and ventilators to combat the pandemic.[21] Taking a fairly standard, right-wing, minimalist federal government approach to the issue, Trump indicated that in his view state governors should be doing the lion's share of the procurement work. While noting that the administration will 'help out wherever we can,' in his view the acquisition of urgent supplies is 'really for the local governments, governors, and people in the state, depending on the way they divide it up.'

One might have thought, given the sentiments expressed in the preceding paragraph, that under Trump the federal government would at least have stayed out of the way of states seeking to acquire their own supplies. But that was far from being the case. On three occasions, the federal government outbid the state of Massachusetts, causing that state's Republican governor, Charlie Baker, to say, somewhat ruefully, 'I've got a feeling that if someone has the chance to sell to you and to sell to me, I am going to lose on every one of those [prospective purchases].'[22] And competing with the federal government also appears to have helped create bitter competition between the states, as well as with them, causing New York's Democratic Governor Andrew Cuomo to complain that trying to obtain supplies was 'like being on eBay with 50 other states, bidding on a ventilator.' Noting that the Federal Emergency Management Agency's bids were pushing the cost of medical supplies higher, Cuomo added, 'I mean, how inefficient. And then, FEMA gets involved! And FEMA starts bidding! And now FEMA is bidding on top of the 50 [states]. So FEMA is driving up the price. What sense does this make?'[23] In a similar vein, an aide to another Democratic governor, who chose to remain anonymous, said 'We are competing against every other state and the federal government' in the bid to obtain critical supplies.[24]

In the face of widespread criticism for his administration's slow and often contradictory COVID supply management coordination effort, Trump turned the issue into a political football, lashing out at his critics as 'complainers' with 'insatiable appetites' for medical and hospital supplies rather than making any kind of serious attempt to improve the situation.[25] The critics included the Democratic governors of Washington, Illinois, Michigan, and New York—four states that were among the country's hardest-hit during the pandemic's first wave. Weary both of Trump's inaction and of his constant attacks on his critics, Michigan Governor Gretchen Whitmer said, 'I've asked repeatedly and respectfully for help. We need it. No more political attacks, just PPEs, ventilators, N95 masks, test kits.'[26] Former director of the Office of Government Ethics Walter Shaub was even blunter in his criticism of Trump's use of the pandemic for partisan political purposes. Describing Trump's series of 'attack tweets' as disgusting, Shaub characterized Trump as '. . .a man desperate to shift blame instead of save a country because he knows he's over his head. He doesn't care who dies, he cares who votes for him.'[27]

Not content to attempt to bully those governors (like Whitmer) who had been among his harshest critics, Trump on July 8 declared his intention to pressure all state governors into ensuring that schools in their state reopened for in-person learning in the Fall, even going to the extent of threatening to 'cut off funding' if they didn't. In addition to being just the opposite of the sort of cooperation and coordination needed to lick COVID-19, the incident amounted to notorious federal overreach into an area of state jurisdiction. Whether he seriously believed he could actually do what he had threatened to do is an open question. Not only is education under state jurisdiction, but all federal monies must be allocated by Congress, and all allocation bills must originate in the House of Representatives. I have never seen any evidence that he actually followed up on his outrageous threat. Most likely, like so many of his other statements, this one was simply meant as political 'raw meat' to his followers, who clearly delighted in seeing him go into attack mode. Still, as if further evidence on the subject were needed, it *was* further evidence of his preference for governing through unilateral fiat rather than through cooperation or negotiation with lower-level officials.[28]

It would be easy to find numerous other instances of Trump's failure to use all the tools at his disposal to combat the COVID pandemic, as well as additional cases in which he tried to shift blame to governors or other lower-level officials. Unfortunately, we haven't the space, here, to cite any more such cases. The overall pattern should be clear from those we have already referenced.

It is impossible to determine what the precise effect of Trump's spotty and frequently misguided coordination efforts would have been on differing rates of COVID in different states. We have no way of discovering which states would have been more or less affected by his mindless antics, though there is anecdotal evidence to suggest that strongly Republican states, particularly those led by a Republican governor, may have received preferential federal treatment in the distribution of medical and hospital supplies.[29] Such behaviour would certainly have been consistent with his overall conduct throughout his time in office. (In this connection, it's probably worth noting that most of his attacks on governors were directed at Democrats such as Whitmer and Cuomo and others in the group just mentioned). What can be said, and this with some certainty, is that his failure with the coordination effort was an important element in the country's appalling COVID showing through the end of his term.

On the day that Trump left office, the U.S. had just seen its 400,000[th] death due to COVID—a figure just short of the 405,000 Americans killed in combat through the entire four years of World War II, and equivalent to the entire population of cities such as Cleveland, New Orleans and Tampa.[30] On that day, there were more than 120,000 Americans in hospital with the virus, and it was killing about 3,300 people per day—far more deaths than had been occurring at the height of the pandemic's first wave during the spring of 2020.[31] Although the U.S. has well below 5% of the world's population, it had, by this point, accounted for nearly one-fifth of world fatalities attributable to the disease.[32] Meanwhile, the number of U.S. cases had reached 24,506,108, over 7% of the country's population.[33] The country's current count stands at 30,926,096 cases and 561,364 fatalities.[34]

A revealing fact about the distribution of U.S. cases is that a clear majority (roughly 60%) of the cases recorded by Inauguration Day occurred between Election Day and Inauguration Day. On the former day, in early November, the case count stood at just over 9.8 million cases—only about 40% of the number recorded on the day Trump left office. Had a larger share of the fatalities occurred earlier, during the first wave, it might be harder to blame Trump for them. The pandemic did take scientists and politicians alike by surprise at first, though Trump's earlier dismantling of the CDC's pandemic unit and reluctance to invoke the Defense Production Act, as noted above, certainly did not help in the country's initial response to COVID.

By November, Trump had had eight months to learn about the pandemic and how best to deal with it. It was no longer a case of the administration's being in a learning curve. The advice from respected scientists and doctors such as Dr Anthony Fauci, the country's leading disease expert, was becoming increasingly consistent and increasingly clear. Had he followed that advice and, equally important, sent a signal to lower-level politicians and ordinary Americans that he was listening to scientific advice about the pandemic and believed other politicians and the general public should do the same, the case and death rates would arguably have been significantly lower than they were.

b) *Setting the Tone*
In addition to coordinating national strategy for dealing with COVID, or any

other national emergency, the President should lead by example, setting a tone, through his personal life and actions, which will inspire ordinary citizens to 'do the right thing' in terms of combating the pandemic.

If Donald Trump's coordination of national strategy against COVID was haphazard and sometimes divisive, the job he did in setting an example to his citizens was nothing short of pathetic. Virtually every time, citizens would have done far better to have done exactly the opposite of what Trump seemed to be recommending through his words and actions.

A President seriously interested in bringing COVID under control would have made his chief medical officer or infectious disease expert a full partner in the fight, giving that expert the lion's share of 'air time' in press conferences and briefings.[35] This was the course of action followed in most Canadian provinces—Nova Scotia comes first to mind here—and in many U.S. states, as well.[36] He would make sure he was always wearing a mask when photographed in public, and would insist that those meeting with him likewise be masked. Certainly, he would require masks at any of his campaign rallies and other campaign functions. Apropos of campaign rallies, he would hold by far the greater proportion of them virtually. Live campaign rallies would be rare, and conducted only under conditions of strict social distancing. He would support the activities of state governors and municipal officials who were trying to control the disease through lockdowns, and would urge citizens to abide by any restrictions those lockdowns might impose. Certainly, he would not recommend reopening a state earlier than a governor was prepared to reopen it. And he would follow the advice of his medical experts regarding the appropriate medications to take to prevent or mitigate the disease. Beyond that, he would at the very least avoid spreading misinformation or outright lies about the disease and what his administration had done to combat it. Finally, were he unlucky enough to contract COVID and to require hospitalization, he would abide by the advice of his doctors regarding medications, staying indoors and the like. He would wait until he had received medical clearance to leave the hospital, and he definitely would not, within two days after his admission to hospital, leave the building to go riding around in a car for a photo-op.

The daily press briefings on COVID, which Trump launched in early March, should have been used as an opportunity to inform Americans about the disease and to provide them with the best available medical and scientific advice as to how to combat it. This was definitely how such briefings were used in most if not all Canadian jurisdictions, and in the more enlightened U.S. states. Instead, doctors and scientists were relegated to the background, with Trump almost always the dominant speaker. In analyzing the content of Trump's briefing speeches from March 9 through April 17, the *New York Times* found that self-praise was the most frequent theme of the briefings.[37]

Not content merely to marginalize the country's leading infectious disease experts and other key scientists and doctors, Trump and the leading members of his administration and political allies started launching attacks on those experts from the pandemic's early days, attempting to have such experts identified in the public eye as part of the 'deep state elite' from which Trump was seeking to deliver the U.S. On April 18, Trump's son-in-law Jared Kushner told journalist Bob Woodward that the President was 'getting the country back from the doctors. Trump's now back in charge. It's not the doctors.' At about the same time, after Dr Fauci had suggested that had the administration 'started mitigation earlier, more lives could have been saved,' his commonsense observation drew an angry response from former Republican congressional candidate DeAnna Lorraine. Lorraine's tweet included a call to 'fire Fauci.' After Trump retweeted Lorraine's post, public alarm was aroused, and Trump was forced to deny he'd ever had any intention of firing Fauci. But to some extent the damage had already been done, as the attack caused Fauci to scale back his TV appearances in May.

Despite the damage the earlier attack had caused to the Trump administration's credibility on COVID, he didn't stop attacking Fauci. On July 1, he would retweet an unscientific social media poll by the organization Act! For America in which Twitter users had claimed to trust Trump over Fauci. And on October 19, during a campaign call, Trump claimed that Americans were bored with hearing about COVID. 'People are saying, "Whatever, just leave us alone." They're tired of it. People are tired of hearing Fauci and all these idiots,' he said, adding that Fauci, 'has been here for 500 years.'

While the main thrust of Trump's attacks on scientists was directed against Fauci, even the soft-spoken Dr Deborah Birx, who was far less willing to stand up for herself than Fauci, did not escape his ire. After Birx appeared on CNN warning of a new surge in cases, she had what she would later describe as a 'very uncomfortable' and 'very difficult' phone call from Trump—a incident she did not reveal publicly until the following year.

One of the best ways for a politician to set a good example is by wearing masks in all public settings. The current President, Joe Biden, has been very careful to do so. But as for Trump, though he has occasionally worn a mask and very occasionally made public statements supportive of mask-wearing, he has for the most part not only avoided wearing masks himself, but has been critical of other politicians (such as Biden) who have worn them.

In May, 2020, Trump didn't wear a mask during a press appearance at a Honeywell factory that produces masks, which in retrospect seems more than a little strange. He also did not wear a mask during a May 21 press appearance at a Ford factory in Ypsilanti, Michigan, although he had worn one earlier during his tour of the plant. Asked why he had removed his mask for the press conference, Trump replied that he 'didn't want to give the press the pleasure' of seeing him wear a mask. On May 26, Trump said it was 'very unusual' for presumptive Democratic Presidential nominee Joe Biden to be wearing a mask at an outdoor Memorial Day ceremony. On that same day, Trump asked a journalist to remove his mask while asking him a question. After the journalist refused, saying he would speak louder, Trump accused the journalist of 'wanting to be politically correct.'

At a campaign rally on September 3, Trump mocked Biden for wearing a mask during *his* campaign appearances, asking 'Did you ever see a man that liked a mask as much as him?' Later, he would go on to suggest that, 'If I were a psychiatrist, I'd say this guy had some big issues.'

Most outrageous of all was his statement, during an October 15 town hall broadcast on NBC TV, that 85% of those wearing masks had contracted COVID. To bolster this outrageous claim, he cited a CDC study, whose results (as per usual) he had totally distorted with an eye to scoring political points.

The instances in which Trump, or key members of his administration, deliberately spread misinformation or even outright lies about COVID-19 and his administration's handling of it are so numerous that we can offer only a very small sample here. These instances began on March 19, when Trump admitted to journalist Bob Woodward, in a private interview, that he had always wanted to downplay the seriousness of the disease, and still wanted to do so, so as not to create a panic among Americans. This assertion was flatly denied on September 9 by his then press secretary Kayleigh McEnany.

On March 30, Trump made the totally absurd claim that his administration had inherited a 'broken test' for COVID-19—a disease that hadn't even appeared on the horizon until he had been in office for nearly three years.

On May 6, he made the equally absurd assertion that if the U.S. had done very little testing, it wouldn't have had the most cases in the world. 'So, in a way, by doing all of this testing, we make ourselves look bad.' The assertion would be repeated at a July 14 press conference during which he claimed that if the U.S. had done half as much testing as it had, it would have half the number of cases that it did.

On May 8, Trump blithely predicted that COVID would go away without a vaccine. Less than two months later, during an Independence Day address, he claimed that 99% of all U.S. COVID cases were 'totally harmless.' Similarly, at a September 21 campaign rally in Ohio, he said that the virus affects 'virtually nobody.'

On October 6, he made what was perhaps his most dangerous misstatement of all, when he claimed in a post made both on Facebook and Twitter that COVID-19 was, in most populations, 'far less lethal than the flu.' This time, he went too far even for the (in my view) excessively tolerant social media giants. Both treated the outrageous post as misinformation, with Twitter placing a warning message over the tweet and Facebook deleting the post outright.

Undaunted by this rebuke, he continued to spread his outrageous and ludicrous lies on the campaign trail. On October 18, at a campaign rally in Carson City, Nevada, he blamed his opponent Joe Biden for the state's stay-at-home orders, referring to them as the 'Biden lockdown' even though it would be another three months before the Democrat would take office. On October 29, Trump said the number of COVID deaths was 'almost nothing,' on a day on which 1,000 people died, and at the end of which the nation's COVID death toll stood at 227,897.[38] And on October 30, at a campaign rally in Michigan, he accused hospitals of artificially inflating COVID deaths, claiming that 'doctors get more money if someone dies from COVID.'

Trump's conduct of his campaign rallies during the 2020 presidential campaign demonstrated his lack of concern for the safety of Americans—even (in fact especially) Americans who were supporting him. Many were held in crowded arenas with poor air circulation, and in most social distancing was not generally adhered to, nor was the wearing of masks the norm. He also held these in-person rallies for a far longer period than did his Democratic opponent, Joe Biden. Although he had suspended in-person rallies from March 3 through June 19, he resumed them with a vengeance on June 20 with a notorious 'superspreader' event in Tulsa, Oklahoma that would wind up claiming the life of at least one well-known Republican politician (Herman Cain) and sickening at least eight Trump staffers—six during the set-up of the event and two after it.[39]

In all, Trump held 67 campaign rallies between June 19 and Election Day, the vast majority being in hotly-contested states. Only two (the Tulsa event and a late October rally in Omaha, Nebraska) were held in solidly Republican states, and none was held in a solidly Democratic state. Over one-fifth (14) of those rallies occurred in Pennsylvania, while seven each were held in Florida, Michigan, North Carolina, and Wisconsin. Six were held in Arizona, four in Minnesota, and three each in Nevada and Ohio. Two were held in Georgia, Iowa, and New Hampshire, while the states of Nebraska, Ohio, and Virginia were each the beneficiaries of a single Trump rally.[40]

There is far from enough space to discuss even a handful of these events, but the first and in many ways most notorious, the Tulsa rally, does warrant brief attention, if only because some of the event's consequences would become immediately apparent. The event was held at Tulsa's BOK Center.[41] Originally, it had been scheduled for June 19, but the date had been pushed back to the 20th because the 19th was a day set aside to honour the emancipation of African-Americans, and organizers realized that to hold it on that day would be seen as insensitive to the Black Lives Matter Movement. It had been expected to draw about 19,000, but actual attendance, as estimated by the Tulsa fire department, would be around 6,200—less than one-third the original estimate. Perhaps the changed date was responsible for the lower-than-expected attendance, or perhaps it was the result of COVID danger warnings emanating both from critics of the event and from local public health officials.[42] It is noteworthy that the event came off despite a recent spike in cases in Oklahoma, a spike which, as we shall see, would worsen in the days and weeks following the event.

Shortly before the beginning of the rally, Trump staffers removed signs from seats that would have promoted social distancing by asking attendees not to sit in the seats in question. Why this should have been necessary or even desirable, in view of the event's low attendance, is not at all clear, especially since the removal of the signs was in direct contradiction to the instructions of the arena's management. I do not know if anyone aside from Herman Cain died as a result of having attended the rally, but many were certainly sickened. In addition to the eight Trump staffers already mentioned, many Secret Service agents were asked to self-isolate, and attendee Kimberly Guilfoyle, girlfriend of Trump's son Donald, Jr, would also come down with COVID not long after the rally. Most tellingly, despite the event's relatively low attendance, in the 30 days following it, the state's daily rate of new COVID cases would triple, to 513 per day. One can only imagine how much the rate would have increased had the event drawn the anticipated number of Trump partisans.

It is not easy or perhaps even possible, to determine the precise effect such campaign rallies would have had on interstate COVID rates. One can, however, make two observations. First, such rallies, particularly when held in closed spaces without proper masking and social distancing precautions, would almost certainly have resulted in increased COVID rates in the states hosting them (as proved to be the case for Oklahoma). Secondly, since the rallies would presumably have brought in people not just from the states in which they were held but other states as well, they would likely have increased COVID rates among Trump supporters generally, since aside from any protesters, who typically would have been expelled from the events forthwith, only Trump's supporters would have been attending the rallies. While Joe Biden did hold live rallies, he held fewer of them, over a shorter period of time, and under far more strictly regulated conditions. Live campaign rallies, therefore, would arguably have resulted in greater numbers of COVID cases in states supporting Trump than in those supporting Biden, and may indeed have been a significant factor in these states' overall COVID rates. Conversely, the fact that fewer campaign rallies were held in solidly Democratic states, and many fewer 'unsafe' ones, may well have been a factor in these states' lower overall COVID rates.

Closely related to Trump's attacks on scientific and medical experts, in fact perhaps the strongest and most bizarre manifestation of his distrust of such expertise generally, were his recommendations that COVID patients use the anti-malarial and anti-lupus drug hydroxychloroquine for treatment of the disease, and that people inject themselves with disinfectants (including chlorine bleach) as a treatment. Along similar lines, he proposed irradiating patient with UV light.

In fairness, Trump may not have been totally off-base in suggesting that hydroxychloroquine might offer promise as a treatment for COVID-19. At the time, the idea was attracting support from people as diverse as his political opponent, New York Governor Andrew Cuomo, and Dr David Juurlink, head of clinical pharmacology at Sunnybrook Health Sciences Centre in Toronto.[43] But his exhortations to medical professionals, issued at a press conference in early April, to use the drug for COVID on the grounds they had nothing to lose[44] were definitely off-base and potentially dangerous, as Mayo Clinic researchers had found an increased risk of heart irregularities in 1% of the drug's users. Moreover, as noted both by Alexander Panetta and Senator Elizabeth Warren (quoted in Panetta's article), the run on the drug created by taking Trump's advice and using it for COVID-19 had created shortages among 'legitimate' users of the drug needing it to treat auto-immune diseases such as lupus and rheumatoid arthritis. Said Warren, 'Medical misinformation is dangerous and Donald Trump has no business giving this advice [to use hydroxychloroquine].' Indeed, even the generally supportive David Juurlink described Trump's promotion of the drug as dangerous, declaring, 'He knows nothing about clinical medicine.'[45] Obviously it is one thing to recommend that a certain drug be tested as a remedy for a certain disease, and to commit federal funds for research on the issue, but quite another to actively promote use of the drug as a cure for the disease before the necessary research has been carried out.

If Trump's promotion of hydroxychloroquine bordered on quackery, his advocacy of disinfectant injections as a COVID treatment crossed all the way over into la-la land. One would have to go back to the days of John (Goat Gland) Brinkley, the so-called doctor who advocated (and practiced) implantation of goat glands as a treatment for male sexual dysfunction, to come up with such a downright crazy idea.[46] The main difference was that while, like Trump, Brinkley was interested in holding public office, unlike Trump, he did not succeed, losing in two campaigns for Governor of Kansas. Having been elected President, Trump was able to use the presidency as a bully pulpit for these and other equally cockamamie medical notions.

On April 23, Trump requested the White Task Coronavirus Task Force to investigate whether a disinfectant could be injected as a treatment for COVID patients, not specifying what type of disinfectant he was referring to.[47] At the same press conference, he also appeared to recommend irradiating COVID patients' bodies with ultraviolet light, a suggestion he said he'd heard from a doctor just a few minutes earlier at the briefing. The response from the medical community was swift and dramatic, with doctors saying that even breathing the fumes from chlorine bleach could lead to serious lung damage, and injecting bleach or disinfectant might lead to death.

Already (in March) there had been a significant increase in accidental poisonings from bleach and disinfectants, owing to their greatly increased use as household cleaners during the pandemic's early days.[48] These poisonings increased after Trump's disinfectant comments of April 23, comments which, as journalist Jeffrey Kluger dryly noted, did not do much for his reputation as a reliable arbiter of public health.[49] Regrettably, as outrageous as Trump's recommendations were, and as strongly as the medical profession warned against following them, a sizable number of Americans did indeed inject or ingest bleach and other disinfectants during the period immediately after his press conference.

Poison control centres across the country saw a marked increase in calls following that press conference.[50] For example, the state of Maryland's health department emergency hotline took hundreds of calls from people asking if it was all right for them to ingest Clorox or alcohol cleaning products. Such phenomena prompted the manufacturer of Lysol to issue a strongly-worded statement saying that the product was not intended for internal use. They also prompted Maryland's Republican Governor, Larry Hogan, to demand that the White House 'communicate very clearly on the facts... because people pay attention when the President of the United States is standing there giving a press conference.' Increases in calls to poison control centres were also reported in New York City and in the states of Tennessee, Michigan, and Illinois; the last of these reported incidents where people had used detergents as sinus rinses, and had gargled with a mixture of bleach and mouthwash. In Kansas, an official stated that a man had drunk disinfectant 'because of the advice he'd received.'

In the face of all the added activity in poison control centres, activity which had the further consequence of making it more difficult for people with legitimate issues to access those centres, Trump denied any responsibility for the situation. Asked by a *Wichita Eagle* reporter about a 'spike in people using disinfectant after your comments last week,' Trump interrupted the reporter, saying, 'I can't imagine why.' When the reporter followed up by asking if Trump took any responsibility, the President replied, 'I don't.'[51] Earlier, he had attempted to walk back the comments by claiming he was being 'very sarcastic.'

Finally, a President during a major pandemic such as COVID-19 has the responsibility to lead through example, first by doing everything possible to keep from getting the disease, and second, should he be unfortunate enough to contract the disease, by setting a good example of how to be a patient to ordinary citizens. Trump, clearly, did neither. His attitude toward masks, which generally ranged from cavalier to downright antagonistic, may well have helped bring about his cases and those of people in his inner circle. So did his holding of large in-person campaign rallies (commented upon earlier). Except for the Sturgis motorcycle rally, which we will comment on in more detail in the next section, it would be hard to find a better example of a superspreader event than a campaign rally of thousands of people, all sitting closely together and most not wearing masks.

Trump's actual conduct as a COVID patient set an equally bad example. Not only did he, as President, receive at Walter Reed Army Hospital the sort of treatment available to few of his countryfolk; he flaunted the fact, later using his relatively quick recovery as an illustration of how the disease wasn't really as serious as most were making it out to be. And his behaviour as a patient at Walter Reed was utterly appalling. Only a very few days after his admission, he left the hospital for much of an afternoon, during which he was repeatedly photographed riding around in a limousine waving to people. Shortly after that, he had left the hospital, well before normal procedure would dictate he should leave. These actions sent the message that if one was in hospital with COVID, it was OK to do whatever one wanted, including leaving the building for the afternoon, as if one had been hospitalized for a broken limb rather than a highly contagious infectious disease. His effectively signing himself out sent the same deplorable message. Like so many of Trump's other actions, it had the effect of downplaying, even minimizing the severity of the disease.

2) Governors

The actions of the governors of the various U.S. states may well have had a greater impact on COVID case rates in their states than those of the President, although they were for the most part less widely publicized. It is the governors who have primary responsibility for setting and carrying out COVID policy within their states. In particular, governors are chiefly responsible for deciding such critical matters as when lockdowns will start, how long they will last, which businesses will be included, what restrictions will be placed on individuals' personal behaviour, and how strictly lockdowns will be enforced. To them falls also the job of deciding which large, potentially dangerous events such as conventions will be permitted to go forward, and which will be ordered cancelled or postponed. Like the President, governors also have an important job to play in setting the tone their jurisdictions will take in the fight against COVID. Will they view their states' chief medical officers as partners in the fight, and take their advice? Will they, a la Trump, ignore or even attack their chief medical officers for providing advice that they think may hurt their states' economies, or their political standing? Or will they, like many governors, end up somewhere in between the two extreme positions listed above?

In some cases, particularly in large cities where conditions may be quite different than in most of the rest of the state, municipal officials such as mayors may also have a significant role to play. The significance of these officials' role becomes more apparent when, as in the case of Atlanta and

Miami during the pandemic's first wave, they are of a different political party than the governor and believe their cities should take a different course on reopening following a lockdown than the rest of the state. The mayors of both the aforementioned cities did not believe their cities should reopen with the rest of the state, during the first wave, and for a time kept their cities locked down after the rest of the state had reopened, generally earning strong public approval for their actions.[52] But at the end of the day, the proverbial buck stops in the governor's office. It is he or she who bears final responsibility for COVID policy. More than once, a governor has overruled a reluctant mayor and ordered a city or certain types of businesses within a city to reopen despite the mayor's objections.[53]

The effect that a governor can have on COVID rates in their state is perhaps nowhere more evident than in the case of large, 'superspreader' events attracting thousands of people. Municipal officials may have some say in whether such events go forward or are postponed or cancelled. But in the final analysis, the decision will be the governor's.

The most obvious example here is the 10-day motorcycle rally held in the small town of Sturgis, South Dakota from August 7 to 16, 2020. Held with not just the approval but the fervent blessing of Governor Kristi Noem, a strong Trump supporter and vocal opponent of lockdowns,[54] the rally, an annual event that had been taking place since 1940,[55] drew some 460,000 people from all across the country to Sturgis, in what *New York Times* reporters Mark Walker and Jack Healy described as a 'Woodstock of unmasked, uninhibited coronavirus defiance.'[56] It is true that some concessions were made to COVID in planning the rally. Ralliers were not permitted to consume alcohol on patios on the town's main street, and certain events such as the traditional opening parade were cancelled.[57] The town's chief health officer was even given the power to stop the rally completely should he feel new COVID cases were getting out of control.[58] But for the most part, to the horror of health officials across the country and many townspeople, and the amazement of observers from other countries, the event appears to have proceeded pretty much as it might have in a more normal year, with much close physical contact and drinking of alcohol and little physical distancing or mask-wearing.

The totally unsurprising result was a significant increase in South Dakota's COVID cases, and COVID cases in other states, particularly those bordering or near South Dakota, in the period following the rally. One quite cautious Center for Disease Control (CDC) study issued in November and focussed on Minnesota linked 86 cases, four hospitalizations, and one death in that state to the rally.[59] While these numbers don't seem especially high, it's important to bear in mind that Minnesota was but one of at least 20 states attributing new cases to the rally.[60] If one were to multiply that number by 19 and then add a greater number of cases for South Dakota, the host state, one would almost certainly emerge with at least 2,000 cases attributable to the rally, along with an untold number of hospitalizations and fatalities. Such numbers are certainly quite horrific enough.

An admittedly less cautious study done through statistical analysis rather than direct observation by a group of University of San Diego labour economists suggested that as many as 260,000 new COVID cases may have resulted from the rally.[61] The study immediately drew the wrath of South Dakota's Governor Noem, who attacked its authors as biased charlatans and invited refutation from honest scholars.[62]

The truth of the matter, as South Dakota Medical Association President Dr Benjamin Aaker suggested, is that it the full extent of COVID spread caused by the virus will probably never be known. 'These people go home and get sick with coronavirus. They don't have any way of knowing whether they picked it up at the rally or back in California,' said Aaker. Similarly, health officials noted that a lack of contact tracing and the sheer scale of the event made it impossible to know how many people were infected directly or indirectly because of Sturgis. (The mind boggles at the thought of even attempting contact tracing for an event of Sturgis' size).

What can be said is that the Sturgis rally was certainly a major factor, and indeed likely the single most important factor, in the extraordinarily high COVID rates experienced in the two Dakotas—the two states with the highest rates in the country, as Table 1 shows—and the unexpectedly high rates in nearby, predominantly agricultural states with low population densities such as Nebraska, Montana, Wyoming and Iowa.[63] These rates are not only far higher than the rates in densely-populated eastern and Pacific Coast states (all primarily Democratic), but even than the rates of densely-populated southern and southwestern states such as Texas and Florida, with high poverty rates and large numbers of immigrants and multi-generational families. In my view, only Sturgis can explain such strongly counterintuitive findings. And only the presence of a strongly [sic] conservative Republican governor in South Dakota can explain how the event was able to happen at all. It is impossible to imagine a Democratic governor—any Democratic governor—allowing such an insane event to occur in their state. Nor can one imagine any sensible moderate Republican of the 'Main Street' variety such as the 'Non-Partisan' anti-Trump Republicans referred to in Table 1 allowing it. That some 460,000 people were allowed to gather in a small town, effectively taking it over for 10 days during which they paraded through it, largely maskless and largely without observing any sort of social distancing, at a time when there was active debate about reopening schools and theatres and allowing weddings and wedding receptions to proceed, defies all logic and all good sense.

In the last analysis, Sturgis is an illustration of partisan politics and crass economism run amok. Although tragic—by March over one in eight residents of both South and North Dakota had officially been diagnosed with

COVID—the results were eminently predictable. One should have expected nothing else in a situation in which public officials rated raw economic gain as far more important than taking even the most rudimentary precautions to protect their citizens' health and safety. To repeat: the role of the governor and the significance of the party label are critical here. Despite Sturgis' near-legendary status as an event that had been taking place for 80 years, had Sturgis been located in Wisconsin or Michigan or Minnesota, all states with Democratic governors, the event would almost certainly not have happened in 2020—and COVID rates both in the host state and across the region and country would have been significantly lower.

The case of Kentucky, governed by an activist Democrat, Andy Beshear, illustrates some of the benefits of having a Democratic governor even in a state with very high Trump support (over 62%, seventh highest in the country) and a political culture inclined to oppose many proposed restrictions on personal freedom and economic activity. It bears mention, as well, that Kentucky is the home state of long-time Senate Republican leader Mitch McConnell, who gave Donald Trump virtual *carte blanche* during Trump's term in office. Despite such indicators, which one would expect to lead to high COVID rates, Kentucky ranked exactly in the middle of the pack—26th of 51 jurisdictions—in COVID rates, with cases reported in 9.22% of the population, only slightly above the national average of 8.79%. (See Table 1.) Despite strong opposition—including a lawsuit against his issuing of pandemic-related executive orders as unconstitutional, a lawsuit which Beshear won—Beshear has stuck to his guns, ordering and then maintaining tight restrictions on businesses, with the result that the state is now in far better shape with respect to COVID than it was when he issued the most recent restrictions, last November, and he anticipates being able to lift most of those restrictions within about four to six weeks.

On November 17, 2020, when Beshear issued the latest round of restrictions, the state was undeniably in a bad way with regard to COVID. On that day, the state's positivity rate reached 9.12%, and there were 2,753 new cases and 15 deaths, including that of a teenage girl.[64] By this point, 106 of the state's 120 counties—nearly 90% of them—fell into the red zone.

Describing the growth in new cases as exponential, Beshear declared (in a dig at some of his many critics) that 'Pretending this virus isn't real is not an option. It's time to do what it takes to finish this fight.'[65] All public elementary and secondary schools in the state were ordered closed to in-person instruction until the end of the semester. Restaurants and bars were closed to in-person dining; with some modifications, outdoor dining was still permitted. Gyms were limited to one-third off capacity, with no group classes or indoor games allowed; masks would be required. Indoor gatherings were limited to two families and a maximum of eight people in all, and weddings and funerals were limited to a maximum of 25 people. Professional service organizations were to have their employees work from home where possible, and their offices were limited to one-third of capacity. A $40 million fund was established to provide relief to affected restaurants and bars.

While probably relatively strict by American standards, these restrictions were mild by most Canadian standards. Still, they aroused fierce opposition among the state's Republicans. State Senate Majority Leader State Senate Majority Leader Damon Thayer, perhaps the harshest of Beshear's critics, predicted in a text to *USA Today* that the governor's latest 'draconian measures' would 'do further damage to our economy and schoolchildren,' adding that Beshear's 'arbitrary rules' would 'continue to bring harm to citizens everywhere and is [*sic*] an affront to the concept of co-equal branches of government.' Thayer and other Republican leaders vowed to respond by bringing in legislation early in the new year (2021) to curb the Governor's powers.

The opposition's partisan attacks notwithstanding, many of the restrictions have remained in place through the present.[66] As unpopular as they may have been, the restrictions appear to have done their job in reducing COVID cases in the state. The test positivity rate, though up somewhat from recent days, is now at 3.16%, or just slightly over one-third what it was on November 17, when the restrictions were initially imposed.[67] The number of new cases (270) is less than one-tenth the number (2,753) on November 17, and the number of new deaths (7) is less than one-half the earlier total. One would have to say that Beshear has done a fine job of bringing the pandemic under control in his state during the past five months.

Like most American governors and Canadian provincial premiers, Beshear expects mass vaccination ultimately to deliver his state from the threat of COVID. Recently (on April 12), he announced that most restrictions could be lifted when the state reaches 2.5 million vaccinations—a figure that is about 60% of the state's 4.48 million population. At present some 1.6 million Kentuckians, accounting for about 35% of the state's population, have had at least one COVID shot. When the 2.5 million threshold is reached, which Beshear anticipates will take another four to six weeks, capacity limits and curfews will be lifted at restaurants, bars, music venues, funeral homes, retail, event spaces, wedding venues, public pools, grocery stores, country clubs, museums, festivals and distilleries, providing these places have 1,000 or fewer patrons. That he has achieved such excellent results with such fierce partisan opposition is even more to his credit.

On the opposite side of the ledger is Arizona, a state narrowly won by Democrat Joe Biden in the Presidential election, but with a long history of being a Republican state and with a Republican governor (Rob Ducey). Recently, it was the home state of the 2008 Republican presidential candidate John McCain, and in the more distant past, it was home to 'Mr Conservative,' Senator Barry Goldwater, the party's presidential candidate in 1964.

Arizona's per capita COVID rate of 11.38% (see Table 1) is about one-third higher than that national average of 8.79%—enough to rank it sixth in the country. As we will see in more detail shortly, the state's political culture has historically been strongly libertarian—a tradition extending back at least to the time of Goldwater. Even as he was taking a fearsome drubbing in most of the rest of the country, the Arizona Senator carried the state, albeit narrowly, in his disastrous presidential run in 1964; it would be the only state he would win outside of the Deep South.

In recent years, a combination of a growing Hispanic population and seniors not unjustifiably concerned about the future of Social Security in Republican hands has moved the state toward the Democrats in national elections. Not only did Joe Biden carry the state in 2020; Democrat Mark Kelly was also elected to the U.S. Senate in that same election. But at the state level, where issues like Social Security are not in play, the libertarian Republican political culture continues to hold sway, albeit by a narrower margin than in the past. Arizona is presently one of 23 states where the Republicans hold a 'trifecta' (control of both houses of the legislature as well as the Governor's mansion).[68] As of the last election, Republicans controlled the state Senate by a margin of 16 to 14 seats; their margin in the state House was 31 to 29. Rather remarkably, the Republicans have controlled both chambers continuously since 1997, with the single and partial exception of 2001-2, when the Senate elections resulted in a tie in that chamber.[69]

Although Arizona and South Dakota both have Republican governors, this has played out in very different ways in the two states. In South Dakota, as in Ron DeSantis' Florida and Brian Kemp's Georgia, the governor, Kristi Noem, is a flamboyant libertarian and Trump supporter arguably well to the right even of many of her fellow Republicans, a fair number of whom did not want the superspreader Sturgis rally to go forward. And, of course, the simple fact of the superspreader rally makes South Dakota a very different case from Arizona, which did not host any such event. Arizona's governor Ducey is a quieter and less flamboyant figure than Noem. While he always supported Trump and was reluctant to impose restrictions, he was eventually willing to impose some, under duress. Within the state's Republican Party, he has ranked as a relative moderate, at times attracting significant opposition on the right from members of his own party who are so strongly libertarian that they view any restrictions on citizens' personal freedom as unconstitutional, no matter how grave may have been the crisis leading to those restrictions.[70]

As *Arizona Republic* journalists Stephanie Innes and Alison Steinbach have noted, there are a sizable number of factors helping to explain Arizona's appalling COVID showing. Only one of those factors, the state's geographic location on the border with Mexico and California, which has inevitably led to consistently heavy cross-border traffic of farm labourers between it and

Mexico, can be regarded as a structural factor effectively beyond the ability of state politicians and health officials to control.

Innes and Steinbach note that rural Yuma County, where agriculture is the major industry, was harder hit by COVID-19 than anywhere else in the state. Its 15.16% per capita COVID rate (as of late January) was roughly twice the national rate of 7.69%.[71] While regrettable, such a high COVID rate can hardly be considered surprising, given the constant coming and going of farmworkers and their families between Mexico, Yuma County, and California—a situation which would provide ideal conditions for rapid spread of the virus. In the words of Amanda Aguirre, president and CEO of Somerton's Regional Center for Border Health, 'The population is huge on the Mexican side and there's a lot of mobility between the families on both sides, going back and forth. Just the nature of people, they want to continue celebrating weddings and birthdays... I think the message was not really resonating with some of the general public.'[72]

State authorities would probably not have had any realistic way of controlling the situation short of imposing a total crackdown of movement between Mexico and Arizona for the duration of the pandemic. Such a crackdown would have imposed terrible hardships on the Mexican farmworkers deprived of their livelihoods, and might also have led to severe food shortages in Arizona. For these reasons, such a crackdown would probably not have been possible, at least not for more than a very short period of time.[73]

Other factors cited by Innes and Steinbach were totally within Arizona state officials' power to control. These included allowing restaurants and bars to remain open through the winter, the lack of a statewide mask mandate, lax enforcement of even such minimal restrictions as were in place, public officials' statements and actions against regulation, and the state's continuing to allow widespread tourism, not just from other U.S. states but also from Canada and Mexico.

Bars, restaurants, movie theatres and gyms all remained open throughout the Fall and Winter, albeit with capacity restrictions. But although Governor Ducey had ordered the bars, gyms and movie theatres, as well as water parks closed on June 29, they would all be reopened at the beginning of September, as the state 'let down its guard,' in the words of Dr Joshua LaBaer, director of Arizona State University's Biodesign Institute. As LaBaer noted: 'At the beginning of September, things looked really good and then we opened everything up again and almost within a month, we saw those numbers start to rise again.'

Stronger language was used by Will Humble, executive director of Arizona's State Public Health Association, who blamed the state's poor COVID-19 showing on 'a lack of evidence-based mitigation efforts by state officials.' In a line strongly reminiscent of a famous speech from Shakespeare's

Julius Caesar, Humble insisted, 'It is not bad luck or fate… It is largely because of a series of bad decisions, misplaced priorities, and an inability to execute core responsibilities.' Humble would go on to describe Arizona's appalling plight at the end of January as a 'consequence of missed opportunities,' adding 'Sadly, many of these COVID cases and deaths could have been avoided if Governor Ducey and Director Christ (state health department director Dr Cara Christ) had implemented evidence-based public health policy interventions and had learned from their successes and mistakes. Because they did not, many thousands of lives have been unnecessarily lost. It is an unimaginable tragedy.'

Even those limited measures that state officials did grudgingly put in place were generally enforced haphazardly, if at all. An *Arizona Republic* analysis of police data through early December found that *no one* (my emphasis) in the Phoenix area's two largest cities, Tucson and Flagstaff, had been cited for disregarding local or county-wide mask mandates in place since June. Other COVID-related enforcement was almost equally haphazard, with only a handful of businesses cited for staying open illegally or not following reopening protocols. During 2020, Phoenix police and the Maricopa County Sheriff's office cited or referred fewer than 75 businesses out of more than 3,500 complaints received—a paltry 2% rate of follow-up. Businesses and homeowners that held illegal gatherings or violated guidelines typically received only a phone call or a warning, rather than a citation, a fine, or notification of closure. In a climate of such lax enforcement, Arizonans would have been entitled to think that since their public officials didn't really take public health guidelines all that seriously, there was no reason they should, either.

With mask-wearing, it was much the same. Arizona had already 'distinguished itself' as being one of only 13 U.S. states not to have a statewide mask mandate.[74] The matter was left for cities and local municipalities to decide for themselves. While some of them did put mask mandates in place, most evidently relied on 'education' to ensure compliance, rather than any sort of enforcement mechanism. This effectively put the onus of enforcement on businesses, which understandably if regrettably, were not always eager to assume such a responsibility. The inevitable result, in the words of Dr LaBear, was that 'Arizona has had its fair share of… crowded businesses and people refusing to wear masks, at a time when public health experts have recommended people stay home as much as possible.'[75]

Perhaps equally damaging were the statements and actions of certain of Arizona's elected officials who publicly downplayed or even denied the severity of COVID, or who repeated Donald Trump's bizarre advice for possible preventive medications (see earlier for details on this last point). One such official was U.S. Representative Andy Biggs, who throughout the pandemic urged Arizonans to flout national and state public health guidelines on the pandemic, at one point going to the extent of urging Arizonans to 'unmask.' Biggs also parroted Trump's dangerous advice about use of hydroxychloroquine as a COVID preventive. State Republican Chair Kelli Ward had her Twitter account suspended in July for allegedly spreading misleading and 'potentially harmful' information about the pandemic in her tweets. And in early January, Governor Ducey's fellow Republicans voted to censure him over his imposition of emergency regulations during the pandemic. Some of those Republicans in the legislature went so far as to take initial steps 'to curb Ducey and future governors' power during emergencies.'

In a classic display of understatement, Dr LaBaer commented, 'Certainly Arizonans, God bless them, there's a little bit of a libertarian streak in them… We're going to do it the way we want to do it. There are many ways in which that kind of mindset is fantastic—it's what makes us special—but when you need everybody to participate in mitigation factors to prevent the widespread exponential growth of a virus, you really need everybody to participate or else the people who don't care are going to spread [the] virus.' Describing the third wave of the pandemic as 'The worst surge Arizona has ever experienced in its history,' LaBaer warned that despite pandemic fatigue, despite even the mental health issues being experienced by those living in isolation, 'Until we get 60, 70% of people vaccinated, we really need to continue following all the guidelines… it's a frustrating time, I know… because we all know that there's a potential for a way out of this, but we're not there yet, so we have to continue doing what we're doing.'

To say that the attitudes and actions of Republican extremists such as Biggs and Ward did little to improve the situation would be to understate things considerably.

Finally, there was the matter of Arizona's continuing to be an extremely popular winter travel destination, despite the pandemic. Not only did state officials do nothing to halt or even reduce the influx of visitors from other U.S. states, Canada and Mexico; they didn't even enforce the 14-day quarantine usually required of arriving visitors, although they did recommend it.[76] Once again, the results were sad, but entirely predictable.

After Trip Advisor, in its November issue, named Sedona and Scottsdale as top Thanksgiving destinations, cases in the state began to spike in the weeks immediately after the holiday. At the very same time, literally hundreds of youth sports teams from Canada and Mexico as well as other U.S. states 'descended on Arizona for soccer, hockey, baseball and basketball tournaments.' Even if the youthful players were careful on the field, court or ice, there was significantly increased risk of COVID spread from their staying in hotels and going out with their families to stores, restaurants, and other places. While public health officials had urged Governor Ducey to halt sports tournaments statewide until the virus was under better control, he and his officials did nothing along those lines, with the result that the tournaments went ahead and COVID rates in the state increased.

At this juncture, it is worth recalling the sobering words of health official Will Humble, quoted earlier in this section. It was not bad luck or fate that had brought Arizona to its sorry state of affairs, Humble said, but misplaced priorities and bad decisions by state officials. It would be hard to find a better example of misplaced priorities and bad decisions than in the state's remaining open to Thanksgiving break tourism and in particular, to the hosting of sports tournaments at that time. Quite simply, Governor Ducey's leaving the state open to tourism during this critical period showed his far greater concern with the potential economic gains to be had than with the risks to public health and safety incurred by allowing it. Whether a Democratic governor would have kept the state open to tourism and allowed Thanksgiving week sports tournaments to go forward is not entirely clear. One can never be entirely sure. But based on the actions of other Democratic governors such as Andy Beshear as well as the northeastern and Pacific Coast liberals attacked by Trump early on in the pandemic, it seems far less likely that a Democratic governor would have kept the state open to tourism at such a highly risky period.

The case of Arizona shows that a state need not permit huge 'superspreader' events to rank near the top of the list in COVID cases, nor need Republican governors be flamboyant extremists of the ilk of South Dakota's Noem or Georgia's Brian Kemp, who was once criticized by Donald Trump himself for reopening his state too soon—a remarkable achievement in its way.[77] If a state's political culture is sufficiently libertarian and anti-regulatory, all that is required for it to 'achieve' high COVID rates is that its governor be a Republican—any sort of Republican, even a comparatively moderate one such as Rob Ducey. Where mask requirements and business closures of any sort are deemed by a large segment of the population to be an unconstitutional infringement on personal freedom, high COVID rates are as inevitable as would be high rates of malaria in a city surrounded by fetid, mosquito-ridden swamps which the authorities refused to drain. In such a culture, there are severe limits to what any Republican governor can do, at least if they want to win their party's nomination in the next election. As half-hearted as Ducey's summer shutdowns might seem to an observer from Canada, or even a more progressive part of the U.S., they were probably the most he could possibly have put in place given his political situation; as was noted earlier, even these modest restrictions aroused significant political opposition on Ducey's right, including threats to rein in his and future governors' ability to regulate future emergencies.

The point is that simply by functioning as a passive enabler of a political culture which makes horrifically high COVID rates a virtual inevitability, a Republican governor can do nearly as much damage—and without attracting anywhere so much negative publicity from outside their state—as a more flamboyant governor like Noem or Kemp could through open flouting of commonsense restrictions. If anything, the party of a state's governor may be an even more important predictor of its COVID case rates than the degree of support shown for Donald Trump, as it is the governor who has final say as to whether a state's COVID policies are designed primarily to protect the health and safety of the state's residents or to minimize the economic damage resulting from the pandemic. The data provide chilling testimony to the effect that far too few Republican governors, other than the 'non-partisan' ones who for our purposes here might as well be Democrats, appear to realize that one cannot maintain a healthy economy with an unhealthy population—particularly an unhealthy work force. Faced with the choice of keeping their states' economies going or keeping their residents healthy, far too many have opted for the former at the expense of the latter.

Conclusion

In this paper, I have tried to show the great importance of partisan political factors in individual U.S. states' experience with the COVID-19 pandemic—an importance far greater than states' relative population density, which would at first have thought extremely important. The extent of states' support for Donald Trump in the 2020 presidential election, and the existence of a Republican as opposed to a Democratic state governor, both appear to be highly significant factors, with the latter of perhaps even greater importance.

What is not clear is whether such a relationship between partisan political variables and COVID-19 case rates would apply universally, or whether in the case of the U.S., it is a product of factors unique to the country. Comparative analysis involving countries outside the U.S. will be necessary to answer this question. Though such analysis must be left to other hands to complete, I may perhaps be able to provide some preliminary hypotheses in my later paper on interprovincial factors affecting COVID-19 rates in Canada.

Vaccination Rates: Coda (June 19, 2021)

We see an even clearer connection between partisan politics and COVID when we look at vaccination rates by state. In some ways, this is a more purely political variable than COVID case rates themselves, as it is more fully within the control of public officials. Here there are few such outliers as we saw with Table 1 in the case of Rhode Island, Alaska and West Virginia. And while a state's COVID case rates might have been significantly increased simply by virtue of its being situated next to a state hosting a superspreader event, as appears to have been the case with states bordering South Dakota, such as Iowa, Wisconsin and Nebraska, no such factors are in play here.

Even the most cursory glance at Table 2, based on vaccination data as of

214

June 16, shows an extremely strong correlation between high vaccination rates and high rates of support for Democrats (and correspondingly low rates of support for Republicans). All 20 of the states with the highest rates of residents fully vaccinated voted for Joe Biden in last year's presidential election. Eighteen of those 20 ranked among the lowest 20 in their rates of support for Donald Trump; the remaining two (Pennsylvania and Wisconsin) were not far behind. As for the state governors' parties in those 'Top 20' states, 15 had Democratic governors, while another three had 'Non-Partisan' Republican governors—Democrats to all intents and purposes when it comes to anything related to COVID. Only one had an ordinary Republican governor, while the 20th jurisdiction, Washington, D.C., doesn't have a governor as such.

The story is pretty much the same in reverse when we look at the 20 states with the lowest vaccination rates. Of those 20, 17 voted for Trump; the three that voted for Biden did so by hairline margins. Sixteen of the 'Bottom 20' states have Republican governors, and 13 of them ranked among the top 20 in Trump support. This latter group includes the six states where Trump drew his highest percentages.

Of special note: the difference in vaccination rates between the highest (all in New England) and the lowest (most in the Deep South) is of the order of 2:1. This disparity far outstrips the relatively minor differences in inter-provincial vaccination rates we see in Canada. The continuing low vaccination rates in the South and in many of the Rocky Mountain states should be of grave concern to President Biden and his public health officials. It will be extremely difficult, if not impossible, to bring the pandemic under control, particularly at a time when new variants, such as the Delta one, are raising fears of a fourth wave, when over 60% of the residents of many states remain less than fully vaccinated.

A number of policy issues cry out for immediate investigation here. One is whether states with Republican governors have had different types of vaccination campaigns from those run by Democratic governors. A second is whether vaccination resistance and refusal is significantly higher in states run by Republican governors and those with high levels of support for Trump. And a third, given that many of the lowest vaccination rates in the country are in Deep South states with very high numbers of Black people, is whether Black people have lower vaccination rates than the general population and, if so, whether this is the result of their reluctance to get vaccinated, or is rather due to racism in ongoing vaccination campaigns.

215

Jon Peirce

State	% age fully vaccinated (rank)	% age popular vote for Trump in 2020 (rank)	Governor (Party)*
Vermont	63.3 (1)	30.67 (50)	R-NP
Maine	59.3 (2)	44.02 (34)	D
Massachusetts	59.1 (3)	32.14 (49)	R-NP
Connecticut	58.2 (4)	39.19 (42)	D
Rhode Island	56.4 (5)	38.61 (44)	D
New Hampshire	54.3 (6)	45.36 (32)	R
New Jersey	53.7 (7)	41.40 (38)	D
Maryland	53.2 (8)	32.15 (48)	R-NP
Washington	51.9 (9)	38.77 (43)	D
New Mexico	51.4 (10)	43.50 (36)	D
New York	51.4 (11)	37.75 (45)	D
Oregon	50.7 (12)	40.37 (40)	D
Hawaii	50.3 (13)	34.27 (47)	D
District of Columbia	49.9 (14)	5.40 (51)	N/A
Minnesota	49.6 (15)	45.28 (33)	D
Colorado	49.4 (16)	41.90 (37)	D
Virginia	49.3 (17)	44.00 (35)	D
Pennsylvania	47.8 (18)	48.84 (28)	D
California	47.5 (19)	34.32 (46)	D
Wisconsin	47.3 (20)	48.82 (29)	D
Delaware	47.0 (21)	39.77 (41)	D
Iowa	46.4 (22)	53.09 (21)	R
Michigan	45.5 (23)	47.84 (30)	D
Nebraska	45.0 (24)	58.22 (12)	R
South Dakota	44.3 (25)	61.77 (9)	R
U.S.	44.10	46.86	D (President)
Illinois	43.7 (26)	40.55 (39)	D
Florida	43.3 (27)	51.22 (24)	R
Ohio	43.1 (28)	53.27 (20)	R
Kentucky	41.6 (29)	62.09 (7)	D
Alaska	41.4 (30)	52.83 (22)	R
Montana	41.2 (31)	56.42 (16)	R
Kansas	40.6 (32)	56.21 (18)	D
Nevada	39.8 (33)	47.67 (31)	D
Texas	39.1 (34)	52.06 (23)	R
Arizona	38.6 (35)	49.06 (27)	R
Indiana	38.5 (36)	57.02 (15)	R
North Carolina	38.2 (37)	49.93 (25)	D
North Dakota	37.9 (38)	65.11 (4)	R
Missouri	37.0 (39)	56.80 (17)	R
Oklahoma	36.6 (40)	65.37 (3)	R
South Carolina	36.5 (41)	55.11 (19)	R
Utah	35.9 (42)	58.13 (13)	R

Table 2, Part 1: State, Percentage of Population Fully Vaccinated (rank), Percentage of Popular Vote for Trump (rank), State Governor by Party.

State	% age fully vaccinated (rank)	% age popular vote for Trump in 2020 (rank)	Governor (Party)*
Idaho	34.9 (43)	63.84 (5)	R
Georgia	34.8 (44)	49.24 (26)	R
Tennessee	34.1 (45)	60.66 (10)	R
West Virginia	33.9 (46)	68.62 (2)	R
Louisiana	33.4 (47)	58.46 (11)	D
Wyoming	33.3 (48)	69.94 (1)	R
Arkansas	32.9 (49)	62.40 (6)	R
Alabama	31.5 (50)	62.03 (8)	R
Mississippi	28.7 (51)	57.60(14)	R

Table 2, Part 2: State, Percentage of Population Fully Vaccinated (rank), Percentage of Popular Vote for Trump (rank), State Governor by Party.

Sources

For COVID vaccination rates, Mayo Clinic: U.S. COVID-19 Vaccine Tracker, by State. Data drawn June 16, 2021.
For U.S. Presidential election results and Governors, see Table 1.

Notes

[1] I'm aware that the District of Columbia is not actually a state. However, for purposes of the present discussion, it can be treated as one.

[2] Data for this point and (except as noted) all other points concerning U.S. data in the first wave were drawn from the Johns Hopkins University web site on the day indicated in the text. Presumably these data were as of April 30 (the day before my download from the Johns Hopkins website).

[3] Population data drawn from *Wikipedia's* census population estimates as of July 1, 2020.

[4] Including the District of Columbia—see Note 1.

[5] Perry, Jack, 'Why Are COVID-19 Rates so High in RI? Here's one doctor's "best guesses",' *Providence Journal*, December 9, 2020.

[6] One such gathering described by another Brown University emergency physician, Dr Rebecca Karb, was a family Thanksgiving gathering of 22, which resulted in all 22 eventually showing symptoms. See Perry, *op. cit.*

[7] As Laura Strickler and Lisa Cavazuti have noted, West Virginia carried out COVID testing of all its 28,000 nursing home residents in two weeks in March, at the very beginning of the pandemic—two full months before the White House was mandating such testing. Strickler and Cavazuti note that West Virginia was actually ahead of much of the nation in its COVID-19 response, right from the very start of the pandemic, due to a combination of careful planning and the state's close-knit small-town culture. In addition to the early testing of nursing home residents, this careful planning included the creation of a 'team of teams,' which leveraged the National Guard early on to come up with and run an operations command center that focused on inter-agency communications and work with the Department of

Health and Human Resources, the governor's office, and the state's health officers. More recently, that careful planning has entailed strong involvement of local pharmacies, which are more apt to be trusted by West Virginians than national chains, in the vaccination effort. See Strickler and Cavazuti's article, 'We Crushed It': How Did West Virginia Become a National Leader in COVID Vaccination?,' *NBC News* (internet), January 31, 2021, downloaded March 29, 2021.

[8] For those wishing to pursue the matter of West Virginia's COVID record further, two points may be worth considering. One is that although the current Governor, Jim Justice, is a Republican, he was elected as a Democrat and only changed parties after his term had started. It is certainly possible that although Justice may have chosen to change parties for political protection in a state that gave over two-thirds of its vote to Trump, he may still be thinking and governing as a Democrat, at least to a certain extent. A second and somewhat related point is that despite its current strong Republican leanings, West Virginia was not always a Republican state. Through the 1980s and into the 1990s, it was a Democratic state—indeed one of the stronger ones, giving its Presidential vote to losing Democratic candidates Jimmy Carter in 1980 and Michael Dukakis in 1988, and backing Bill Clinton in both his Presidential runs (1992 and 1996). Historically, support for large-scale federal government initiatives was strong in West Virginia, a state whose poverty left it badly in need of federal assistance. It may be that a huge crisis such as the COVID pandemic triggered, particularly among older West Virginians, memories of positive government by FDR, JFK, and LBJ, thus increasing West Virginians' support for the state's quite sweeping COVID initiatives.

[9] The state's previous Republican governor, Sam Brownback, was generally acknowledged (even by many Republicans) to have been a disaster, leaving the state awash in red ink and its education system in shambles. Kelly's opponent, Kris Kobach, had been Secretary of State under Brownback. Had he been elected, he could have been expected to continue Brownback's policies or even make them worse in such areas as voter suppression and treatment of immigrants. Kobach was widely regarded as too extreme for many Kansans. Indeed, a sizable number of current and former Republican office-holders in the state endorsed Kelly, believing that only she of the candidates for the job could restore some measure of political balance. Among those endorsing her was former Republican governor Bill Graves, who said that Kelly was the first Democrat he had supported in his entire life. (Most information in this paragraph, including the statement from Graves, is drawn from the *Wikipedia* article on Laura Kelly, downloaded March 27, 2021). Thus, while Kelly's election was not really surprising, it was also not an event that would necessarily be repeated.

[10] The District of Columbia, treated as a state here, does not have a governor.

[11] The New Hampshire governor immediately preceding the current Republican governor, Chris Sununu, was Democrat Maggie Hassan, who now serves in the U.S. Senate. Indeed, both of the state's U.S. Senators are Democrats—a fact which hardly points to a solidly Republican political culture.

[12] Jacobs, Andrew, 'Despite Claims, Trump Rarely Uses Wartime Law in Battle Against COVID,' *New York Times*, September 22, 2020, updated January 20, 2021, downloaded March 30, 2021. Except as otherwise noted, all materials for the discussion about Trump's coordination of federal government strategy against the pandemic have been drawn from this article.

[13] Jacobs, *op. cit.*

[14] Jacobs, *op. cit.*

[15] Quoted in Jacobs, *op. cit.*

[16] *ibid.*

[17] See, among others, Riechmann, Deb, 'Trump Disbanded NSC Pandemic Unit that Experts Had Praised,' *Associated Press* news story, March 14, 2020, downloaded April 6, 2021. See also Tracy, Abigail, 'How Trump Gutted Obama's Pandemic Preparedness Systems,' *Vanity Fair*, May 1, 2020, downloaded April 6, 2021.

[18] Riechmann, *op. cit.*

[19] Quoted in Riechmann.

[20] Tracy, *op. cit.*

[21] Forgey, Quint, '"We're Not a Shipping Clerk," Trumps Tells Governors to Step Up Efforts to Get Medical Supplies,' *Politics*, March 19, 2020, downloaded April 3, 2021.

[22] Fabian, Jordan, 'Trump Outbid Governors on Coronavirus Supplies after Telling Them to Buy Their Own,' *Fortune*, March 19, 2020. Downloaded April 1, 2021.

[23] Allen, Jonathan, 'Trump's War Between the States Creates eBay-like Fight for Aid,' *NBC News* (internet), March 31, 2020, downloaded April 1, 2021.

[24] *ibid.*

[25] Jackson, David, 'Trump Calls Some Governors 'Complainers' as He's Criticized over Delivery of Coronavirus Supplies,' *USA Today*, April 2, 2020, downloaded April 1, 2021.

[26] *ibid.*

[27] *ibid.*

[28] 'Trump Administration Communication on COVID-19,' *Wikipedia* review article, downloaded April 6-8, 2021.

[29] See, for example, Von Wagtendonk, Anya, 'The Government is Distributing Emergency COVID-19 Supplies. But Some States Are Losing out,' *Vox*, March 29, 2020, downloaded July 1, 2021. Among other things, Von Wagtendonk notes that while Florida had received all the supplies it had requested, Massachusetts had received just 17% of its request. Michigan was another Democratic state experiencing severe shortfalls at the hands of the federal government.

[30] Geller, Adam and Hur, Janie, 'Shameful: U.S. Virus Deaths Top 400,000 as Trump Leaves Office,' *Associated Press*, January 19, 2021, downloaded April 6, 2021. See also Alex Ortiz, 'Blood on His Hands,' in *USA Today*, January 17, 2021, downloaded April 6, 2021.

[31] Geller and Hur, *op. cit.*

[32] *ibid.*

---

33 Miller, Sam and Wu, Jizchuan, 'Coronavirus in the U.S.: Map of How Many Cases Have Been Confirmed Across the Country by State,' *NBC News*, downloaded April 6, 2021. (The map is updated daily).

34 *ibid.* Data are as of April 6, 2021.

35 I use 'his' because, to date, there have been no women elected President of the U.S. Hopefully this situation will change during my lifetime, at which point I shall be delighted to adapt my syntax accordingly!

36 In Maine, daily COVID briefings have been conducted by Dr Vijay Shah, the state's chief medical officer. The state's Democratic governor, Janet Mills, has generally remained in the background during these briefings. It may or may not be coincidental that, as Table 1 shows, Maine ranks near the bottom in COVID rates nation-wide.

37 'Trump Administration Communication on COVID-19,' *Wikipedia* review article, downloaded April 6-8, 2021. Except as otherwise noted, all information in this section is drawn from this compendious article.

38 Death toll drawn from Johns Hopkins Interactive Map for October 29, downloaded April 8, 2021.

39 '2020 Trump's Tulsa Rally,' *Wikipedia.* Downloaded April 11, 2021.

40 'List of post-2016 Election Donald Trump Rallies,' *Wikipedia,* downloaded April 11, 2021.

41 Except as otherwise noted, all information in this discussion of the Tulsa rally has been drawn from '2020 Trump Tulsa Rally,' *Wikipedia,* downloaded April 11. 2021.

42 It remains a mystery to this writer why the Mayor of Tulsa or the city's or state's chief public health officer did not simply order the event cancelled or postponed.

43 Alexander Panetta, 'Trump's touting of an unproven COVID-19 drug is unusual. We'll soon see if he's right,' *CBC News* (internet), April 8, 2020. Except as otherwise indicated, all the information in this paragraph has been drawn from Panetta's article. For a more complete discussion, see the *Wikipedia* review article cited earlier.

44 Cited in Panetta, *op. cit.*

45 Cited in Panetta.

46 Sifakis, Carl, *American Eccentrics* (Facts on File: 1984, no publication place given). This book was subsequently reprinted under the title of *Great American Eccentrics*, with no change in its content.

47 'Outcry after Trump Suggesting Injecting Disinfectant as Treatment,' *BBC News*, April 24, 2020. Except as otherwise noted, all information in this paragraph has been drawn from that BBC article.

48 Kluger, Jeffrey, 'Accidental Poisonings Increased after Trump's Disinfectant Comments,' *Time,* May 12, 2020.

49 *ibid.*

50 Information for this paragraph and the next one has been drawn from the *Wikipedia* review article cited earlier.

51 See note 274 of the *Wikipedia* review article for the full source of the *Wichita Eagle* citation.

[52] See, for example, Reimann, Nicholas, 'Miami Will Keep Issuing Citations for Covid Violations—Defying DeSantis' Order,' *Forbes,* March 18, 2020, downloaded July 1, 2021, and Amanda Holpuch, 'Georgia Mayors Alarmed by Governor's "Reckless" Plan to Reopen the Economy,' *The Guardian,* April 21, 2020, downloaded July 1, 2021.

[53] This has been particularly true with respect to mask mandates. In July, 2020, Georgia Governor Brian Kemp sued the city of Atlanta over its mask mandate, claiming that Mayor Keisha Lance Bottoms lacked the authority to implement the mandate. Earlier that week, Kemp had issued an executive order voiding all mask mandates across the state. See 'Coronavirus: Georgia Governor Sues Atlanta Over Face Mask Rules,' *BBC News,* July 17, 2020, downloaded July 1, 2021.

[54] Walker, Mark and Healy, Jack, 'A Motorcycle Rally in a Pandemic? We kind of Knew What Was Going to Happen,' *New York Times,* November 6, 2020.

[55] *ibid.*

[56] *ibid.*

[57] Cherney, Andrew, 'Is the Sturgis Motorcycle Rally Still Happening for 2020?,' *Cruiser* news story, July 24, 2020, downloaded July 1, 2021.

[58] *ibid.*

[59] 'COVID-19 Outbreak Associated with a 10-Day Motorcycle Rally in a Neighboring State—Minnesota—August-September 2020,' *CDC Morbidity and Mortality Weekly Report,* November 27, 2020.

[60] Walker and Healy, *op. cit.*

[61] AFP Staff, 'U.S. Biker Rally May Have Led to 260,000 New Covid Cases: Study,' AFP Staff, September 8, 2020.

[62] 'S.D. Governor Disputes Report Tying COVID-19 Case Surge to Motorcycle Rally,' *Insurance Journal,* September 8, 2020. (No author given). In one of her milder remarks, Governor Noem dismissed the report as 'fiction.'

[63] In fairness, many of these states also have large number of slaughterhouses, businesses which have also experienced numerous COVID outbreaks. But Sturgis would have dwarfed any of the other outbreaks, significant though they may have been.

[64] Schneider, Grace and Austin, Emma, 'As Cases Soar, Gov. Andy Beshear Unveils New Coronavirus Restrictions for Kentucky,' *Louisville Courier-Journal,* November 18, 2020.

[65] *ibid.*

[66] This is being written on April 13, 2021.

[67] 'Ky Gov. Beshear Announces Lifting COVID Capacity Restrictions/Curfews when State Reaches Vaccine Milestone,' *WSAZ News,* April 12, 2021. Except as otherwise noted, information in this paragraph and the next have been drawn from this news item.

[68] Source: *Wikipedia,* downloaded April 14, 2021.

[69] Source: *Wikipedia* article on the Arizona Legislature, downloaded April 14, 2021.

[70] Innes, Stephanie and Steinbach, Alison, 'Why is Arizona Worst for COVID-19 Nationwide? Here Are 7 Contributing Reasons,' *Arizona Republic,* February 1, 2021,

updated February 2, downloaded April 13, 2021. Except as otherwise indicated, information on Arizona in the following discussion is drawn from this article.

[71] Source for these COVID rates: Centre for Disease Control (CDC).

[72] Cited in Innes and Steinbach, *op. cit.*

[73] It is important to note that there have been problems with Mexican farmworkers bringing COVID into Canada, as well—albeit on a far smaller scale than would be the case in Arizona.

[74] As of the time of publication of the Innes and Steinbach article.

[75] Cited in Innes and Steinbach, *op. cit.*

[76] One can only imagine how many tourists might have complied with the toothless voluntary recommendation. Let's see… how many fingers do we have on both hands…

[77] See, among many others, Gregorian, Dareh, 'Trump Reverses Course, Says It's "Too Soon" for Georgia Gov. Kemp to Reopen State,' *NBC News*, April 22, 2020, downloaded July 1, 2021.

Politics and COVID II
Causes of Canadian Interprovincial Variations in COVID Rates
An Interview with Jon Peirce

Roving Reporter

Good day. This is your roving reporter, broadcasting from the Erewhon Studio somewhere in central Canada. As part of our ongoing weekly series on the COVID-19 pandemic, we're interviewing people who have studied different aspects of that pandemic. Today our guest is Jon Peirce, co-editor of *Plague Take It!* a COVID almanac written from elders' perspectives. He'll be speaking to us from his cozy duplex near the banks of the Gatineau River in western Quebec. Mr Peirce has provided me with explicit tables of data and footnotes to back up his statements, and I have printed these at the end of this document.

Jon, when you started writing about COVID last spring, did you think that the pandemic would still be going on 13 months later?

Yours Truly

Thanks for having me on your show, R-squared. In answer to your question, I suspect that I thought there would still be some cases, but nothing like the situation we have now, which in most of Canada is some orders of magnitude more serious than what we saw during the first wave. But perhaps we should have been prepared for something like this, given that the 1918 flu pandemic, so often wrongly referred to as the 'Spanish' flu, followed a similar pattern in much of North America, with subsequent waves often worse than the first. Those who don't learn the lessons of history are doomed to repeat them, etc.

Roving Reporter

I love history, too, but let's start with something that's in the news today,[1] as we speak. Just yesterday, Ontario Premier Doug Ford, who had earlier requested help from the federal government, withdrew his request on learning the province would be getting increased vaccine shipments from Pfizer. This suggests that Ford sees a connection between increased vaccination rates and lower rates of COVID-19 cases. What do you make of that?

Yours Truly

This *sounds* plausible, but if you scratch beneath the surface, you'll soon see that Ford is completely off base. If you start by looking just at Canada, you will see pretty minimal variation in vaccination rates among the provinces.[2] With vaccines, at least up to this point, having been distributed on a per capita basis, the administration of those vaccines has basically followed suit. Right now, Saskatchewan leads the pack, with 27 jabs administered per 100 people. Close behind is Quebec, with 26 jabs per 100 people. Bringing up the rear is Nova Scotia, with 20 jabs per 100.[3] These are not the kind of variations that lead to much, if anything, in the way of statistical significance. And interestingly enough, Nova Scotia, with the lowest vaccination rate in the country, also has amongst the lowest rates of COVID-19 cases, both overall and over the past seven days.[4]

Roving Reporter

But really, is Mr. Ford so off base as you suggest? Isn't vaccination the way to bring the pandemic under control?

Yours Truly

Ultimately, yes. But it's a long-term solution. It will take weeks if not months for it to have any real effect on COVID rates. With its 4,000-plus new cases per day,[5] Ontario has grave problems in the here and now. Bringing in paid sick leave, as not just the opposition parties but also the medical profession have been urging Ford to do for weeks, is the best way to cut new cases in the short term. With paid sick leave, workers in essential businesses who are sick won't feel compelled to go in to work, sick or not, because they have to pay the rent. *That* would get something done quickly. Ford's inability to distinguish between the long term and the short term is really quite pathetic.

Roving Reporter

That Nova Scotia finding you mentioned a moment ago seems a bit strange. How might we explain that?

Yours Truly

If this finding has any significance at all—and again, note that I hesitate to ascribe any significance in a case with this little overall variation within the sample—it would be that the authorities in Nova Scotia, which has had many fewer COVID cases than provinces in central and western Canada, feel somewhat less urgency about vaccination than do the authorities in most of the rest of the country. You can get a much better illustration of this phenomenon from looking at Australia and New Zealand, two countries where, to all intents and purposes, COVID has been effectively wrestled to the ground. There, the per capita number of doses administered stands at 5.6 and 2.8%, respectively.[6] A good example of causation moving in the opposite direction from what one might have predicted, as low incidence of the disease has evidently created a climate in which there is little urgency about people getting vaccinated. And this can also work in the opposite direction, with high vaccination rates going along with high case rates. We see this in the state of Maine, to give just one example with which I'm quite familiar because I have a close relative living there. There, the unusually high case rates, which I must say came as a shock to me because throughout most of the pandemic Maine was the third or fourth lowest COVID state in the U.S., have arguably driven an extra push toward vaccinating as many people as possible.

Roving Reporter

That's really interesting, and may bear further investigation. But turning back to Canada again…

Yours Truly

Well, as we've already seen, the top-to-bottom interprovincial variation in vaccination rates is roughly one-third.[7] But the top-to-bottom interprovincial variation in COVID-19 cases is huge, whether we look at the per capita rate of new cases—those reported just in the past seven days—or the per capita rate of total cases throughout the pandemic.

Roving Reporter

Just how big are those differences?

Yours Truly

Starting with the new cases, Alberta today shows 212 per 100,000 residents. Close behind is Ontario, with 204 per 100,000.[8] At the other end of the spectrum, you have Newfoundland, with just 2.7 cases per 100,000, followed closely by PEI, with 3.1 cases per 100,000. Haul out your third-grade arithmetic book, and you'll see that this makes for a top: bottom difference of the order of about 80:1!

Roving Reporter

Astounding!

Yours Truly

It really is, and with total cases it is pretty much the same. Quebec 'leads,' with 3,896 total cases per 100,000, with Alberta close behind at 3,789 cases per 100,000. At the bottom of the list is Prince Edward Island, with 105 cases per 100,000. The largest figure you will see anywhere in the Atlantic region is New Brunswick, with 226 cases per 100,000. The top bottom difference between Quebec and Prince Edward Island is about 37:1.

Roving Reporter

Have there been any significant changes in the provinces' relative ranking between the first wave, last year, and the present?

Yours Truly

Oh, indeed there have. As you may recall, the first wave was really all about Quebec, and, to a lesser extent, Ontario and Alberta. Cases were low in the Atlantic region and generally low in the West, except for Alberta.

Roving Reporter

Just how much *did* Quebec dominate the national scene during that first wave?

Yours Truly

To an unbelievable extent. For instance, on April 10, 2020, CBC COVID-19 Tracker[9] data showed Quebec with 10,912 total cases—somewhat over half of the national total of 20,716. The province had also had 216 deaths, or about 40% of the national total of 544. This despite the fact that Quebec has less than a quarter of Canada's total population. Ontario had slightly more deaths (235), but only slightly more than half as many (5759) cases as Quebec, despite having nearly double Quebec's population. By April 13, just three days later, Quebec had taken the lead in fatalities, with 360, about 45% of the national total of 799. Driving the fatality figures were numerous deaths in long-term care homes, whose condition was a scandal all across Canada, but nowhere more so than in Quebec.

Quebec would continue to lead the country in COVID indicators throughout the Spring. On May 8, for example, the province had 36,150 cases, amounting to about 55% of the national total of 65,400, and 2725 deaths, or nearly 62% of the national total of 4408. Unsurprisingly, its recovery rate, meaning the number of recovered cases as a percentage of all non-fatal cases, lagged far behind that of other provinces and the country as a whole. On May 8, the national recovery rate stood at 49%. Without Quebec's abysmally low 27% rate, it would have been about 75%. By this time, no province other than Quebec had a recovery rate below 63%. I remember having a very hard time understanding how Quebec's data could be that bad. It almost seemed more like an American state, in that regard, than a Canadian province.

226

Roving Reporter

Is it true that in those days, a good many people, including some of totally different political persuasion from Doug Ford, were saying he was doing a pretty decent job of handling the pandemic?

Yours Truly

Yes—and I (a near-lifelong New Democrat) was one of them. I was wondering if Mr Ford was the same man who had gotten elected after campaigning as an outright, proud supporter of Donald Trump! Slightly over three in eight (about 38.6%) of Canadians live in Ontario.[10] If you look at the data for April 8, 2020 that we were discussing earlier, you'll see that as of that date, Ontario had about 44% of the country's COVID deaths, a figure slightly higher than the national per capita rate but not out of line with it. Quebec's 40% of deaths must be seen against its 22.8% share of the national population. In other words, Quebec's *per capita* death rate was nearly twice the national average. With regard to case numbers, the contrast between Canada's two biggest provinces was even greater. With nearly 40% of the country's population, Ontario had had just 28% of its cases, giving it a per capita case rate well below the national average. Quebec, on the other hand, had about 52.5% of the country's total cases, despite having less than 23% of its population, for a per capita case rate of about two and a third times the national one.

Beyond the numbers, the situation seemed to be pretty well in hand in Ontario. For the most part, Ontarians seemed to be at least fairly satisfied with how the Ford government was handling the pandemic. With the exception of the long-term care homes—a huge exception, to be sure—we weren't hearing much coming out of Ontario. All the big noise was coming out of Quebec, the condition of whose long-term care homes was in many cases beyond appalling, and to a much lesser extent Alberta, some of whose slaughterhouses and packing plants became small superspreader venues during the first wave.

Roving Reporter

But the third wave has been different...

Yours Truly

Just a bit.

Roving Reporter

And Mr Ford isn't doing so well...

Jon Peirce

Yours Truly
Not quite.

Roving Reporter
While M Legault (Francois Legault, Premier of Quebec), on the other hand…

Yours Truly
Has improved immensely. Of all the country's premiers, I would have to give him the prize for improvement since the first wave, just as I would have to give Doug Ford the booby prize for deterioration.

Roving Reporter
Can we just have a quick look at the big picture before we start taking a more detailed look at the third wave's numbers?

Yours Truly
By all means. During the first wave, it was all about Quebec, and to a lesser extent Alberta. This time, it's all about Ontario and Alberta,[11] with the other western province playing a strong supporting role. Quebec is now out-performing the national average with respect to virtually all the COVID-19 indicators.

Roving Reporter
What about the Atlantic provinces?

Yours Truly
Well, they have been the one constant throughout this whole pandemic. During the first wave, their case and death rates were far, far below those in the rest of the country—so far below that they almost seemed like a different country. And the same has pretty much been true this time around, though there have been a few small-to-medium-sized outbreaks in New Brunswick, particularly in the western parts of the province such as Edmundston and Campbellton, which border on Quebec.

Roving Reporter
How do you explain the continuing low rates in the Atlantic region?

Yours Truly
I think you need to start with their comparative geographic isolation from

228

the rest of the country. If you look at the region as a whole, you'll see that two of the provinces (Newfoundland and PEI) are islands, while a third, Nova Scotia, is a peninsula, with land entry possible from only one other province. Internationally, the countries that have consistently had the lowest rates are generally islands; Australia, New Zealand, and Iceland are three that come to mind. It's really no secret why islands have lower rates than other places. Normally (Prince Edward Island's bridge is the one exception I'm aware of) there are a limited number of ways to get onto these islands; one can generally do so only by plane or ship. This makes it much easier for governments to control entry and to keep out potential sources of infestation.

Roving Reporter
Interesting. Anything else that would help explain those low rates?

Yours Truly
I think there is, although this factor might be harder to quantify. What I'm talking about is the high degree of social consensus you tend to see in this region, as compared to other parts of Canada. It would be fair to describe all four Atlantic provinces as more or less traditional societies, marked by a generally high degree of deference to government and other constituted authorities. In more normal times, this is a trait that some of us (including me) find more than a little irritating. But it's a useful trait for a society to have during a pandemic. In my experience living through the first wave in Nova Scotia, there was a general consensus that government orders and directives around COVID were to be obeyed. The two cases I can recall where people didn't obey those orders involved a woman walking her dog in Point Pleasant Park and a boy shooting baskets in a playground that had been closed. Both incidents made the newspapers, and both individuals received fairly hefty fines. At the time, though I thought the $700.00 fines excessive, I agreed with the actions overall. Now I would say those were serious instances of overkill. The risk of any sort of transmission in such outdoor settings is pretty near zero from all I can tell. And in fact, as many people including some scientists and public health officers have been suggesting recently, it's healthier for people to be outside, getting some exercise, breathing fresh air, and getting out of their own psychological ruts than it is for them to be sitting indoors all the time. This isn't really rocket science, but it was one of those obvious facts that people tended to overlook in their initial panic over the disease.
The truth of the matter is that during the first wave, regulations were a matter of trial and error (though nobody was saying that, then).[12] No one had seen anything remotely like this pandemic at first hand, although some of our more historically aware politicians might have browsed through some old newspaper clippings to look at some of the approaches taken during the

1918/19 pandemic. The result was that (in Nova Scotia, at least—I can't speak for other parts of the country), we were all pretty much terrified into complying with the restrictions, which were really pretty draconian, because none of us knew much of anything about the virus and most of us were as scared as hell. All somebody would have to do, in those days, was mention 'COVID,' and at least 95% of the population would immediately comply with the order or directive, no matter how asinine or nonsensical it might have sounded on the surface. Those were the days of innocence, for sure! All you need to do now is look at the anti-mask protests that have become far too common pretty much across the country (except perhaps in Atlantic Canada), or even at the sneaky, law-circumventing actions of normally responsible, law-abiding citizens, to see how far we have come from those early days.

Roving Reporter

Are you suggesting, then, that somewhere between the first and third waves, the pandemic became politicized in Canada?

Yours Truly

That's exactly what I'm suggesting. In my view, the main reason why the first wave was, by and large, handled so well across Canada was that the pandemic was *not* politicized. There was generally a pretty minimal difference between the approach taken by politicians of the left, like B.C.'s John Horgan, politicians of the right, like Doug Ford and Jason Kenney, and politicians of the centre, like the Atlantic premiers. To the extent that there were differences—leaving Quebec aside as a special case here—they had to do with the timing of measures and the speed with which they were introduced, rather than with the actual measures themselves.

When people abide strictly by the laws and directives, and the laws and directives have been at least somewhat intelligently formulated, the result is very likely to be a much lower incidence of cases. That's exactly what we saw in Nova Scotia, with the single, tragic exception of the Northwood long-term care facility in Halifax, where the vast majority of the province's fatalities and a sizable share of its cases occurred. We certainly saw it in the other Atlantic provinces. Hell, through the first wave, Prince Edward Island not only didn't have any COVID-related deaths; it hadn't even had any *hospitalizations* resulting from the disease. If you look at how the pandemic played out across the rest of North America during the first wave, you'll see that that's a truly extraordinary achievement.

Given Donald Trump's virtually continual politicization of the pandemic throughout his last year in office, it was probably inevitable that some of that politicization would spill over into Canada, particularly into provinces such as Alberta where a larger share of the population would have been sympathetic to Trump's approach to politics overall. And some politicization would likely have occurred even without Trump, even if the U.S. had had a calm professional like Hillary Clinton or Joe Biden in charge in 2020. But probably nowhere near as much as we got, with right-wingers in Alberta and rural Ontario consciously modelling themselves on the Trumpsters in the U.S.

Roving Reporter

Do different types of restrictions and lockdowns explain the variation in COVID rates we saw in different provinces during the first wave?

Yours Truly

Not really—at least, not to any great extent. I was paying close attention to how the different restrictions were evolving at that point,[13] and what surprised me then and still surprises me now is how similar the restrictions and lockdowns were across the country. So similar, in fact, that even minor variations, such as whether or not to allow public parks to remain open, became quite conspicuous. Other variations included whether or not to allow cannabis stores to remain open—Nova Scotia did but Ontario initially did not—the allowable size of private gatherings, whether indoors or outdoors, and the strictness with which restrictions were enforced. In Nova Scotia, as already noted, the restrictions tended to be quite strictly enforced. In other provinces, however, notably Alberta, enforcement often took the form of 'education' around the restriction or restrictions in question, such as regulations banning parking in public parks.

I did notice some variation in how quickly tough restrictions were enacted following the initial reporting of COVID cases in the different provinces. In Nova Scotia, where I then lived, lockdown restrictions were being announced before the province had officially reported even one single case. And on Sunday, March 22, by which time the province had 14 confirmed cases, its restrictions were identical to those of B.C., which by then had around 200 cases.[14] The Atlantic provinces appeared to be somewhere between five days and a week ahead of most of the western provinces in enacting restrictions, despite their later start with cases and overall lowercase numbers. And later, there would be differences over closing the schools, and reopening them. But again, most of these differences had to do with timing, rather than with the measures themselves.

Roving Reporter

What about interprovincial travel restrictions? Those did seem to vary quite a bit, as I recall...

Yours Truly

Yes, you're certainly right about those. By early April, there was a definite east-west pattern to those, with the eastern provinces having tougher restrictions and the western provinces (except for the Territories) having laxer ones. In a small way, this was a foreshadowing of the type of pattern we've been seeing lately, during the third wave.

Roving Reporter

Would you mind getting a little more specific here?

Yours Truly

Not at all. By the beginning of April, Quebec had set up checkpoints, both at its borders with Ontario (including those falling inside the National Capital Region) and at other provincial borders, with the aim of halting all non-essential travel into the province.[15] By this time, a similar ban was in place in the Northwest Territories and Nunavut. The Atlantic provinces hadn't yet started turning people away outright, although New Brunswick later would, in the case of those without what it deemed to be a valid reason for entering the province. But all four were by this time requiring visitors to self-isolate for two weeks upon entry, as was the Yukon. In the West, Manitoba was recommending that same period of self-isolation, though it was not requiring it. The remaining western provinces had at that time no interprovincial travel restrictions at all.

Roving Reporter

Do you think those interprovincial travel restrictions had any effect on COVID rates in different Canadian provinces?

Yours Truly

That's really hard to say. We need to bear in mind that the motivation for these restrictions was different, particularly as between Quebec and the Atlantic provinces. In Quebec, the restrictions were brought in to try to help prevent a bad situation from getting worse. In the Atlantic region, their purpose was to try to keep a good situation from suddenly turning ugly because of an influx of travel-related cases.

For Quebec, I have absolutely no idea whether the restrictions did any good or not. That province's first wave was so heavily dominated by cases (and deaths) coming in great clusters from long-term care facilities and other seniors' residences that I don't know if people coming in in ones and twos really would've made much difference—especially since Quebec's rate was then already significantly higher than that of any other province.

232

For the Atlantic region, and especially for New Brunswick, there's some evidence, albeit of an indirect nature, to suggest that the restrictions might have helped. You may remember that case last spring where a doctor from Campbellton drove across the Quebec border on essential family business, picked up his kid, and then drove back home. Right after he got back home, he went back to work at the hospital, without self-isolating at home at all, despite provincial regulations which dictated two weeks of self-isolation after travelling outside of the Atlantic region. He wound up working for about a week before he and the kid both got COVID...[16]

Roving Reporter

I do vaguely remember that case. . .

Yours Truly

Well, right after that doctor and his son got COVID, so did a whole bunch of other people in Campbellton. Initially, the outbreak was blamed on him. He was suspended from his job at the hospital, and even had to go into hiding after numerous threats were made against him. Contact tracing would later establish that the doctor in question was *not* the cause of the outbreak. But at the same time, about 20 essential healthcare workers had entered New Brunswick from outside the province, some coming from as far away as Montreal. They, too, had not self-isolated. Given the high likelihood that it was one of *these* workers who was the cause of the outbreak, there is reason to believe that the provincial restrictions were in fact useful, since had they been adhered to by the out-of-province health care workers, the outbreak would likely not have occurred.

Roving Reporter

Now, if I've understood you correctly, what you're telling me is that ideological issues such as the party in power in different provinces or the particular character of a given premier's actions did not in fact have much to do with how the first wave was handled and played out. Is that right?

Yours Truly

That is pretty much the case—except for Quebec.

Roving Reporter

What about Quebec, then?

Yours Truly

Quebec's first wave experience was definitely different from that of any other province. Though this is hard to remember now, when Quebec is outperforming the national average with regard to almost all the COVID indicators, during the spring over half the cases and three-fifths or more of the deaths were occurring there. But I don't think any sort of conventional ideological factors, certainly not those of the kind we saw in the U.S.[17] or even in Ontario or Alberta, will be helpful here. While Quebec's current CAQ government is generally classified as being on the right, or at least centre-right, there is a tradition of *dirigisme* in Quebec that cuts across party lines. Like virtually all Quebec premiers, Premier Legault has throughout his term gone in for a degree of intervention that right-wing English Canadian politicians would find totally unacceptable, and that would give even many English-Canadian politicians of the centre-left pause. *(Pause)* But as for his handling of the pandemic during the first wave, the only word I can find to describe it is 'bizarre.' Totally and utterly bizarre.

Roving Reporter
Please explain.

Yours Truly
I'll try, but actually I find it very difficult to explain or even to understand just what M Legault was doing, or trying to do, during that first wave. On the one hand, Quebec had some of the toughest lockdown restrictions in the country, including checkpoints to keep people from entering from Ontario, Manitoba, New Brunswick, and the U.S. On the other hand, big box stores like the Dollar Stores stayed open throughout the first wave. At one point, Quebec had a maximum allowable *outdoor* gathering size of one, meaning that a married couple couldn't legally go for a walk—and certainly not without keeping a six-foot distance from each other. I believe I read an article last year about a married couple being arrested and fined for taking a walk and holding hands in one of the province's big cities. All this while the parking lots were full outside the Dollar Stores, and the stores themselves were busy all day. And then there was the matter of reopening the schools. While couples couldn't take a walk together, the government apparently saw no problem with reopening the schools, bringing hundreds of children and adult teachers and staff together in close quarters for six or seven hours a day, five days a week. If memory serves, the Premier did finally back off on reopening the schools before September in Montreal, after strong protests from teachers' unions and school boards, among others. But the schools were reopened in most if not all of the rest of the province. And for all the personal and travel restrictions Quebecers were faced with, Legault was quite quick in trying to reopen stores, even in malls. After a while, I gave up even trying to make sense of his approach.

Roving Reporter

But perhaps there was some method to all of this apparent madness...

Yours Truly

I don't think so. Quebec's first wave performance was as appalling as Alberta's or Ontario's third wave performance. As we've seen already, despite having less than a quarter of the country's population, the province was consistently reporting more than half of Canada's COVID cases and about three-fifths of its COVID deaths. I don't know about you, but to me that was a sign that there was something very, very wrong with Quebec's approach to the pandemic. If that constituted some sort of 'method,' I shudder to think of what an *unmethodical* madness might have looked like! Fortunately for all of us in Quebec, M Legault appears to have learned from his many first wave mistakes, to the point where Quebec is consistently outperforming all provinces to the west of it in almost every COVID-related indicator.

Roving Reporter

What else was different about the first wave, as compared to what we're seeing now?

Yours Truly

Aside from the lack of politicization, three things come fairly quickly to mind. The first is the nature of the virus itself. A year ago, we were dealing with what appeared, at least, to be a single strain of the COVID-19 virus. Now, in addition to the 'main' strain, we have variants from the U.K., South Africa, Brazil, and most recently India, to name but a few. This makes controlling the disease a good deal more difficult.[18] While the three main variants, those from the U.K., South Africa, and Brazil, have been reported all across Canada, they have been most prominent in Alberta and Ontario. Taken together, those two provinces now account for over 80% of the total number of variant cases reported in Canada.[19]

Roving Reporter

What is the second key difference?

Yours Truly

The age distribution of reported COVID cases. The first wave had a disproportionately heavy effect on seniors over 60, especially those living in nursing homes and other long-term care facilities. This was certainly one reason for the high rate of fatalities as a proportion of cases during the first wave. Older people have always been more likely to die from COVID than younger people. This is especially true of those in nursing homes and other long-term care facilities, who probably were not the healthiest to begin with—otherwise they wouldn't have been in those facilities in the first place. It's important to bear in mind that standard public health measures used during the first wave such as lockdowns, business closures, and travel restrictions would not have done much to help those in long-term care facilities. The vast majority of them weren't going to be going anywhere anyway. But once the disease got established in a given facility, which often happened as a result of staff members on part-time contracts bringing it in from one of the other facilities where they worked, it could spread very rapidly, soon affecting a majority of the facility's residents.

The third wave has been totally different with regard to age distribution. Table 1 (appended to this interview) shows that about 81% of the cases in Canada as a whole and 78% of those in Quebec have been in people under age 60. This means that most cases are now among people of working age or less, people who by and large are still working, raising children, or going to school.

Roving Reporter
How would this play out in terms of differing effects from COVID this time around?

Yours Truly
On the one hand, it could mean a lower hospitalization rate and almost certainly has led to a lower rate of deaths from COVID, since younger people are probably less likely than older ones to require hospitalization and are definitely less likely to die from COVID. But on the other hand, it has almost certainly led to a greatly increased spread of the disease. It's a matter of simple mathematics. The more people one comes into contact with during the course of a day or week, the likelier one is to contract COVID. Those who are working, especially people like essential workers who can't work from home, and those who are going to school, as well as those teaching them, have many more contacts with others, comparatively speaking, than seniors confined to a home. Thus, community spread is increased—sometimes dramatically, as appears to have been the case in Ontario and Alberta.

Roving Reporter
Do the variants play into this?

236

Yours Truly

They may well, although at this point it is hard to know for sure. It's a very significant finding, I think, that over 80% of the cases involving the three major variants have occurred in Ontario and Alberta, the two provinces currently showing the highest rate of new cases. So, I think the issue definitely bears further investigation. Knowing even what I know, I wouldn't bet against it!

Roving Reporter

Any idea what might account for the different age distribution of cases now as opposed to a year ago?

Yours Truly

First off, there has been the vaccination campaign. To date, this has focused primarily on people over age 60. Access to vaccines has been based primarily on an age-related system. Vaccinations began with those over age 80 (or in some cases even older) and gradually worked down in five-year or ten-year increments. While no vaccine offers 100% protection, overall widespread vaccination of seniors has led to a major reduction in the incidence of COVID among seniors. This in turn has led to a preponderance of cases occurring among those under 60, who for the most part have not been able to get vaccinated yet, though the new Astra-Zeneca vaccine has lately become available to younger, working-age Canadians.

Secondly, during the first wave most non-essential workers did stop working, at least for a time. A generous federal benefit (the CERB program) guaranteed a living income for those stopping work because of COVID. Later, this was even extended to self-employed individuals. With most workplaces closed, restaurants and bars closed, and schools in most (though not all) of the country closed, the likelihood of community transmission was greatly reduced. Granted, there were still some cases among essential workers such as bus drivers, hospital staff, and those working in grocery stores or slaughterhouses. But on the whole, so long as working-age people abided by the restrictions and did not participate in illegal gatherings such as private parties or large in-person religious services (a number of which would turn into superspreader events), they would have been relatively unlikely to contract COVID. These days, with most schools having (at least until very recently) generally been open, more workplaces open, and, to be quite frank, a greater carelessness around COVID, a working-age or younger person is quite a bit likelier to be exposed to the disease, whether at work, on the way to and from work, at school, or (as in the case of stay-at-home parents) as a result of direct contact with people who have been regularly been going to work or school.

Roving Reporter
And the third key difference?

Yours Truly
The existence of a vaccine, or, more properly, at least four of them which have been certified as safe to use in Canada. In addition to affecting the age distribution of COVID cases, as we saw earlier, the existence of vaccines gives people (and politicians) more hope that the pandemic may also, finally, be brought under control. But there's also something we might call an unintended negative consequence.

Roving Reporter
What would that be?

Yours Truly
A certain carelessness among large segments of the population, particularly people who have received one jab and are waiting for their second. Some of these folks, as I've seen in articles on the internet, evidently think 'Now that I've been vaccinated, I can go and do whatever I want. The vaccine will protect me.' And it isn't true. While one shot provides significant protection, it is not total protection, particularly not against the kind of concentrated exposure you would get from being part of a large crowd. We learned that early on, in the aftermath of the attempted coup in Washington on January 6. As you may remember, a whole bunch of U.S. Representatives, Democrats and Republicans alike, were huddled together on the floor for safety for some time. While virtually all the Democrats wore masks, many of the Republicans were not doing so. At one point, a Democratic Congresswoman even gathered up a whole bunch of masks and offered them to her Republican colleagues who were without one. Many of them refused her offer. So as a result, you had a huge number of people huddled together in the closest possible proximity to each other—forget about anything even remotely related to social distancing—with a lot of those people not wearing masks. Ideal conditions for the spread of a virus like COVID-19, and indeed, not long after this horrific event, another Democratic Congresswoman, an older woman of around 70, contracted the disease even though she'd been vaccinated a few weeks earlier. The vaccine did help. Thankfully, her case was mild, and she recovered quickly. Still, the case offers a useful lesson for anyone in Canada who thinks they can do whatever they want just because there's a vaccine out there, or just because they've had their first jab. Not so. At least until you are two weeks past your second jab, at which point you can be considered as fully vaccinated, you still need to take the same precautions

you've had to take all along. That means avoiding crowds and large gatherings whenever possible, staying six feet apart from people not in your household or bubble, washing your hands frequently, and wearing a mask in all public indoor settings, at the very least. We are not out of the woods yet, by any means.

Roving Reporter

Anything else you can think of, in terms of differences between the first wave and the third wave?

Yours Truly

One thing you certainly can't disregard is COVID fatigue. By this point, most Canadians have been cooped up to a greater or lesser extent for more than a year. The mental stress is real, particularly on those who were living in isolated circumstances already and those under especially heavy stress, such as working mothers of young children forced to do two-and-a-half jobs at once when the schools close, or those working as caregivers for elderly or infirm family members.

All of us, from age three to 93, have suffered and continue to suffer from COVID fatigue. But younger people, having more energy and perhaps being more inclined toward active rebellion, are more likely to do things like go to crowded indoor parties without their masks—things that put them at significantly higher risk of contracting the virus. Given that many of these younger people are still working, and thus also exposed to the virus in the workplace and (if they use public transit) traveling to and from work as well, they face a sort of 'double whammy.' And given the active, busy lives many of these young people live, they tend to come into contact with many more people each day than do the older retirees who made up the bulk of first wave cases. As a result, community spread of the disease is increased still more.

Roving Reporter

What about the vaccines?

Yours Truly

That's certainly a major difference. During the first wave, all people could do was hope that a vaccine would be discovered and put on the market as soon as possible. The very fact of waiting for a vaccine may have made people a little more careful. I mean, why take chances when it's likely that before too long there will be a vaccine and all our troubles will be over? That seems to have been the attitude of most reasonably sensible people a year or so ago.

239

Now that we have vaccines, it seems that people may be getting a bit more complacent about their personal behaviour, knowing that a vaccine is there to protect them. And, yes, in the long run, vaccination is what will deliver us from this plague—providing that the overwhelming majority of Canadians are willing to be vaccinated. The jury is still out on that one. Even leaving aside the question of resistance to being vaccinated, no vaccine is a 100% solution. What many Canadians apparently don't realize (and some have learned to their great regret) is that it takes a vaccine injection at least two weeks to take effect. And if that injection is your first, even once it has taken full effect it still won't be 100% effective. The figure I've seen most often is 80%, but the estimates I've seen range from 65 to 85%. And it's entirely possible that, given the new variants we're now seeing in Canada, these numbers might be even lower. The long and the short of it is that at least until you are two weeks past your second jab, you still have to maintain pretty much all the same precautions you did earlier.

Roving Reporter
Speaking of masks, we got through the first wave pretty much entirely without masks, except as something you needed to wear to the doctor's or dentist's office. Why are they still needed now?

Yours Truly
That's a most interesting question. And yes, it's true that during the first wave, at least in Nova Scotia where I was then living, you didn't see all that many masks—not even indoors, let alone out of doors. The only place I ever saw very many of them outside was along Spring Garden Road in Halifax. Being the city's main drag, Spring Garden was often a busy place, even during the pandemic, and it could sometimes be hard to maintain a six-foot distance from other people there. Rarely if ever did you see a mask outside in Dartmouth, and even in the grocery stores, only a minority of people were wearing them, many of those being older or infirm people with some sort of pre-existing condition that put them at special risk. It's hard to believe this now, but during the pandemic's first month or so, the medical profession itself was divided on the usefulness of mask-wearing. No less than Dr Theresa Tam herself, Canada's Chief Medical Officer, on more than one occasion expressed open skepticism about the value of masks.[20]

All of that said, the first wave lockdown restrictions were extremely strict in all other respects, and because so many cases were occurring in long-term care facilities, community spread was relatively limited compared to what it is today. Given the strictness of lockdown restrictions generally, masks may not really have been necessary for most people.

Mask requirements in most Canadian provinces came in during the late spring and early summer—a time I have referred to, in another essay in this anthology, as the 'Mid-Cycle Thaw.' This was generally a time of very low case rates, both in comparison to the first wave, and in comparison to the third wave we're now experiencing. At first glance, it might seem odd that this new restriction, which had not generally been applied during the first wave, should have been introduced at a time of general reopening of the country, and a time of such low overall COVID case activity. But in retrospect, it makes perfect sense to me, particularly given that by this time, the medical profession was in general agreement that masks were a useful way of helping prevent the virus' spread. First off, the mask requirement allowed for widespread reopening of the economy while significantly reducing (if not eliminating) the risks posed by that reopening. Secondly, the mask requirement sent Canadians what I consider to have been a useful psychological signal. While things may have opened up somewhat, enough to allow most people to live some semblance of a normal life, COVID was still a threat which we all needed to guard against. Each time someone entered a store or restaurant or some other type of indoor business, the mask was there as a reminder not to let down our guard.

Roving Reporter

Interesting. But of course, since then, for many people—including a great many Americans but also a growing number of Canadians—masks have taken on quite a different symbolic meaning.

Yours Truly

That, unfortunately, is true, and may perhaps be an inevitable result of the far greater politicization of COVID that we've been seeing this time around. For this, we largely have Donald Trump to thank. We might still have a small, vocal minority refusing to wear masks if Trump had not been in power, but as my American interstate piece shows conclusively, Trump did a huge amount to inflame public opinion against mask-wearing, even going to the extent of criticizing his Democratic opponent, Joe Biden, for always wearing masks at his public speeches and rallies. The worst effects of this were felt in the U.S., where at times there were even acts of violence perpetrated against insistent mask-wearers, in stores, by those who viewed masks as an unwarranted interference on personal freedom.[21] But there is no firewall between Canada and the U.S. when it comes to political behaviour, and so it was more or less inevitable that some of Trump's anti-mask sentiments would spill over into Canada, particularly into provinces like Alberta, where support for Trump and his world view tends to be strongest, as well as rural Manitoba, Saskatchewan, and even parts of Quebec.[22]

Nor have those anti-mask and anti-lockdown sentiments been confined to provincial politics. As this piece was being written, I became aware of a Global News story stating that federal MP David Sweet, representing the Ontario riding of Flamborough-Glanbrook just outside of Hamilton, had apologized after issuing a tweet the previous night in which he claimed there was 'no evidence' that COVID-19 lockdowns work and decried the lockdowns as the 'single greatest breach of civil liberties [in Canada] since the country's World War II internment camps.'[23]

When combined with a growing reluctance on the part of Canadian police forces to enforce regulations with which they may not personally agree,[24] such anti-mask and anti-lockdown sentiments create an increasingly serious risk of an anti-mask or anti-lockdown demonstration turning into a superspreader event. Not to mention that the police's growing reluctance to intervene in such events has started to breed a climate of growing public disrespect for the law and the people paid to enforce it. A serious situation, on all fronts! The fact that these demonstrations have been allowed to continue and are even, apparently, becoming more frequent should be a matter of grave concern to anyone working in public health in Canada.

Roving Reporter
Just how politicized has the COVID pandemic become in Canada, would you say?

Yours Truly
To quite a considerable extent, I'm afraid. Granted, we haven't gone quite as far as our friends south of the border did last year. At least not yet. We haven't had a Prime Minister or provincial premier attacking his own medical advisors, as Trump fairly consistently did to poor Dr Fauci. We haven't had a major political figure recommending that people use unproven medications intended for other purposes or drink or inject outright poisons, as Trump did, presumably in an attempt to downplay the seriousness of the disease to Americans.[25] We also haven't had major political figures condoning, let alone promoting, major superspreader events, as South Dakota's Governor Noem did last year with the Sturgis rally.[26] Nor have we had major political figures challenging COVID-related data not to their liking, as Trump did more or less consistently and as Governor Noem did in the case of some studies that appeared in the aftermath of Sturgis. Finally, and thankfully, resistance in Canada has thus far stopped short of the violence that has become all too frequent in the U.S. in disputes over masks and lockdowns. We haven't had the awful spectre of armed men storming the Parliament buildings or provincial legislative buildings *en masse* in a bid to take over the building or kidnap or otherwise harm a premier, as was the case in Michigan when a gang of thugs stormed the state capitol and tried to kidnap Governor Gretchen

Whitmer, who had imposed the lockdowns these men disagreed with. And we also haven't had many (or perhaps any) of the sort of altercations that have become all too frequent in the U.S. over the wearing or non-wearing of masks in busy, crowded stores like Wal-Mart. Thank God for all that!

Roving Reporter
Still…

Yours Truly
Still, the U.S. is a very low bar indeed. A country could be doing a lot better than the U.S. and still not be doing very well at all. As, I fear, is the case with Canada with regard to COVID generally, and particularly with regard to political resistance to COVID-related restrictions such as lockdowns and mask requirements. As you think about the resistance to COVID, please bear in mind one simple fact. The U.S. has now had over 31 million cases reported.[27] Even assuming that there haven't been any additional cases that have gone unreported, which is probably an optimistic assumption, this means that nearly one American in 10 has had the disease. Nearly one in ten! To me, this is beyond appalling.

Roving Reporter
Would you mind giving some examples of how the resistance to government regulations around COVID has played out in Canada?

Yours Truly
Not at all. Moving west to east, CBC News recently had a story about a restaurant in Vancouver's Kitsilano district that has not only continued to operate despite repeated closure orders and formal suspension of its business license, as well as a province-wide ban on indoor dining in effect through the end of May, but on the night of Friday, April 23 held a rally with dozens of unmasked protesters blocking the sidewalk and the street.[28] An angry Vancouver Mayor Kennedy Stewart declared in a tweet that the decision by Corduroy Restaurant owners 'to continue to [sic] flaunt[29] public health orders despite the city suspending their business license is unacceptable. I am exploring all avenues to bring a stop to this—including a court injunction.' Owner Rebecca Matthews' actions drew down on her the fire not just of Mayor Stewart, but also of the president of the B.C. Food and Beverage Association, Ian Tostenson, who said he'd warned Matthews earlier in the month that her course of action would 'not end well' for her if she continued with it, adding 'The fact is that the way she's conducting herself is not going to do her any favours, and I don't want it to represent the hard work of thousands of

businesses that have done it the right way.' I'm sure you'll agree that things have reached a pretty sorry state when business owners feel they can defy suspension orders and shutdowns of their entire sector.

Roving Reporter

Indeed. So (continuing our move west to east), what about Alberta?

Yours Truly

In this historically right-wing, libertarian province, resistance has entered the formal political arena. Now, Jason Kenney is arguably the country's most right-wing premier, and you might find it hard to believe he could have attracted significant opposition from the right. But that's exactly what has happened, by golly. After Kenney, in the face of spiralling case numbers, including many cases involving the new variants, ordered a relatively moderate set of restrictions, including closure of restaurants to eat-in dining and reduction of capacity of gyms and retail stores,[30] 16 of his own United Conservative Party (UCP) MLAs—a quarter of the total UCP caucus— signed a letter decrying the restrictions. Signatories included the current House Speaker and a former cabinet minister.[31] The letter said that issuing the restrictions listed above was 'the wrong decision' and would move the province backward. Striking a pure libertarian note that Ayn Rand herself might have applauded, the letter-writers went on to say, 'We have heard from our constituents, and they want us to defend their livelihoods and freedoms as Albertans. For months, we have raised these concerns at the highest levels of government and unfortunately, the approach of the government has remained the same.'

In a cosmic piece of irony, on the same day the dissident MLAs' letter was issued, the province recorded 1,351 new COVID cases, its highest level since New Year's Eve, including 575 cases (nearly half the new total) involving variants of concern.

CBC columnist Graham Thomson suggested that the far right might have been feeling betrayed by Kenney, who last year had 'called COVID-19 the "flu," downplayed its lethality, defended the right of anti-maskers to hold public demonstrations, and made it easier for people [including members of his own caucus, who soon took full advantage] to fly to vacation hot spots.'[32] What will happen to the dissident MLAs who signed the letter is not yet clear. What is clear is that Kenney is faced with a horrendously difficult choice, between saving his citizens' lives and his own political survival.[33] As little as I like him, I don't envy him that choice.

Roving Reporter

So, what exactly has Kenney done about the public health laws since he received that letter?

Yours Truly

As late as Monday, Kenney was rejecting calls for stricter laws, saying all that needed to be done was to enforce existing regulations more strictly.[34] But by the end of the week, a continuing rise in cases forced him to take stronger action. Both Thursday and Friday saw the province record more than 2000 new cases—nearly twice as many as were being recorded in Quebec, a province with nearly twice Alberta's population. Worse yet, over 60% of Alberta's active cases have been identified as being variants of concern. And ICU utilization in hospitals has risen to record levels.[35] If you look at the tables at the end of this paper, you will see that Alberta is at or near the high end in just about every COVID indicator. It ranks highest in case positivity (Table 2), second only to Ontario in number of variant cases (Table 3), and highest in both per capita new cases and per capita total cases—and all this before the last week, which has seen a still further increase in cases. All totally predictable, of course. As Calgary emergency room doctor Joe Vipond said, the continuing rise in COVID cases is a clear reflection of government policy failure. 'We've avoided making the hard decision of putting in strong restrictions... and this is what you get... exponential growth.' Quite simply, the pandemic in Alberta is now completely out of control.

Roving Reporter

And Kenney's response has been...

Yours Truly

To bring in new, 'targeted' measures. Don't laugh. That is what he has done. With what are now by far the worst numbers in the country, Alberta's restrictions are still less severe than those of Quebec, whose numbers in the third wave are better than the national average. What is most noteworthy, perhaps, is what he didn't do. No province-wide lockdown. No province-wide curfew. No province-wide travel restrictions. And diners can still eat outside on restaurant patios, providing they do so in groups of a single household per table. (Wonder how restaurant staff are supposed to enforce that). Such as they are, the new 'targeted' restrictions apply in communities with more than 350 active cases per 100,000 population and at least 250 active cases in all.

Roving Reporter

Looks like he's trying to let rural areas off the hook...

Yours Truly

Yes, it looks that way to me as well. In any case, the affected communities include Edmonton, Calgary, Fort McMurray, Red Deer, Grand Prairie, Airdrie, Lethbridge and Strathcona County. The new restrictions are for a minimum period of two weeks. All primary and high schools in the affected communities have been moved to at-home learning. All gyms and indoor fitness centres have been closed, and scheduled surgeries (presumably not of an emergent nature) have been cut back by up to 30% in the two major centres and in the North to make room for a possible influx of COVID patients into the hospitals. And that, my friend, appears to be about it.[36]

Roving Reporter

If that's what the new, restrictive regime looks like, I hate to think of what the previous one looked like. Whew! That Dr Vipond sure said a mouthful there. In any case, now on to Saskatchewan...

Yours Truly

Where Tommy Douglas is at this moment spinning alarmingly fast in his grave at the sight of what has happened and is happening to his beloved province.

Roving Reporter

Are you by any chance referring to the children's anti-mask festival that was scheduled for Saskatoon for April 24?

Yours Truly

That's definitely one of the things I was referring to. By the way, the festival did go ahead as scheduled on the 24th, despite a personal plea from the city's mayor that people stay away, and despite warnings and pleas from local officials and a justice studies professor at the University of Regina. About 100 people, many of them children and virtually all of them maskless, attended. There was face painting as well as various other games designed specifically to attract kids.[37]

Roving Reporter

Sounds bad enough. But there's more, you say?

Yours Truly

Oh, definitely. A whole lot more. First off, I'd say it speaks volumes that, given all his misgivings about the festival, which he went so far as to describe as 'insane,' in an interview earlier in the week, the city's mayor didn't simply order it cancelled or postponed.

Roving Reporter
Fear of backlash from the far right, perhaps?

Yours Truly
That's entirely possible. But I really have no idea. In any event, both this event and a similar one held the week before in Prince Albert raise larger issues around police enforcement of public health restrictions—or the lack thereof.

Roving Reporter
Can you give some details about how police enforcement seems to be working in Saskatchewan?

Yours Truly
The short answer is that to all intent and purposes, it's not, because there really isn't any. Even after the children's festival, Saskatoon police said that they had issued only 11 tickets to protesters throughout the entire course of the pandemic.[38] In many other Canadian cities, particularly those in eastern or central Canada, a single demonstration might well have resulted in a greater number of formal charges than that. The minuscule number of tickets issued lends strong credence to University of Regina justice professor Michelle Stewart's assertion that protesters are operating in 'a culture of impunity' because police are quite simply refusing to act.

In Stewart's view, police inaction is itself a serious threat to public health and safety. Speaking of the two events to be held in Saskatoon on April 24, she said: 'These have all the potential to become superspreader events. It's quite concerning. We are trying to figure out how to get ahead of COVID, not to spread it around.' By in effect looking the other way at demonstrations involving large numbers of unmasked people, the police, in Stewart's view, are simply not doing their job. During a pandemic like COVID, she said, 'The role for police and politicians and other leaders is to say, "These events are not welcome. You cannot gather." And the public health orders need to be enforced more rigidly.'

Roving Reporter
Sensible advice, but not really rocket science, would you say?

Yours Truly
Not exactly. But advice which, for whatever reason, the citizens, police forces, and elected officials of Saskatchewan seem to have found extremely difficult to follow.

Jon Peirce

Roving Reporter

I notice that you used a past tense, or, more precisely, a past perfect tense in your last statement. Did you mean to suggest by this that lax enforcement in Saskatchewan is a phenomenon that was going on for some time even before the Saskatoon events were planned?

Yours Truly

That's exactly what I meant to suggest! At least three months before the Saskatoon events, a Saskatoon psychiatrist named Tamara Hinz was making a very similar point to Stewart's with regard to local bars' open flouting of closing hour restrictions. Said Hinz at the time, 'We can't have a conversation about rule compliance without enforcement.' She added, quite tellingly, I thought, that 'It would help if people start[ed] thinking of the pandemic as a group effort.'[39]

Roving Reporter

Why did you find Hinz's statement so significant? Isn't it, like Stewart's statement, not much more than simple common sense?

Yours Truly

It is… but again, in certain populations 'common sense' can be quite rare indeed. What her statement tells me is that many if not most of her fellow Saskatchewan residents hadn't been seeing dealing with the pandemic as a group effort, and were in fact approaching things from a highly individualistic 'me first!' kind of attitude. In a nutshell, it sums up the approach that far too many westerners and Ontarians have been taking toward the pandemic, at least throughout the third wave, after things had become more politicized.

Roving Reporter

So, what you're saying is that through their inaction, the province's police are providing some sort of at least *de facto* endorsement of the prevailing radically individualistic political philosophy?

Yours Truly

Exactly—and, again, the consequences of this are potentially really scary. In a nutshell, at a time when many if not most citizens view pretty well any restrictions on their personal freedom as unwarranted, and the police effectively go along with such a view by not enforcing public health regulations regarding masking and public gatherings, such gatherings will continue, as they have in Saskatchewan, more or less unchecked—and COVID cases will rise dramatically.

Roving Reporter

Are there at least some residents of the province who don't agree with the police's hands-off approach to demonstrations and other violations of the public health laws?

Yours Truly

Oh, there definitely are some. One of them, for sure, is a guy named Kelly Munce, who was lying in a hospital bed in Regina with severe COVID at the time when the Saskatoon festival was going on. Munce was outraged on learning that a health inspector had shaken hands with the organizer of an out-of-province convoy during a stop in Maple Creek and then invited the man to stay a while.[40]

'That was like he just spit in my face. I'm lying in hospital with COVID-19 and he's... going up to a guy who's claiming it's fake and doesn't exist, claiming "freedom" and "don't wear masks." I was just dumbfounded by that,' Munce said in a phone interview from his Regina General Hospital bed this week.[41]

'I'm starting to think it's a symbol they're not enforcing the rules,' said Munce, adding that it had become increasingly clear that people wouldn't listen to polite requests to stop breaking the laws, and would only stop doing so if made to by some kind of authority.

Munce's outrage is shared by University of Saskatchewan infectious disease expert Andrew Potter, who said police must break up the gatherings, or at least ticket everyone there on the spot. What has happened instead is that police have escorted protesters and blocked off road and park access to the public during these illegal gatherings and marches, only occasionally issuing tickets following events. (According to another CBC story, 11 tickets were issued following the Saskatoon festival—a number representing a mere fraction of those in attendance.)

'The way it comes across is that the police are, in fact, protecting the protesters, not protecting the vast majority of the province of Saskatchewan,' Potter said. 'That's just not right. We have public health orders on the books and they need to be enforced. If they're not enforced, it's a farce.'

Just how many Saskatchewan residents share the views of Munce and Potter is anybody's guess. The fact that ultraconservative Saskatchewan Party leader Scott Moe saw his government re-elected last year, during the pandemic, with a big majority, is not a good omen for the future in this regard.

Roving Reporter

Do Saskatchewan's COVID case numbers lend some credence to this?

249

Yours Truly

I think they do, though precise connections may be difficult to establish here. We'll be taking a quite detailed look at the numbers shortly. For now, suffice it to say that despite its lack of any big cities, the province ranks third worst in new cases per capita, behind Alberta and Ontario, and third worst in total per capita cases, behind Alberta and Quebec. Its test positivity rate (as a percentage of completed tests) is a troubling 7.1%. So, yes—and I do think my U.S. paper shows this as well—there does seem to be a connection between a jurisdiction's libertarian, individualistic political philosophy (and that of its political leaders) and high COVID rates.

Roving Reporter

Continuing our eastward swing, what about Manitoba?

Yours Truly

We haven't heard as much about Manitoba as we have about some of the 'flashier' western provinces. But some of the stuff that's been going on there is quite amazing—even stranger, in its way, than the stuff we were just discussing from Saskatchewan.

Roving Reporter

Do tell. Inquiring minds need to know.

Yours Truly

To give just one example, there was recently (on April 17) a rally protesting the province's public health orders.[42]

Roving Reporter

That in itself doesn't sound so surprising. These rallies are being held pretty well all across the country these days.

Yours Truly

True. But there were some special features about this rally that bear close attention.

Roving Reporter

Such as?

Yours Truly

To begin with, its size. A CBC videographer on the scene estimated there were 300 people in attendance. The fact that a CBC videographer made the estimate cited in the piece may itself be of some significance.

Roving Reporter
Why is that?

Yours Truly
Because such estimates normally come from the police or other authorities supervising the rally.

Roving Reporter
So?

Yours Truly
(Patiently, but with a patience that's beginning to fray a bit)
What does it tell you when there's no police estimate of the rally's size? What this tells me is that police probably weren't there at all. And this indeed appears to have been the case. Unless the police were there in plain clothes, which seems rather unlikely. That same videographer saw no sign of either police or public health officials at the rally. Which is really surprising, in fact even shocking, given many of the features of the rally.

Roving Reporter
Well, what about those features, in addition to its size?

Yours Truly
The size itself is highly significant. As the story's subhead tells us, public gatherings in Manitoba are limited to a maximum of 25. This gathering had 12 times that number of people, which should itself have been a trigger for some kind of official action.

Roving Reporter
What else?

Yours Truly
Most of the protesters weren't wearing masks, and they were definitely not practicing any sort of social distancing. As you can see from the picture included

251

with the internet news story, they were gathered together across the grounds in good-sized clumps.

Roving Reporter *(wearily)*
Anything else?

Yours Truly
Indeed, there is. Some of the featured guests were high-profile, to the point of outright notoriety. One was Patrick Allard, who has organized anti-mask protests and runs a Facebook group espousing 'freedom of speech' and 'freedom of choice' messages. Another was Tobias Tissen, minister of the Church of God in Sarto, Manitoba. His congregation has been fined many times for holding large, in-person gatherings in violation of public health orders, and members of his congregation have also clashed with police and other enforcement officers. Guys like this don't come to a little place like The Forks to view the scenery. They mean business. They're bad news. Stepping aside when they are known to be coming to town would be akin to the sheriff's booking off for vacation when John Dillinger had just been spotted in the area.

Roving Reporter
Yet in the face of all this, the authorities apparently did not send so much as one cop or public health official, even to observe what was going on, let alone put a stop to it. Is this what you're telling me?

Yours Truly
That's exactly what I'm telling you.

Roving Reporter
Why, given all the violations of public health orders and the very real likelihood of a serious confrontation, did the authorities *not* have police on the scene?

Yours Truly
I wish I knew. Unfortunately, I'm not privy to what goes on inside these people's heads, so I don't have an answer for you. Laziness, perhaps. Cowardice, very possibly. Simple incompetence carried to an extreme. An unspoken belief—common in the west and even more common in much of the U.S.—that anything that goes on is OK so long as it has a 'church' label to it. The fact that many of the authorities actually agreed with the protest. Possibly even all of the above.

Roving Reporter

So, would you say that this situation was even worse than the Saskatchewan one we were talking about earlier?

Yours Truly

I would, actually. There, as the stories noted, police were at least on the scene, if only to 'observe and escort.' That isn't in my view the role they *should* have been playing, but at least they were there. Had the situation got out of hand, they'd have been able to put a stop to it. The fact that police and public health officials were not even there heightened the already great danger the event posed to the public. It also sent the ominous message that anyone else planning to hold such an event could feel free to proceed, that the authorities would almost certainly look the other way, as they had at The Forks.

Roving Reporter

Did the CBC ask local or provincial officials about the lack of police presence at the protest?

Yours Truly

They did. Specifically, CBC News asked the provincial government if enforcement officers had been aware of the rally ahead of time. The reply they got was not, to say the least, reassuring.

Roving Reporter

What was that reply?

Yours Truly

The provincial government spokesperson to whom they talked said that any updates with regard to enforcement would not be made available until the following Tuesday—three full days after the rally! Not to be cynical, but to me it sounds very much as if the province felt it needed three days to pull together some kind of story to cover their backsides in the face of what had amounted to, at the very least, severe negligence on the part of enforcement officials.

Roving Reporter

And now for the sixty-four-thousand-dollar question: How have Manitoba's case rates been trending lately, in the wake of this possible superspreader event?

Jon Peirce

Yours Truly

Glad you asked that question. As it happens, new cases in Manitoba are rising at an alarming rate. At a time when many provinces' new case rates[43] are going down, and the national rate of new cases is down about 8%, Manitoba's rate is up by more than half, at 53%. Only Nova Scotia, among the provinces, has a higher rate of increase, and its circumstances are special given the exceptionally low base it was starting from. Moreover, if you look at the province's test positivity rate, it is not reassuring either. That rate (see Table 2) is an alarming 8%, third highest in the country behind Alberta and B.C. Given that the test positivity rate is a sort of 'lead indicator' pointing the direction for cases in any given jurisdiction for the next week or two, Manitoba authorities should be very, very worried. I wish I saw more signs of concern coming from them.

Roving Reporter

Do you think that that April 17 protest might have had something to do with these high rates?

Yours Truly

Well, you can't attribute higher case rates throughout a province entirely to a single event, however big that event may have been. But it almost certainly had some effect—just how big an effect may take some time to figure out. And, if I can just rephrase a point I made earlier, it may have had as big or even bigger an indirect effect than the demonstration's direct event, by sending Manitobans the message that they could hold protests with impunity and that, indeed, they could pretty well do whatever they wanted, because enforcement officials would almost certainly be looking the other way whatever they did. Everyone knows that a law that isn't enforced is not worth a hill of beans, however reasonable and sensible may have been its design.

Roving Reporter

This is all starting to look like a pretty grim picture. I almost hate to ask you what's going on in Ontario, but duty compels me...

Yours Truly

So much to be said here that I hardly know where to begin. But since we were already on the subject of lack of enforcement, we may as well begin with a church service that took place recently in Aylmer, Ontario. As has often been the case with anti-mask and anti-lockdown events in rural Ontario, maverick redneck MPP Randy Hillier was at the heart of it. You may remember, he was the one who was kicked out of the provincial

Conservative caucus a while back...

Roving Reporter
Yeah, I seem to remember that name. So, what's Randy been up to this time?

Yours Truly
Along with Kingston-area MP Derek Sloan, another renegade Conservative who's been kicked out of his party's caucus, he's been charged for taking part in a large, indoor church service earlier this month at the Church of God in Aylmer, a place that has become notorious for violating COVID-19 restrictions on indoor worship service size. The maximum under current Ontario law is supposed to be 10, but this service was believed to have had about 100 in attendance. The sermon, preached by pastor Henry Hildebrandt, was a fiery defence of civil disobedience and non-violent resistance to provincial COVID restrictions. Calling other pastors who wouldn't open their churches 'noodle-backs,' Hildebrandt said, 'people say to us, "Why can't you just be kind, wear a mask? Is it that hard?" It's not about that. It's not about the mask... We will not kneel down. Every single person in this room, I admire you for taking a stand in this time.' Hildebrandt went on to call Sloan, Hillier, former neonatal nurse Kristen Nagle, and an off-duty police officer up to the pulpit, praising them by saying 'This is what leadership looks like in 2021.'[44]

Roving Reporter
What else has Hillier done?

Yours Truly
Among other things, he and his sons were charged in connection with a brawl in Perth earlier this spring. He was also charged in connection with an illegal demonstration at a brew pub in Kemptville.

Roving Reporter
So, given that the man seems to have no respect whatever for the law, and keeps on attending and even leading illegal demonstrations no matter how often he has been charged and fined, why is he still at large?

Yours Truly
I've often asked myself that same question. To me, locking him up or revoking his driver's license would appear to be a no-brainer. But with him, as with so many people and illegal demonstrations in the western provinces, the authorities simply seem reluctant to act, or at least to act decisively enough that trouble-makers are deterred from continuing to make trouble.

Roving Reporter

How exactly does that reluctance show itself?

Yours Truly

There are a number of different ways, depending on where one is and what kind of authority is being referred. If we could return to Aylmer for a moment, that community's approach appears to have been characterized by what its police chief Zvonko Horvat has referred to as an 'educative' approach toward violations of the public health ordinances. While admitting that in this case, 13 months of the 'educative' approach had failed, leaving him with no choice other than to lay charges, he said Aylmer police had taken and would continue to take a 'gradual' approach toward education and liaison with the church and the community in cases involving non-compliance with COVID rules. In a truly astounding statement, Horvat added, 'From my perspective, I hope and wish that people would understand the current situation that we were in however we can't control their actions.'

Roving Reporter

Thereby suggesting that, for whatever reason, Aylmer police have all but given up on strict enforcement of the COVID rules, at least for townspeople?

Yours Truly

Exactly. This sends the message that, particularly if you live in Aylmer, you will not be punished, at least not by anything more than a slap on the wrist, for violating the public health restrictions. Hardly the right message to be sending at a time of continuing high caseloads, including a great many involving the new variants. (As Table 3 shows, Ontario has more of these than any other province in the country).

Roving Reporter

But what's wrong with educating people about the law? Isn't that more constructive than moving in with heavy-handed enforcement measures?

Yours Truly

With respect, I would say that Chief Horvat appears to have misunderstood the appropriate role for education in law enforcement. Education is appropriate when new measures are first brought in. It should be used for a relatively brief period, to allow people to become familiar with those new measures. But it should be an introduction and a complement to enforcement, not a substitute for it. After a certain length of time—say, a month—the educational phase of enforcement needs to end, and fines, jail terms, and other penalties issued. If this doesn't happen, people will get the impression that the authorities simply aren't serious about enforcement—and will go on doing what they've been doing. The fact that there have been numerous illegal services at that church in Aylmer speaks volumes. After the first service, yes, warnings could have been issued, as an educational measure. But after the second and certainly after the third illegal service, fines and other penalties should have been levied. And if the church had continued its illegal services with impunity after a couple of rounds of fines, the authorities should have concluded that the pastor and other church leaders had no intention of complying with the law, and ordered the church padlocked, permanently if necessary, and the pastor and other church leaders jailed. That is the only effective way to deal with people who repeatedly flout the law.

Roving Reporter

So why *didn't* the Aylmer police deal with the church as you've suggested they should have?

Yours Truly

Again, I have no idea. Cowardice. A reluctance to lay criminal charges against one's friends and neighbours. The knowledge that at least some police force members sympathized with the pastor's approach.[45] Whatever the reason, the approach clearly hasn't worked. I would suggest that if the local police force can't or won't take the appropriate enforcement measures, it may be time for the OPP to step in. Perhaps even past time.

Roving Reporter

Do you think Doug Ford would've been willing to send in the OPP?

Yours Truly

Quite honestly, I've no idea. He might have been more willing to call in the provincial police force than Jason Kenney would have, but that's a pretty low bar. Perhaps the main difference between the two is the political context in which they operate. Despite Rachel Notley's surprise win a few years ago, Alberta is, overall, a pretty solidly right-wing province. Ontario is more to the centre—a bit right of centre, but pretty much middle of the road overall. So, while some of Kenney's most serious opposition may be coming from the right, Ford's is definitely coming from the left. And he is definitely in trouble heading into next year's election, which makes his current course of action (or inaction) even harder to explain.

Roving Reporter

How would you sum up Ford's overall approach to the later waves of the pandemic?

Yours Truly

The sad thing for me is that unlike his neighbour, Premier Legault of Quebec, he appears to have learned nothing from the pandemic's first wave, and indeed seems to have retrogressed quite badly, from a respectable performance to second worst in the country, behind only Alberta.

The one consistency in his strategy—if we can say he even *has* a strategy—is his inability and/or unwillingness to address larger structural issues, such as the condition of the province's long-term care homes or the lack of sick pay for workers. (True, he finally may be doing something about the latter, but he has had to be dragged, kicking and screaming, to take the very modest steps he appears finally to be ready to take, in that direction). I'm not sure whether his failure to deal with structural issues such as these arises from his inability to conceptualize how to deal with them, or from his unwillingness to spend money—admittedly, large sums of money, in the case of the LTC homes—which in his view would be far better spent giving tax breaks to his millionaire friends.

Aside from that, his 'strategy' appears to be pretty much reactive. When the medical and scientific community put heat on him to bring in more restrictions, he responded by shutting down things like playgrounds, which were about the only places where poor kids living in apartments or projects could get outdoor exercise. Then he backpedalled on that, with a tearful apology. With the checkpoints it was much the same. First, they were going to be there, and enforcing entry strictly, and then he backtracked on that after public criticism, saying the checkpoints would be operating only selectively. The result is that the general public is confused, not knowing, almost literally from one day to the next, what they can and can't do. And the constantly changing regulations pose serious difficulties for those charged with enforcement, as well. Because people don't know what his overall plan is, or even if he has a plan, they have started to use their own judgement and to pretty much do what they like. The lack of a clear overall strategy has definitely bred in Ontarians a disrespect for the law and for the government that is supposed to be making and enforcing that law. And that isn't in any way a good place to be.

Roving Reporter

Some have characterized Ontario's third wave pandemic performance as a 'preventable disaster.' Would you agree with that characterization?

Yours Truly

I certainly would! Far-sighted people, like Timothy Ellis,[46] have seen this coming for some time. And so have I. Yet Ford has continued to do pretty much the opposite of what a true leader would have done in the same situation.

Roving Reporter

What are some examples of what he's done—or not done?

Yours Truly

Got another four hours? Seriously—there's so much I *could* say that I hardly know where to begin. But a great deal of it can be summed up like this: failing to use the advice his medical and scientific advisors have given him in formulating a pandemic strategy. No, he doesn't go around attacking those advisors the way Donald Trump did when he was in power. This is, after all, Canada, and such tactics wouldn't play well here—not even in Kenney's Alberta. But he does have a bad habit of ignoring or misconstruing a lot of what his advisors are telling him, and then doing pretty much what he pleases when it comes time to formulate new strategies.

Roving Reporter

Again, some examples would be helpful here.

Yours Truly

I think we've already talked about paid sick leave. This was something his medical and scientific advisors had been urging him to bring in—or bring back, since he had actually cancelled a paid sick leave program instituted by a previous government—for some time. His initial failure to do this, combined with what some saw as a lack of equity in his initial approach to vaccination, led the Director of Ontario's COVID-19 Scientific Advisory Table, Dr Peter Juni, to seriously consider resigning.[47] But this was far from the first time that Ford had failed to listen to his scientific advisors. In early November, he introduced new guidelines for COVID restrictions, claiming to have consulted public health professionals in devising the guidelines. However, the guidelines had thresholds for activation that were four times higher than public health doctors had actually called for. In essence, Ford was lying to Ontarians about his use of scientific advice.[48]

Roving Reporter

Anything else?

Yours Truly

As Ellis has pointed out, he's refused to offer supports for small businesses or employees, passing the buck to the federal government. He also refused to adequately support schools, and was tardy about closing them when they proved to be vectors for transmission. The one thing he's good at—and this is something he *does* have in common with Donald Trump—is blaming other people and other levels of government for his own government's failings. His focusing attention on the apparent lack of vaccine in Ontario was one example of this. Since the federal government is responsible for distribution of vaccine to the provinces, this was something he thought he could blame the federal government for, even though there was no evidence at all that Ottawa had treated Ontario unfairly. More recently, he's been hammering on the need for tough travel restrictions, with the same idea in mind—shifting blame away from his government and its failed policies to the federal government, which is responsible for international travel regulation. And yes, it's true, a certain number of cases have been brought into Canada through people who travelled here from other countries and should not have been allowed to do so. But overall, Canada has been regulating international travel quite strictly, with its recent outright ban on flights in from India, quarantine regulations, and so on. Arguably far more cases have resulted from the lack of paid sick leave, which has forced workers who are sick to continue working so they can pay their basic bills, or from keeping the schools open longer than they should have been, or from lax or tardy enforcement of the laws as they apply to churches, many of which have proven to be superspreader venues.

Roving Reporter

So, you're saying, then, that Ford's failure to use his scientific and medical advisors' advice, coupled with his inability or unwillingness to address longer-term causes of the pandemic, like lack of sick pay or the condition of the province's long-term care homes, are likely to have led to a significant increase in COVID activity in Ontario?

Yours Truly

How could anyone doubt it? When a province is allowed to stay open too long because its premier gives the economy higher priority than the health of its citizens, many people will get sick as a result and, regrettably, some will die. The fact that death rates as a percentage of cases are lower, now, in the third wave because most of the people contracting COVID are younger must not blind us to the fact that many of these people have required hospital-ization and some have died, and are continuing to die. I would say Timothy Ellis got it completely right. Doug Ford is guilty of gross negligence and serious incompetence in his handling of the pandemic. During the past couple of weeks, he has also been guilty of confusing both the general public and the police and others charged with enforcement by changing his mind so often on important issues such as the closing of playgrounds.

Roving Reporter

That sounds pretty final. Now, what about Quebec?

Yours Truly

I have been saying some pretty glowing things about that province's third wave performance, but before we start talking about them, we need to discuss something that happened just yesterday in Montreal, something that concerns me greatly, as a resident of Quebec.

Roving Reporter

Would that be the anti-lockdown demonstration outside Olympic Stadium?

Yours Truly

Yes, it would. Frankly, given how strict M Legault has been in most other areas of pandemic management, I was surprised, even shocked that the thing was allowed to go forward.

Roving Reporter

Why? Shouldn't people demonstrating against government COVID policy have the same rights as anyone else?

Yours Truly

That's a tricky question, actually. I can only say, yes and no. Bear in mind that freedom of speech is not, or at least should not be an absolute. Your freedom of speech (and action as well) ends where it impinges on mine. In particular, freedom of speech does not justify actions that endanger public health and safety. And I do believe this demonstration did.

Roving Reporter

Why would you say that?

Yours Truly

In the first place, we must consider its size. According to *Montreal Gazette* reporter Katelyn Thomas, who covered the event,[49] over 30,000 people had indicated, on Facebook, that they would be attending. In Thomas' view, the estimate was pretty accurate, although the Montreal police declined to issue

Jon Peirce

a figure of their own. Even if this figure is a significant overstatement, even if only half that many attended, it is still a huge number, especially considering the fact that most did not wear masks and few (if the picture accompanying Thomas' article is any kind of indication) were practicing social distancing. Any gathering of that size, whether for a good cause or a bad one (which in my view this was), has the potential of causing hundreds if not thousands of unnecessary COVID cases. The fact that people were generally not masked and generally not practicing social distancing only aggravates the potential problem here.

Roving Reporter
Is the fact that People's Party head Maxime Bernier was among those attending of significance, do you think?

Yours Truly
Well, I guess M Bernier has as much right to demonstrate as anyone else, but I do find his attending quite significant. It points to a significant politicization of the anti-mask, anti-lockdown, anti-vaccination movement in Quebec, as well as the Western provinces and Ontario.

Roving Reporter
What else bothers you about the demonstration?

Yours Truly
You mean, aside from the fact that it should never have been allowed to proceed in the first place? What I find both shocking and bitterly ironic is that the demonstration was held directly outside the city's largest vaccination site, Olympic Stadium, where the Expos used to play baseball in pleasanter times. The choice of venue forced those in charge of scheduling vaccinations to move people scheduled to have their jab yesterday afternoon to other times or venues. So, in other words, the demonstration had two different types of negative effect. The first was its likely direct effect as a superspreader event. The second was its indirect effect, in disrupting the COVID vaccination effort. Even given that the thing was going to be allowed, which as I said I don't think should have been the case, at the very least the demonstration organizers should have been forced to move their event, to make way for the people who had a fully legitimate reason to be there and who indeed were doing their fellow-citizens a service by being there. Making those coming to be vaccinated move or reschedule sends absolutely the wrong message. In a way, it's a bit like enabling a bully.

Roving Reporter

How concerned are you by the 'more aggressive' group who did things like throw smoke bombs at police?

Yours Truly

Frankly, not very. Now don't get me wrong. I don't and would never condone such actions. But in the larger scheme of things, a couple dozen people throwing smoke bombs at police at the end of a demonstration involving 30,000 really isn't all that important. It definitely should *not* have been in the story's headline. Things like that almost always happen at almost all kinds of demonstrations. Putting this into the headline is by way of normalizing a right-wing, anti-government demonstration that put many people's health and lives at risk, caused the disruption of many scheduled COVID vaccinations, and has the potential of undoing all the good work that Montreal has done in dealing with COVID. The headline should have had something to do with the 30,000 people gathering without masks, or the forced move of the vaccination clinic, or the fact that one of the key movers and shakers in the demo is the head of a national political party, albeit one still (thankfully) on the fringe.

At least they didn't put the number of arrests into the header. According to Katelyn Thomas, there were 28 people arrested for violating provincial laws, and other six for violating municipal laws.[50] That's a total of 34, or just over 0.1% of those attending, assuming the 30,000 figure is accurate. I daresay that if you'd had that number of people driving into Montreal to shop or watch a hockey game, you'd have had more traffic tickets and arrests for minor moving violations than that. Clearly enforcement of this event was a joke, as we've already seen has been the case with so many similar events in provinces west of Quebec.

What is it I'm missing here? I can't take my girlfriend out to our local bistro for pasta and wine on Saturday night even wearing a mask, or even see her in her home or mine, for fear of COVID, but 30,000 mostly unmasked people can troop through the province's largest city arm-in-arm with impunity? Is it that people can do whatever the hell they like so long as there's a good right-winger associated with their cause and there are enough of them to make the police afraid? I guess respect for the law doesn't mean what it did when I was growing up.

Roving Reporter

So, if there were so many things wrong with this demonstration, why was it allowed to go forward?

Jon Peirce

Yours Truly

Beats me. The fact that demonstrations are legal in Quebec. A misguided interpretation of what constitutes free speech and expression. Fear. Cowardice. Secret sympathy, on the part of many of the authorities, with the cause. Whatever the reason, it was a most horrendously wrong decision, which I can only hope will not be repeated any time soon. *(Pause)* For the demonstration proviso to be at all realistic in the current high-risk situation, there must at least be a numerical threshold in place. I wouldn't want to see 30,000 gathered together in the streets for a dog show or antique car show, never mind an anti-mask, anti-lockdown demonstration. As I think I said before, free speech can never be an absolute right; it needs to be constrained by things like consideration for public health and safety. When free speech and free expression are absolute rights, as the people at that demonstration were calling for, what you have is anarchy—or maybe something akin to Hobbes' state of nature, where life is brutish, and above all, short. Regrettably, lots of innocent lives could be shortened if the authorities don't get a grip on these demonstrations PDQ.

Roving Reporter

I understand there are other, similar demonstrations scheduled in the near future across Quebec…

Yours Truly

There are, and I think the authorities must act now to stop them if they don't want to see a fourth wave of cases in the province even worse than the third.

Roving Reporter

So, what I'm hearing from you is that this demonstration is likely to lead to a spike of cases in and around Montreal in the near future.

Yours Truly

Absolutely, and it's really too bad, because the provincial and municipal authorities and Montrealers themselves had, up to that point, been doing a really fine job of bringing the pandemic under control. As of this past weekend, Gatineau was under a stricter lockdown than Montreal, based on various case measures. Who'd have believed that could ever happen? I think the question now isn't *whether* there will be a spike, but how big it will be, and whether it will be confined to the Montreal area. If we're lucky—and if there are no more such demonstrations in or around Montreal this spring and summer—the spike will be held to a couple of hundred additional cases and won't go much past the Metro area. The province could recover from this, albeit with some difficulty. If we're not so lucky, we could see a mini-Sturgis,[51] with cases spreading to other parts of the province or maybe even to Ontario as protesters return to their home towns. Only time will tell which of these two scenarios is likelier to unfold.

Roving Reporter

Now, what about Premier Legault? Would you say his reputation has taken a hit as a result of this demonstration?

Yours Truly

Oh, no question. Here again, as with the spike in cases, the issue isn't *whether* his reputation has taken a hit, but how *big* a hit it has taken and whether he will be able to recover from it.

Roving Reporter

What should he do now, by way of damage control?

Yours Truly

First off, he should say straight out that he made a mistake allowing such a huge demonstration to take place, and that he certainly won't be allowing another. Either he must ban these demonstrations completely, which would be my preference even though such a ban would raise civil liberties issues, or at the very least restrict them to the number of people allowed to gather outdoors for other purposes, such as sporting events or religious services. And the same rules regarding mask-wearing and maintaining of social distance must apply as apply to these other events. In this way, the risk of major COVID spread would at least be minimized. If I were Legault, I would also say that I recognize the current curfew hours are too early for the spring and summer months and are not, in fact, realistic. An 8:00 p.m. curfew means one thing in February, when it's dark by 5:30, and quite another in May when there is still daylight at that hour. I would move all curfew times back two hours, not as a sign of relaxation but in recognition of the fact that summer hours need to be different. This would tell people that he's been listening, and might possibly cool the ardour for future demonstrations.

Up to now, I think Legault has maintained quite a good rapport with his citizens through the third wave. One reason is that he has been honest about his limitations and his mistakes. I personally liked the fact that he admitted the curfew was a trial, that he didn't know whether it would work or not but nonetheless thought it was worth a shot. That was honest, and it turns out that the curfew has also appeared to have worked. I also liked it when, apropos of some COVID issue that I no longer remember, he said, 'This

Jon Peirce

doesn't come with an instruction manual.' With this bit of dry humour, he allowed his citizens to put themselves in his shoes for a moment. Because of Legault's good rapport with most of his citizens, at least as regards COVID, most have trusted him and been willing to go along with his restrictions, painful and difficult though they may have been. The sentiments of the demonstrators in Montreal clearly were not those of the majority of Quebecers.[52]

Given all of this, I would say that if he admits his mistake this time, along with adjusting the curfew for summer daylight hours, he has a chance of pulling through with his reputation largely intact. But if he doesn't, and particularly if another large, superspreader demo is allowed to go ahead while ordinary people still can't go to restaurants or the movies or even to a Staples store for office supplies, I would say he is done. In that case, his credibility would be finished... he would be on the way to becoming just like one of the western premiers, or Doug Ford.

Roving Reporter
Yet up to now, you say, he has done a pretty good job overall with the Third Wave. What's the evidence on that?

Yours Truly
Take a look at the numbers in Tables 2 through 4. You will see that up to this point (bearing in mind that these numbers do *not* reflect last Saturday's demonstration), Quebec is outperforming both the national average and all provinces west of it in just about every current (third wave) indicator. Its test positivity (Table 2) is less than half the national average, at 3.0%, and lower than that of any province west of it. With regard to the variants (Table 3), Quebec accounts for only a little over 4% of them, despite having nearly a quarter of the country's population. And the vast majority of variant cases it has experienced are of the U.K. variant, which would arguably be the easiest to control, if only because it has been around longer. Moving on to Table 4, we see that Quebec's rate of new cases is half again below the national average and lower than that of any province west of it; only B.C. is even close. Its percentage drop in new cases over the previous week (26%) is also far greater than the national average percentage drop of 9%. And the province's drop in total hospitalizations over the past week, 13.6%, is, again, nearly twice the national figure of 7.6%.[53] This is a truly impressive record—one which suggests that the general public have been on board up to this point. It would be a terrible shame to spoil all this good work, and to destroy the public's trust, for the sake of one or two mindless right-wing-led demonstrations. To put it another way, should Legault be listening to the vast majority of his citizens or to a guy (Bernier) whose party got about 3% of the vote in the last

federal election? At this point, one can only hope that Legault recognizes the fact himself, and will act accordingly. My fingers are crossed.

Roving Reporter

Believe me, so are mine. In any event, we've now, at long last, reached Atlantic Canada. Earlier, you mentioned some special features of this region that might have helped explain its excellent COVID performance up to this point. Those features include geographic isolation (two of the Atlantic provinces are islands and a third is a peninsula), a relatively small and close-knit population, and a high degree of social consensus. But now, just these past few weeks, we've seen a big surge in cases in Nova Scotia—the biggest single surge any of the Atlantic provinces has seen throughout the pandemic. Given this sudden third wave surge, do your earlier points still apply?

Yours Truly

I think they do. Most of these features haven't changed. The region is still relatively isolated, and relatively quite easy to shut off from outside 'contamination.' The population is still relatively small and close-knit, which in turn leads both to the high degree of social consensus we've mentioned before, and to a relative ease in tracking cases. The two main differences now are the availability of vaccination, and the existence of several COVID variants.

Roving Reporter

But don't you think that the size of the surge in Nova Scotia, particularly in Metro Halifax, runs the risk of putting the province into the same category as those provinces west of New Brunswick?

Yours Truly

No. Not really. The number of new cases is certainly worrisome—there were over 100 such cases on at least two days in the past week—but there have been surges in all of the Atlantic provinces at some point or another through the pandemic. And these surges were generally brought under control quite quickly, through some sort of circuit-breaker lockdown, either province-wide or targeted to a particular area. Nova Scotia's new premier, Iain Rankin, acted quickly to impose a circuit-breaker lockdown on the entire province. The chief health officer, Dr Strang, is completely on board with it, and so, I suspect, are the vast majority of the province's citizens.

Roving Reporter

Even though there was a 'demonstration for freedom' on Citadel Hill last weekend?

Yours Truly

Yes, even despite that demonstration. Of course, this demonstration wasn't much like the one in Montreal.

Roving Reporter

Please explain.

Yours Truly

For one thing, it was small. Probably no more than a couple of hundred people in attendance. For another thing, at least if the photos are any indication, demonstrators were practicing social distancing. The police's attitude was different, as well. Although no tickets were issued, the police worked proactively with organizers to stop a planned march, which almost certainly limited any possible risk from the event. A police statement issued after the event stated: 'HRP officers were present throughout the event, [and] used their best judgment to contain the event, averting a more widespread public safety challenge.' The police statement concluded by noting that at future gatherings, gathering size limits and social distancing requirements would be enforced, with fines for any violation $2,000.00 for individuals and $7,500.00 for businesses and organizations.[54] And the police backed up this warning by issuing 37 tickets at five different gatherings across Metro Halifax over the weekend.[55] All of this suggests to me that local police are monitoring protest activity quite strictly and will not be allowing it to get out of hand.

Roving Reporter

Anything else different about the Nova Scotia situation, despite the high case numbers.

Yours Truly

In the bigger provinces, contact tracing of all cases would be extremely difficult if not impossible to carry out, given the large number of cases, even during relatively 'slack' times. Whether or not Nova Scotia is still doing contact tracing on all cases, as it attempted to do during the first wave, it is certainly doing it on a great many of them. And health authorities are also being extremely proactive in notifying the public about possible exposure sites. On May 2, CBC Internet News published an exhaustive listing of all potential recent COVID exposure sites in the province. The first list, for Metro Halifax, lists nearly 50 locations as possible exposure sites. All individuals who visited those sites on the date and time listed are advised to apply for a COVID test and to self-isolate while awaiting their test results. In the case of a second, shorter list (7 locations), individuals are advised to apply for a COVID test and then self-isolate even if their results are negative. There are other lists pointing out possible exposure sites on Halifax Transit busses, Maritime Bus busses, and planes arriving at Halifax Airport. Finally, the lists are not confined to Metro Halifax. At least a dozen other Nova Scotia communities, including Antigonish, Truro, Sydney, Yarmouth and Glace Bay have their own lists. It would be hard to imagine any other jurisdiction doing a more exhaustive job of tracing possible exposures than this.

Roving Reporter

Very impressive indeed. So, I take it that you think that such exhaustive tracing of possible exposures, together with much more active enforcement of the laws than we've seen in most other provinces and the ongoing circuit-breaker lockdown, will keep the current Nova Scotia surge from getting out of hand.

Yours Truly

I do. It's by no means a given, and all sorts of things could still happen to aggravate the current situation. But it's clear from what we've seen so far that the government, police, and health authorities have taken the situation firmly in hand and will do their level best to prevent things from getting worse. That's all you can expect any jurisdiction to do, and more than most Canadian jurisdictions outside Atlantic Canada have done, quite frankly.

Roving Reporter

What about the 'variants of concern' in Nova Scotia?

Yours Truly

Well, as chief provincial health officer Dr Strang has suggested, they are certainly of concern. But so far, they don't seem to have hit Nova Scotia very hard. Table 3 showed only 79 cases of the variants in the province, with the vast majority of those being of the U.K. variety. A check of more recent data from the federal government's daily epidemiology report showed only seven more cases since April 22, when the data in Table 3 were collected. All seven of those were of the U.K. variety. In contrast, there have been huge increases, and by huge, I mean in the thousands, in the number of variant cases in Ontario and Alberta.

Roving Reporter

Do you see a connection between strictness of regulations and enforcement and incidence of variant cases?

Yours Truly

I think there may well be such a connection. What makes me think there probably is one is the apparent relationship between high recent case rates and high incidence of variants. The two provinces with the highest recent case rates, according to Table 4, are also the two accounting for the vast majority of variant cases, according to Table 3. But why don't you hold that thought while we try to put together the big picture summarizing the findings we've been discussing up to this point?

Roving Reporter

Summing up the situation in the Atlantic region, would you say that despite events like the recent demonstration in Halifax, the pandemic still hasn't really been politicized in that part of the country?

Yours Truly

Yes, I would say that's true. So far, I haven't seen any evidence of any Atlantic Canadian politician trying to score political points through their handling of the pandemic, as Trump so often did and as premiers like Jason Kenney and Doug Ford have. I also haven't seen any evidence, there, of politicians pandering to particular groups or interests, as Premier Legault seems, regrettably, to have done with regard to the recent demonstration in Montreal. All the evidence I've seen to date suggests that enforcement in Atlantic Canada has been tough but even-handed.

Roving Reporter

And would you say that that comparative lack of politicization is reflected in the region's relatively low case rates?

Yours Truly

Absolutely. When restrictions are consistent and comprehensible and are enforced even-handedly, the public retains its trust in politicians and government and generally complies with the restrictions, which in turn leads to a better outcome in terms of case numbers.

Roving Reporter

Looking at Canada as a whole, what conclusions would you draw from the cross-country journey we've just taken?

Yours Truly

To begin with, the third wave has been driven by the West, along with

Ontario, in sharp contrast to the first wave, which was driven primarily by Quebec and to a lesser extent Alberta. A combination of traditional western alienation from central Canada combined with increasingly prevalent right-wing, libertarian, individualistic political views has created a perfect storm in Alberta and, to a lesser extent, Saskatchewan and Manitoba. Even as Alberta reports record numbers of new COVID cases, with per capita numbers exceeding those of any other jurisdiction in North America, and even as people like the province's former chief medical officer of health, Dr. James Talbot, are calling for a hard lockdown,[56] there continue to be elements in that province protesting the relatively modest restrictions thus far imposed by Premier Jason Kenney; protests over the first weekend in May included a rodeo in Bowden and anti-mask demonstrations across the province.[57] It seems clear that politicization of COVID in Alberta has reached the point where it is seriously interfering with efforts to control the pandemic.

To a lesser extent, the same appears to be true with the other western provinces, with the partial exception of British Columbia, which is both a western province and (for now at least) a socialist province. In my view, it is because the province's NDP government is more willing both to impose and to enforce COVID-related restrictions than the Conservative governments in place in the other western provinces that B.C. has both a lower total number of cases per capita and a lower per capita rate of new cases, with a sharper decline in new cases, than any of the other western provinces. Quite simply, the evidence we've examined suggests that Conservative governments outside of Atlantic Canada impose restrictions later, lift them sooner, and enforce them more sporadically and less stringently than governments of other political stripes. Regrettably, the result has been generally higher COVID numbers in almost all categories.

In Quebec, whose premier, Francois Legault, cannot be neatly character-ized according to any conventional sort of left-right rubric, politicization of the pandemic has generally been avoided during the third wave. For the most part, Legault has laid down tough but fairly consistent restrictions and has enforced them fairly consistently, as many party-goers across the province have recently learned, to their regret. And this approach has paid off. Through May 1 (see Tables 2 through 4), Quebec had a better record with regard to almost all new case numbers, including the crucial variant number, than any province to its west. But his government's failure to crack down on the huge May 1 demonstration in Montreal casts a dark shadow over what would otherwise be a solid record of achievement. It remains to be seen whether Legault's reputation can recover from the serious blow it undoubtedly took by allowing that demonstration. Much will depend on whether the province allows future demonstrations of this sort, and how strictly it enforces its outdoor gathering regulations with regard to such demonstrations.

271

Jon Peirce

As for Atlantic Canada, it would appear that by generally avoiding politicization of the COVID pandemic, with no discernible difference between Liberal and Conservative governments' handling of the pandemic, it has managed to keep most citizens 'on side' with regard to observance of restrictions. When the recent surge hit Nova Scotia, its current premier, Iain Rankin, was as quick to clamp down with circuit-breaker lockdowns as had been his predecessor, Stephen McNeil, during the first lockdown. Even though that latest surge in Nova Scotia is the largest the Atlantic region has thus far experienced, I would predict that thanks to the provincial government's swift action in locking down the province and continued strong efforts in contact tracing, it will be brought under control relatively quickly. I would also predict that the region will continue to maintain remarkably low numbers of per capita cases and deaths both by Canadian and by international standards, thanks to the above-mentioned factors as well as the small population of the Atlantic provinces and the high degree of social cohesion mentioned earlier.

Roving Reporter

Sorry it has taken so long to get this interview to get to air, Jon. But since we still have a wee bit of time, before I let you go, one more question. What do you make of Dr Anthony Fauci's recent (July 20) statement to the effect that politics is the reason why Canada has surpassed the U.S. in COVID vaccination?[58]

Yours Truly

That's a really good question, R-squared. Frankly, I'd have to say there's more here than meets the eye.

Roving Reporter

Mind elaborating on that?

Yours Truly

Not at all. If you're talking just about vaccination rates, the statement is largely true. Nationally, just over 70% (70.1%) of the entire population have had at least one shot, according to today's CBC Vaccine Tracker. The range is from 76.8% in PEI to 63.6% in Alberta and 63.8% in Saskatchewan.[59] In other words, it appears there are about 13% more people not wanting to get vaccinated in Alberta and Saskatchewan than there are in Prince Edward Island. I'm not happy about this but I think we can live with it. Barely.

272

Roving Reporter

So, what's the problem, then?

Yours Truly

What concerns me is that the learned doctor—a man I very much admire, by the way—like many decent, educated, well-meaning Americans—appears to be viewing Canada through rose-coloured glasses, at least to some extent.

Roving Reporter

Can you elaborate a bit on *that?*

Yours Truly

Certainly. In the interview that CBC quoted in its news story, Fauci said, 'Canada is doing better not because we are trying any less than they are trying. It's because in Canada you don't have that divisiveness of people not wanting to get vaccinated, in many respects, on the basis of ideology and political persuasion.' To me, with respect to the good doctor, this is just too simplistic. In the first place, Canada isn't a monolith. Not by any stretch. If anything, it is a more heavily regionalized country than the U.S., with arguably more matters left to the provinces than are left to U.S. states. As we've already discussed at some length, we have one COVID story in the Atlantic region, another, very different one in the West, particularly in the Prairie provinces, and different stories yet in Quebec, B.C. and Ontario. Secondly, Fauci's statement fails to recognize the very real spillover of American Trumpite politics into parts of Canada, particularly Alberta, Saskatchewan and Manitoba. As I told you earlier, there were a sizable number of Jason Kenney's own MLAs opposing him from the right, basically arguing that Albertans should not have any restrictions at all on their personal freedom or on businesses' ability to operate. If that isn't politicization of the pandemic, I don't know what is. The result, as we pointed out earlier, has been a huge difference in overall COVID case rates and variant case rates between the provinces run by right-wing Conservatives and the rest of the country. And there have been large numbers of anti-mask, anti-lockdown rallies across Canada, certainly in all the provinces west of Quebec and to some extent in Quebec as well. While these events have not resulted in bloodshed, as has sometimes been the case in the U.S., it doesn't mean they haven't happened. What's worried me the most is that, as we have also seen, the authorities' enforcement of the sorts of measures that would have kept these events from happening has been spotty at best, sometimes all but non-existent. If public health measures like lockdowns are not going to be enforced, they won't be of much use in combatting COVID. We've seen—at some length—how authorities in

Jon Peirce

Saskatchewan, in Manitoba, and in Ontario turned a blind eye to demonstrations and church services involving far larger numbers of people than were supposedly allowed to gather publicly. What this indicates to me is significant politicization of the pandemic. Regrettably, it has also resulted in higher than necessary case levels in the jurisdictions where such events were condoned. What I'm saying is that, except for Atlantic Canada, where lockdown and public gathering measures have been enforced pretty evenhandedly, COVID *has* been politicized in much of Canada. The difference between Canada and the U.S. is one of degree, not kind. And I think that if Dr Fauci were to dig down beneath the surface, and look at the case numbers for different provinces, and the numbers for different variants in different provinces, he would recognize this himself. There is really no firewall between the two countries, much as some might like to believe there is one.

Roving Reporter
Whew! Thank you very much. And I'm pleased to report that we will be running this interview quite soon.

Yours Truly
And thank you for your patience. Next time we get together, I hope we'll have something pleasanter to talk about.

Age Group	Quebec	Canada
0-19	20.1	17.9
20-29	15.4	18.9
30-39	14.3	16.1
40-49	15.0	14.7
50-59	13.1	13.3
60-69	8.1	8.4
70-79	5.2	4.6
80+	8.8	6.0

Table 1: Age Distribution of COVID-19 Cases, Quebec and Canada (% in each age group)

Sources for Table 1

For Quebec: 'Donnees COVID-19 par age et sexe au Quebec,' Figure 1.3, 'Repartition des cas confirmes de COVID-19 au Quebec selon le groupe de l'age.' Data current as of April 22, 2021 at 11:00 a.m. Downloaded April 22, 2021.

For Canada: 'Government of Canada COVID-19 Daily Epidemiology Update,' Figure 3. Data current as of April 16, 2021. Downloaded April 22, 2021.

Jurisdiction	# Tests Conducted	# Tests Positive	% Tests Positive
Canada	137,021	8373	6.4
British Columbia	10,113	1006	10.0
Alberta	18,414	1857	10.1
Saskatchewan	3706	254	7.0
Manitoba	3248	261	8.0
Ontario	51,877	3682	7.1
Quebec	41,971	1248	3.0
New Brunswick	1202	19	1.6
Nova Scotia	4562	38	.8
Prince Edward Island	843	1	.1
Newfoundland	866	3	.35

Table 2: COVID-19 Tests Conducted, No. of Tests Positive, and % Positive, Canada and Provinces[60]

Source for Table 2

For number of tests conducted and number of tests positive: Government of Canada Daily Epidemiology Update. Data as of April 22, 2021, 7:00 p.m. Downloaded April 23, 2021. Percentage of tests positive: author's personal calculation (which should be considered unofficial—I may be off by a bit, though I'm probably not off by much).

Jurisdiction	Var. B.1.1.7 (UK)	Var. B.1.351 (S. Africa)	Var. P.1 (Brazil)	Total Variants
Canada	75,413	463	2853	78,729
British Columbia	4041	76	2062	6179
Alberta	20,654	59	548	21,261
Saskatchewan	2046	9	5	2060
Manitoba	727	20	2	749
Ontario	44,205	113	218	44,536
Quebec	3304	169	16	3489
New Brunswick	180	4	0	184
Nova Scotia	66	12	1	79
Prince Edward Isl.	10	0	0	10
Newfoundland	178	1	0	179

Table 3: Incidence of COVID-19 Variants of Concern: Canada and Provinces[61]

Source for Table 3

Government of Canada Daily Epidemiology Update. Data as of April 22, 2021. Downloaded April 23, 2021.

Jurisdiction	New Cases per 100k	% Change in New Cases over Past 7 Days	Total Cases per 100k
Canada	146.1	-9%	3101.9
British Columbia	91.7	-34%	2405.0
Alberta	248.7	+11%	4105.7
Saskatchewan	150.6	-4%	3390.1
Manitoba	104.3	+52%	2724.9
Ontario	192.5	-7%	3022.8
Quebec	91.6	-26%	4020.7
New Brunswick	8.1	-5%	236.4
Nova Scotia	25.1	+531%	209.7
Prince Edward Isl.	3.1	-38%	109.6
Newfoundland	2.7	+7%	200.0

Table 4: New Cases per 100k, % Change in New Cases, and Total Cases per 100k, Canada and Provinces.[62]

Source for Table 4

CBC (Internet) COVID-19 Tracker, data through April 25, 2021, downloaded April 26.

Jurisdiction	Population	% of Total Population	# COVID Cases	% COVID Cases	COVID Intensity Rate (rising or falling)
Canada	38,048,738	100.0	1,187,918	100.0	1.0
Ontario	14,755,211	38.78	448,861	37.78	.974 (rising)
Quebec	8,575,944	22.54	345,697	29.10	1.291 (falling)
British Columbia	5,135,039	13.54	126,249	10.63	.785
Alberta	4,436,258	11.66	183,301	15.43	1.323 (rising)
Manitoba	1,380,955	3.63	37,802	3.18	.876 (rising)
Saskatchewan	1,178,832	3.10	40,176	3.38	1.09 (rising)
Nova Scotia	979,449	2.57	2119	0.18	.070 (rising)
New Brunswick	782,078	2.06	1854	0.16	.078
Newfoundland/Labrador	520,438	1.37	1046	0.08	.058
Prince Edward Island	159,819	0.42	177	0.015	.036

Table 5: Population of Canada and Provinces, % of Population in Each Province, No. of COVID Cases in Each Province, % of COVID Cases in Each Province, and COVID 'Intensity Rate in Each Province.'[63]

Sources for Table 5

For population, Statistics Canada Table 17.10-009-01, Population Estimates by Quarter, Q1 2021. For % of total population, *Wikipedia,* downloaded April 27, 2021, using the same Stats Can data as that just cited.

For number of COVID cases, CBC COVID-19 Tracker, downloaded April 27, 2021. Data as of April 26. For % of COVID cases by province and COVID intensity rate, personal calculation by author.

Notes

[1] For the record, 'today' was April 17, 2021.

[2] This discussion leaves aside the territories, which are so small and whose circumstances are so peculiar to them that in my view they can't meaningfully compared to the ten 'old line' provinces.

[3] Source: CBC Vaccine Tracker, downloaded at 12:00 noon, April 17, 2021.

[4] This was true as of April 17, 2021, when this passage was written. I recognize that the situation in Nova Scotia is now (April 25) somewhat different, but the fact does not negate my main point here.

[5] As of April 17. After two weeks of intermittently strict lockdown, the case numbers have dropped somewhat, but are still well over 3500/day on average—a rate that is still dangerously high.

[6] CBC Vaccine Tracker, 'Vaccinations around the World,' downloaded at 12:15 p.m., April 17, 2021.

[7] Now (as of June 28) it is significantly less than that.

[8] Information drawn from CBC COVID-19 Tracker, at 1:00 p.m. on April 17, 2021, and with three digit or larger numbers rounded to the nearest whole number.

[9] Except as otherwise noted, all historical data in this section have been drawn from this source.

[10] Source: Statistics Canada, 'The Daily,' population estimates for 2018, downloaded April 20, 2021.

[11] Again, this is of late April. As of today (June 28), Manitoba and Saskatchewan would have to be ranked among the leaders.

[12] Quebec Premier Legault, whom we will discuss in more detail later, has said this on at least two later occasions, once during the second wave and once during the third.

[13] For more detail, see my *Field Notes: Journal of the Start of a Plague Year.* Publication forthcoming.

[14] From *Field Notes.* Data for *Field Notes* were drawn from CBC Internet News, except as otherwise indicated.

[15] MacGregor, Sandra, 'Canada's Provinces Introduce New Coronavirus Travel Restrictions to Limit Domestic Travel,' *Forbes,* April 3, 2020. Except as otherwise noted, material for this paragraph has been drawn from MacGregor's article.

[16] See, among many others, Brown, Laura and Van Horne, Ryan, 'Campbellton Doctor Blamed for Cluster of COVID Cases Won't Be Charged,' *CTV Atlantic News*, July 8, 2020. Except as otherwise noted, all information about this case is drawn from the Brown and Van Horne article.

[17] See my 'Politics and COVID I: Interstate Variations in COVID Rates in the U.S.' This essay appears elsewhere in this anthology.

[18] See Table 2 for more details.

[19] Again, see Table 2.

[20] See, among many others, Kay, Jonathan, 'The Case for Wearing Face Masks during COVID-19 Was Obvious a Month Ago,' *National Post*, April 4, 2020, downloaded June 29, 2021. Kay notes that through the beginning of April, 2020, Tam was offering 'no fewer than four reasons why asymptomatic Canadians shouldn't wear masks when they left the house.'

[21] See, among many others, Pawloski, A., 'Why We Hate Being Told What to Do: Psychologists Explain the Battle over Masks,' *Today*, July 7, 2020, downloaded June 29, 2021. Among the incidents chronicled by Pawloski were a shoving match in a store in Florida, the issuing of 'terroristic threats' in a store in New Jersey, and a woman in Texas flinging groceries from her cart after being told she had to keep her mask on.

[22] Later sections of this essay will discuss anti-mask, anti-lockdown demonstrations in the West and in Quebec in much more detail.

[23] Gilmore, Rachel, 'Tory MP Sorry after Calling Lockdowns Greatest Civil Liberties Threat since WW II Lockdowns,' *Global News*, April 24, 2021, downloaded that same day.

[24] See, among others, Warick, Jason, 'Public Health Orders Need to be Enforced': Sask. Officials Beg Police to Act Against Anti-Mask Protesters,' *CBC News* (internet), April 23, 2021, downloaded April 24, 2021. Most alarmingly, Warick points out that Saskatoon anti-mask events planned for the weekend of April 24-25 included a children's festival featuring face painting and other games designed to appeal to kids. The Saskatoon children's festival, which did in fact take place as scheduled on April 24, is discussed in more detail in a letter section of this piece.

[25] For much more detail on these points, see my essay 'Politics and COVID I: the United States' which appears elsewhere in this anthology.

[26] *ibid.*

[27] As of late April. The figure now (as of June 29) is 33.2 million, or a full one-tenth of the U.S. population, according to 'Coronavirus: A Timeline of how the Deadly COVID-19 Outbreak is Evolving,' *Pharmaceutical Technology*. Data through June 28, 2021. Downloaded June 29, 2021.

[28] 'Vancouver Mayor Calls for Court Injunction to Close Restaurant "Defiant" in the Face of COVID Restriction,' *CBC News* (internet), April 24, 2021, downloaded April 24. Except as otherwise indicated, all information about the Corduroy Restaurant and its owner have been drawn from this article.

[29] The proper word would be 'flout.'

[30] The fact that the gyms were allowed to remain open at all suggests that the restrictions were moderate by typical Canadian standards. In most provinces under lockdown, gyms have been closed down altogether.

[31] Johnson, Lisa. 'Quarter of UCP MLAs Speak Out Against Alberta's Latest COVID-19 Restrictions,' *Edmonton Journal*, April 7, 2021, downloaded April 24.

[32] Thomson, Graham, 'Not so United Conservatives: Kenney Being Punished Politically for Doing the Right Thing,' *CBC Internet News* opinion piece, April 9, 2021, downloaded April 24.

[33] See Thomson, 'Not so United Conservatives,' *op. cit.*

[34] See Bennett, Dean and Krugol, Lauren, 'Banff, Fort McMurray Await Details before Deciding on COVID-19 Curfews., *Canadian Press*, April 30, 2021, downloaded May 1.

[35] *ibid.*

[36] See 'Everything You Need to Know about COVID-19 in Alberta on Friday, April 30,' *CBC News* (internet), downloaded May 1, 2021.

[37] See Warick, 'Public Health Orders Need to be Enforced…' *op. cit.* Except as otherwise noted, all information about the Saskatoon rallies has been drawn from this article.

[38] Warick, *op. cit.*

[39] Anton, Jessie, 'Sask. Doctors Push for Tweaks to COVID-19 Restrictions, Stronger Enforcement,' *CBC News* (internet), January 20, 2021, downloaded April 24.

[40] I have used the neutral wording 'on learning…' because I don't know how Munce found out about this—whether from watching TV in his hospital room or from being told.

[41] See Warick, Jason, 'COVID-19 Patient Has Message for Sask. Police, Officials: Enforce Public Health Laws,' *CBC News* (internet), April 30, 2021, downloaded May 1.

[42] 'Hundreds Protest Manitoba's COVID-19 Public Health Orders at The Forks,' CBC News (internet), April 17, 2021, downloaded April 25. Except as otherwise indicated, all information about this rally at The Forks has been drawn from this CBC article.

[43] Defined as the rate of new cases within the past seven days. Source for this discussion on new case rates, CBC COVID-19 Tracker, downloaded April 28, 2021, covering data through April 27.

[44] Dubinski, Kate, '2 Politicians among Aylmer, Ont. Church-Goers Charged for Defying Pandemic Rules,' *CBC News*, April 27, 2021, downloaded April 29. See also Jabakhanji, Sara, 'Charges to be Laid after "One of the Largest Services" Held at Aylmer, Ontario Church on Sunday,' CBC News, April 25, 2021, downloaded April 26.

[45] This is strongly suggested by the fact that an off-duty officer was called up to the pulpit by Hildebrandt and praised during the church's most recent illegal service, as noted in the Dubinski article cited earlier.

[46] See Ellis' 'Doug Ford: Resign for Gross Negligence in a Pandemic.' Original written in February, 2021, updated April 16, 2021. Internet campaign.

[47] For a moving interview with Dr Juni, see Jason de Souza, CBC Interview on YouTube video, conducted April 17, 2021. During the interview, Juni confessed to feeling terrible, said he had a serious crying fit the day before, and said he had stayed on because many friends and professional colleagues had implored him to do so.

[48] For more detail on this, see Ellis, *op. cit.*

[49] 'Protest against COVID-19 Measures in Montreal Ends with Tear Gas and Arrests Due to "More Aggressive" Smaller Group,' *Montreal Gazette,* May 2, 2021, downloaded May 2.

[50] 'Protest against COVID-19 Measures in Montreal…' *op. cit.* See also Isaac Olson, 'Demonstrators, Many Maskless, March in Montreal against Public Health Restrictions,' *CBC News* (internet), May 1, 2021, downloaded May 3.

[51] This refers to the giant motorcycle rally held in August, 2020, in Sturgis, South Dakota, which attracted some 200,000 people to the small town and proved to be a giant superspreader event across the entire Upper Midwest of the U.S.

[52] Again, see Thomas, *op. cit.*

[53] Hospitalization data drawn from CBC COVID-19 Tracker on May 3, 2021.

[54] See April, Allan, 'Halifax Police Issue Statement Addressing "Freedom Rally" Held Saturday on Citadel Hill,' *CTV News*, May 3, 2021, downloaded May 3.

[55] April, *op. cit.*

[56] 'Former Alberta Chief Medical Officer of Health Calls for Hard Lockdown in Province,' *CBC News* Network Video, May 3, 2021, downloaded May 4, 2021.

[57] 'Hundreds in Alberta Defy Public Health Orders as COVID-19 Cases Surge,' *CBC News* Network Video, May 2, 2021, downloaded May 4.

[58] Panetta, Alexander, 'Politics the Reason Canada Has Surpassed U.S. on COVID Vaccines, Fauci Says,' *CBC News* (internet), July 20, 2021. Downloaded July 23, 2021.

[59] Data for July 22, 2021, downloaded July 23, 2021.

[60] For present purposes, I have excluded the Territories.

[61] Again, the Territories have been omitted from this table (and also from Table 4)

[62] Note: 'new cases' refers to cases reported within the seven days previous to the download.

[63] The 'COVID Intensity Rate' is the percentage of COVID-19 cases reported in each province divided by the percentage of the country's population living in each province. If, for example, a province had 50% of the reported COVID cases but only 25% of the country's population, its COVID Intensity Rate would be 2. If the preceding numbers were reversed, the COVID Intensity Rate would be 0.5.

COVID, Social Responsibility and 'The Next Times'
Alan Lennon

'It was the best of times, it was the worst of times.' These words of Dickens have been used to describe a variety of times since he first penned them in 1859. The time of COVID-19 (and its variants) will no doubt be described in this way and indeed may well be the most critical of all such times.

Today our world is linked together more closely than at any other time in history. In this 'global village,' we have experienced the lives of all people, regardless of race, colour, creed, religion, gender and nation, put on hold, disrupted and threatened in a way never experienced before. Much has been written about 2020 and likely much more will be written, but this best of times and worst of times should teach us valuable lessons about ourselves and our future.

In the following, I share my thoughts on how we, as societies, have responded to COVID-19 and how we, as individuals, may have failed in that response, with consequences for the very future of our societies. The 'next times' may be even darker than the 'worst of times' as the problems underlying the weakness of our pandemic response are exacerbated.

'The Best of Times'

On the bright side, we as individuals have generally acted well. We have socially isolated ourselves according to the guidelines, worn masks, stayed at home and tried to the best of our ability to limit the virus. Beyond that, we have recognized and saluted those who were on the front lines in caring for victims of the virus, recognized and saluted those who worked in essential services, recognized and supported those who were more susceptible to infection, and tried to help each other out in a variety of ways.

In our neighbourhoods, we came out at sunset to bang pots and pans in honour of health care workers. We cheered them on sight. At grocery stores, we let seniors and health care workers have their own time in the store to help ensure their safety and to recognize their vulnerability or their contributions to our general wellbeing. We shopped for those unable to do so for themselves, to help minimize their risks. We even (though not often enough) followed the directions on the floor in store aisles.

We held impromptu concerts and street parties without getting close to each other. We learned new skills—baking, cooking, cutting hair, and playing musical instruments—and, perhaps most important of all, we learned how to Zoom!

We all have stories or examples of how we behaved during the pandemic as responsible citizens. We put aside our rights—our right to travel, to visit, to shop—because we decided that the end of the pandemic was worth the inconvenience.

The idea from the experts was to limit, if not stop, the spread of the virus. Socially responsible behaviours such as those listed above were encouraged in order to slow the spread by isolating those who carried it or might be carrying it. Clearly, what we did, did not work, even though by and large we did what we were asked to do. We freely took responsibility for our own safety and the safety of others. Overall, we have behaved as citizens, taking responsibility and contributing to keeping the pandemic at bay. Clearly it has not been enough; now the virus is more widely spread amongst us than at any earlier time. This raises the thorny and difficult question: what should we have done? What else could we have done to alter the outcomes?

'The fault, dear Brutus, lies not in our stars but in ourselves for we are underlings.' Cassius (or Shakespeare) was both right and wrong. The fault does not lie in our stars or our fate. It does lie within us but not because we are underlings. We are not underlings, and the pandemic shows that. We didn't do the 'right' things because we are underlings, obedient to our masters, but because we are citizens. We freely took responsibility for our safety and for the safety of others, so if the fault doesn't lie within ourselves, where does it lie? One view might be that not enough of us behaved as we should. We didn't achieve any level of social immunity because of that; too many people decided not to be inconvenienced to allow the rest of us to contain the virus. But this is not a question of a few bad apples but of what constitutes a significant number of such apples. Once that is established, the implications go much deeper… right to the very roots of society.

'The Worst of Times'

While not forgetting how so many of us demonstrated our citizenship and social conscience, we cannot ignore those of us who were not so community-spirited in their behaviour.

Who can forget the outrage the majority felt when last Spring people crowded into parks to catch a few rays, refusing to wear masks and generally behaving as if there were no pandemic. And we should not forget those who denied the science, and ignored the public health guidelines, flaunting their freedom while threatening ours.

The second wave, starting in the Fall of 2020, seemed to increase both the case numbers and the virulence of those acting on their own. While people were asked to stay home for the holidays, as time passed the number ignoring that advice seem to climb. People were asked not to undertake international travel—particularly to the south for the winter—but they went anyway. Businesses decided to stay open or reopen even in the face of laws shutting them down for public health reasons. It was as if the virus had taken control of them and demanded they do what it wanted to make its spread easier and people complied with the virus. But these people were not victims controlled by the virus or anything else. They acted not as underlings but as autonomous individuals.

Over Christmas and New Year's, the second wave ushered in what may have been 'the worst of times.' There was a significant increase in socially irresponsible behaviour. People who ignored the request to stay home went south 'because they could' and then complained about being penalized through having to get tested before returning, or having to quarantine in a hotel at their expense before they were allowed to return to their homes. Some churches demanded the right to hold services in person in defiance of the public health guidelines. Petitions proliferated to reopen businesses and services even while case numbers skyrocketed and people continued to die from the virus. Lawsuits were filed claiming the Charter of Rights and Freedoms protected individuals from these kinds of limitations on their 'freedom.'

We were faced with a group of people—some of them the very leaders who had asked us to stay home and self-isolate—who stood on their freedom, their 'right' to do as they wished. For them, rights meant freedom and freedom meant licence: I have a right therefore I can do as I please. The anti-social minority, in essence, threatened the rest of us because it was their 'convenience,' which they understood as their freedom, that they felt was being undermined.

When we talk about society and rights, implicit in the discourse is also the notion of social responsibility. If we want the right to drive a car, we have a responsibility to others to do so safely. If we want the right to have safe food, we have a responsibility to pay our share of food inspections at all stages of production and distribution. And so on. Similarly, if we want the right to run a business or an organization, then we have a responsibility *not* to run that business in a situation where it cannot be done safely for customers or employees.

We have a society in which goods and services are distributed via markets. During the pandemic, we let businesses decide if and how they would 'work' the market. Some rewarded workers, albeit temporarily, for the risks they had to take at work. Some provided special access to certain groups for the purpose of shopping. Some created new businesses—food delivery, for example—to meet perceived needs.

Others, however, set up businesses to help people avoid or get around the public health guidelines. Some went so far as to 'price gouge' in various ways because the market would not punish them for it. As time passed, some businesses even took money from the government earmarked to help workers, or to provide additional services for safety needs and gave it to their shareholders.

And What of the 'Next Times?'

Early in the pandemic, we heard a lot about 'herd immunity.' It seemed to mean that the overall society would be safe once the necessary percentage of the population (the herd) was safe due to having the appropriate antibodies through having had the virus or through having been exposed to it. This inevitably would involve a great deal of suffering for those who contracted the disease but, for some, it seemed a price worth paying. However, as the death toll rose and there seemed to be no 'herd immunity' coming, this approach lost much of its rather small amount of appeal.

But there is another kind of immunity: immunity for a society overall if—and as we know it is a big if—people take extraordinary precautions and act in a socially responsible manner.

A combination of a sufficiently high rate of vaccination *plus* following public health guidelines will provide that immunity, just as it does with other viruses such as the seasonal flu. But if some people don't get vaccinated, don't follow public health guidelines, then what?

With the seasonal flu, this results in a certain number of cases (some more severe than others) and, most commonly amongst seniors, death. We seem to find this acceptable. But this is not an acceptance based on any actual decision-making. There has been no examination of the questions: 'Is this level of illness and death acceptable? And, if not, what, if anything, can be done to lower the rate of death and what are the consequences of taking such actions? These are important issues that need to be addressed but it seems the effects of seasonal flu have simply been accepted by our society.

With COVID-19 and its variants, the stakes are much higher. The risks created by people behaving unsafely as well as not getting vaccinated are much greater. In moving forward, we have to rethink what we want the balance between rights and responsibilities to be. How much death is acceptable to maintain how much convenience for the living? This is, admittedly, a stark question but, in the world of COVID-19 and its future, it is a necessary one.

We must face the reality that, as anti-social behaviour increases, it puts us all at higher and higher risk for another wave of COVID-19 and its variants. It also lowers the bar around socially responsible behaviour in the face of social threats in the future.

The pandemic has cast light on the inequities of our society. The toll has been disproportionate for groups who had been left behind or cast aside by society in pre-pandemic times. The old, rather than those in their prime years, have died at an appalling rate. Women suffered much more of the economic fallout of the pandemic than men. People of colour and First Nations faced

Alan Lennon

the same fate in relation to white people. The rich got richer and the super-rich got away with billions. There has been little recognition that the market, which drives the distribution of goods and services, has dealt these already disadvantaged groups a disproportionate share of the COVID pain. And there seems to be no plan to change that. Privilege has its price, but it appears it will be paid by the less privileged rather than the privileged.

Most important of all, the failure to address these inequities or even to talk about a plan to do so undermines the fabric of society. If people see that others' convenience is more important than their safety, if people see that others can act selfishly and be allowed to let other people take the risks and the pain in order to protect themselves, then why should they continue to act in a socially responsible manner?

Nothing undermines social norms faster and more insidiously than the realization that a 'privileged' group can get away with not following the rules and norms. The future of our societies rests on the end of privilege provided to individuals because 'they want it' or 'it is convenient for them.'

The pandemic has done many things to our society. Among other things, it has taught some of us our interdependence, and has shown some of us our vulnerability. But it has also, with the connivance of a relatively small group of individuals, undermined the social responsibilities that we all have. Without those responsibilities, we will either slowly or quickly decline into a Hobbesian state of nature and life will become increasingly 'nasty, brutish and short.'

For all of us.

SECTION 7

COVID
and
Working

*T*his section is of special interest to me because I have been a student of the world of work for several decades. As my bio points out in more detail, many of my publications have been in this area.

Like the other sections of this almanac, 'COVID and Working' offers a broad range of perspectives on the pandemic's effects on how people have gone about their work. In 'Back to (pre) School,' Elizabeth Barnes expresses considerable satisfaction at having been enabled to find her true calling—that of nurturing pre-school age children—thanks largely to the pandemic. In 'An Inhospitable Season,' long-time Michigan hotelier Rodney Clough describes the travails he and his wife Linda Jo went through trying to keep their business alive during the pandemic. As Clough sees it, there was a silver lining at the end of all the stormy weather. He and his wife have learned to see their surroundings differently, in particular more fully appreciating the natural wonders those surroundings afford, which in turn has helped them to refocus their business.

It's important to note that COVID has had many significant effects on people's volunteer work, as well as on work done in the paid labour market. In 'Fundraising Amidst COVID,' Andover class agent Bill Hartman, after pointing out some of the numerous ways in which the pandemic has made life at the venerable boarding school more difficult, concludes that COVID has been 'a curse that is being transformed into a positive unifier for good. It shows us how globally interconnected we are and illustrates the necessity of unifying and working together.' Unlike Hartman, my Amherst class secretary, Lee Keener, has experienced little COVID-related change in his work for Amherst. Most of that work, Keener notes, was being done online anyway. He found far greater effects on his other volunteer job, as a board member for the Canadian Pacific Mountain Region of Hostelling International, and on his family's ability to travel as they normally would.

Going back to graduate school for serious study of Icelandic history, language and culture would be a strenuous enough endeavour for a septuagenarian in relatively normal times. What would it be like to do so during the COVID pandemic? Not all that different from what it would have been like at any other time, concludes Fran Ota in her inspiring memoir, 'Sudden Turns.' Ota's advice is that her readers step out without knowing and tackle something new and different. 'Even mid-pandemic, learn as much as you can and have as many new experiences as you can. Life is still good!'

Two different perspectives on the impact of Zoom and other new technologies on their work are offered by economics professor Betsy Hoffman and end-of-life physician Bill Newmann. For Hoffman, who suffers from Parkinson's Disease, virtual teaching via Zoom has been a 'boon,' which has likely extended her teaching career well beyond where she would have been able to take it 'live.' For Newmann, on the other hand, having to do his end-of-life work virtually instead of meeting with family members and attending at physician-assisted deaths in person has made him feel far less engaged in his work than he did prior to the pandemic.

Psychiatrists, psychologists, and other mental health professionals have been under exceptional stress throughout the pandemic. Psychologist Ruth Hawkins' short but powerful memoir, 'It's OK if I'm Not OK,' offers an ultimately positive and reassuring answer to a question many of us have had: what happens when things get to be too much for our healers?

Our two French pieces are inspiring illustrations of the work being done with seniors in West Quebec during the pandemic. Physiotherapist Camille Pellerin-Forget provides a moving description of her work with a recovering COVID patient in her memoir, 'Un petit récit, pour se sortir des statistiques…' It is with a mix of joy and relief that we learn, near the end of her memoir, that her patient has been cured. For their part, Yves Rochon and Julie Fortin describe the good work done by the staffers of Logements de L'Outaouais in providing the facility's residents, whose average age is 74, with an environment that's safe and secure but at the same time stimulating, even during the heart of the pandemic.

The section concludes with my former colleague Denise Giroux's sometimes angry, sometimes mournful, but always powerful and moving memoir, 'Zooming Our Way into Oblivion.' After noting that the pandemic robbed her work with union members of much of the satisfaction she formerly took from it, Giroux concludes that even long after the pandemic has ended, the ways in which it has changed how work is done will remain the subject of discussion and debate for many years to come. I would hazard the guess that few readers of Giroux's essay—or of the others in this section—would be inclined to dispute her.

Back to (pre) School
Elizabeth Barnes

I have gone back to school several times in my life, but the most important time was the time during the COVID-19 pandemic, when, unbeknownst to me at the time, I was an elder/crone-in-training. The first few times back at the books were for the usual things: to finish a university degree or to further my professional development. This time, even though I was the teacher, I learned more about myself during this time than at any other life stage. Since that first day, when the seed of the Grandma School idea grew like a weed in my head, I thought I might be onto something. A school where learning was combined with love, the outdoors was our classroom, and children could learn in a safe environment during a world-wide pandemic.

It all started with my senior kindergarten-aged grandson not returning to school in September 2020 due to the uncertainty surrounding what a typical kindergarten class of thirty students might look like in the middle of a pandemic. My son and daughter in law decided the risks were too high for a five-year-old, their family and extended family. There is also a little brother. They had a little friend in the same situation. That's three! Good enough for a class!

From there, I decided to offer a school-like setting three days per week. We would do circle time, learn about days of the week, do science, French, music and art. Hot homemade lunches and wholesome snacks were supplied. It was a school where boo boos were kissed and sandwiches never had crusts. If we needed to break from the routine for an hour of story time snuggled under a blanket, we did. We visited ponds, bee hives, toboggan hills and bakeries. We learned how to play hockey, how to put on plays, and sing all the nursery rhymes. By the end of the first month of Grandma School, I could feel my own personal growth and I could see the kids' incredible social, emotional and academic progress. 'What if,' I thought, 'Grandma School became a real thing?' I had never felt so vibrant, energetic, alive and happy in my life. This was when I knew I had found my true calling.

Being with three- to five-year-olds all day was better therapy than anything I could have found on my own. I believe that Grandma School helped me and my mental health as much as it helped the children.

I'm constantly amazed by the chord my little school has struck with people. Other grandmas saw what I was doing on social media and started dropping off amazing things for my classroom. I could feel the grandma-to-grandma love and support for what I was doing. I knew my posts and updates were bringing happiness and joy to people during a very challenging and often lonely time. People would send me craft ideas and ask for updates and pictures. I scoured buy-nothing groups for furniture and supplies. I refinished and painted tables, chairs and shelves. I had never understood the concept of 'she has found her calling' until Grandma School. Never have I felt so content, confident, relevant, happy, and useful. People started hearing about what we did every day. I started getting interest from people who were not my grandchildren.

I began to feel like an ambassador for the phrase 'It takes a village to raise a child.' My village was showing up for me and my little charges, and I felt I had a duty to honour that. I took great pride in my Grandma School. I figured out that while I was physically speeding up every day to keep up with the preschoolers, I was slowing down each night to be with myself. Having recently come through a serious illness, I found the combination of physical activity and rewarding days exactly what I needed to heal and move forward.

A year ago, I might have been appalled to consider myself an elder, or a crone. Now I can only hope that I fulfill my role of being an elder in a meaningful way. I'm certain now that because of the interruption in day-to-day life that COVID-19 has created, nurturing children aged three to five is both my therapy and my path forward to full crone/elder status.

An Inhospitable Season:
What we learned from this terrible chapter in human history
Rodney Clough

My wife and business partner and I own and operate a group retreat/family vacation rental in Southwest Michigan. In one form or another—we previously marketed our property as an inn—we have been in the hospitality business for 13 years. Our opening, May 15, 2008, was auspicious. Three months later Lehman Brothers collapsed and like others, we suffered through the Great Recession. Yes, financially speaking our timing for opening an inn in 2008 was a bit off. But onward we persisted and challenged by the fickleness of the hospitality industry, morphed into an Airbnb-type property rental in 2014. As was the case with most small mom-and-pop businesses, January 2020 found us muddling through, paying off debt, borrowing from family, booking Spring and Summer reservations and denying the voraciousness of a distant exotic virus percolating in Wuhan, China.

And now, here we are.

Don't ask, tell

Our avoidance-amidst-denial—'is this really happening to us'—unfortunately was echoed in the public sphere. So, belatedly our first lesson from COVID-19 was 'we are alone' and also 'we are not alone.' Denial, it has been proposed, deprives the carrier of this dual acknowledgment: the feeling that we are alone and that we are not alone. We had a property to maintain, so denial was a luxury we could not afford. This was the first lesson from COVID-19.

The second lesson from COVID-19: 'Don't ask, tell.' We got straight with our guests. We did have a choice: to avoid our customers or to level with them, about their reservation deposits, about their concerns over occupying our property, about their future travel plans. It wasn't about the money, yet it was about the money. We struggled to assure our guests, but also not to mislead them. We tried to anticipate our guests' concerns, avoiding the inevitable questions and innuendos. We didn't wait for our guests to ask... we related to their concerns.

Fortunately, though we couldn't control the public messaging about the impact of COVID-19, our Governor, Gretchen Whitmer, was telling it straight to Michigan residents, so we could calibrate our messaging with her news conferences. This helped as we moved into and out of the state's March and April stay-in-place restrictions. Our guests and their groups, most of whom were traveling to Michigan, needed to be informed and kept up to date. We attempted to address their concerns with a broad brush and then individually by e-mail. We are a small business and we wanted to build on that advantage to stay in touch with our customers. We sent out two group e-mails. Some triggered cancellations, which we had expected. Some triggered renewed commitments, which we didn't expect. A few reluctant cancellations came in—'maybe next year'—which, though well-intentioned, didn't help our bottom line.

(We were rejected for receiving disaster relief. Being self-employed we are 'our payroll,' so were excluded from PPP relief. We are a mom-and-pop hospitality business so were not deemed necessary for disaster relief, as presumably our business would simply bounce back once the disaster part went away and we returned to normalcy.)

We turned smallness to our advantage. We began to move incoming reservations away from third party booking agencies to booking directly, thereby saving our guests third party booking fees. We revised our cancellation policy. We talked through our layout and public areas with our guests, assuring them manageable distancing as well as two private acres to roam. We enhanced our outdoor living amenities: a new barbecue, a new fire pit, additional landscaping. We didn't promote these improvements; we simply made our arriving guests aware of them.

Reinventing Outdoorsy-ness

In December, 2020 we sent out a teaser to our guests about our location and the ease of 'getting into nature.' This e-mail invitation to visit Rabbit Run seemed appropriate, given the uncertainty about how best to sample our neck of the woods during the time of the pandemic and recovery:

Getting away is half the fun… getting into nature is the rest!

Rabbit Run is near hiking trails, like Warren Dunes, Deer Creek, Robinson Woods—all within fifteen minutes from Rabbit Run; near hiking destinations, Grand Mere State Park, Chikaming Park and Preserves; near recreational opportunities, like kayaking through Sima Marsh, solitary fishing in a nearby pond, biking through vineyards.

Rabbit Run is your 'jumping off place' for spring to winter recreation! Bring your serious boots, your bikes, your fishing gear, your binoculars, your camera and step off our porches: an outdoor world awaits!

What we took for granted about our property, we were reminded of by a comment following this post. Our property, slightly under two acres, is near Warren Dunes State Park, an eight-mile stretch of sandy beach fronting Lake Michigan with trails up and down a string of glacial dunes. This is what our commenter recalled about our property: its proximity to Warren Dunes and the joy of trekking out the door to a remarkable landscape and watery horizon.

Back at the property, we have a variety of outdoors access points, from room suite outdoor decks (four), a main deck with barbecue and umbrellaed lounge area, an open space—southern exposure—with Adirondack Chairs, a pond side outdoor gazebo, a fire pit area. And the property's two acres is an important resource. Not so much for the size or scale, but for the space. We bought sweeping lawns as well as woods and a pond. We had lost sight of, or ignored, or taken for granted, the spatial openness until recalled by returning guests.

In the wake of a terrible tragedy, we saw our surroundings differently. This was lesson three.

Another Inhospitable Season?

2021 compared to 2020 changed the pace of our reservations. Whereas 2020 was a season of flux and churn—many cancellations, a late season and Fall increase in bookings—2021 is trending with fewer cancellations and a slower pace in bookings. People are waiting to receive their vaccination(s), navigating the modifications in airline travel, and trying to match family get-togethers with school openings. With a new administration in place in Washington and on damage mitigation, we feel like we are holding our collective breath.

The Final Lesson

New visitors to Rabbit Run experience temporary disorientation. The buildings have multiple entrances (five) and French doors (four), arranged to open the interior to the Michigan Dunes landscape. There is no front door, no hierarchy of entries. Hence, the exterior is not an external, but an invitation to the outside and is a fitting window into this inhospitable time we inhabit. We find ourselves taking solace in nature's assets, open space, seasonal light change.

And to what we cannot lay claim.

Fundraising Amidst COVID
Bill Hartman

In early 2020, COVID emerged at first as a distant event, but it was one that soon spread. For me, COVID struck home when my sister contracted the virus. She had been living in a nursing facility for a couple of years, and had become bedridden with various ailments. Then, on April 10, she tested positive, and on the 18th she died. She was the first case at the nursing home, but within weeks dozens of other residents and staff had succumbed. COVID was real.

Over the ensuing months, the disease spread and became a global pandemic. COVID posed a new threat, akin to 9/11's shattering a long-standing sense of invincibility, but one that was invisible and widespread. The media published developments with an emphasis on the number of new cases and deaths, along with their locations. There were also numerous human-interest features of heroic efforts to save lives and portrayals of horrendous personal suffering and loss amidst a shuttered economy. A lack of preparedness, a disorganized response, and extensive disinformation led to a morphing of the pandemic into an abstraction as numerical tracking of new cases and death produced a numbness in the general public. Various attempts at preventative health protocols along with an early pursuit of testing, vaccinations and other treatments were reported and updated as understanding of the disease progressed and as mutations unfolded.

Many facets of daily life were affected, including transportation, communication, work, and education. There were numerous restrictions and other considerations for a fall opening of school campuses. My school, a large New England boarding school for which I am class agent, had the challenges of a delayed opening, limited and staggered on-campus living, an abundance of new health protocols, and new psychic stresses. Admirably, the school kept parents, alumni and others current on developments.

Notwithstanding COVID, the school continued to emphasize its primary mission of educating youth from every quarter. But it also recognized that many people were suffering financial hardship, and deemphasized fundraising. Although my school is a well-established institution with a large endowment, its need-blind admissions policy relies on annual contributions for support, especially as revenues fall while new costs arise.

As logistics were worked out, fundraising was renewed, but with a high level of sensitivity. While facing one's own hardships, it can be difficult to muster enthusiasm to solicit funds; the needs of today's students and the institution, however, offered encouragement. Fortunately, many alumni identified with the school's situation and contributed with little or no coaxing. As former students, we had benefited from our forebears. As one classmate wrote, there is 'an obligation for all to keep the institution doing its ever-changing job!' Then something unusual happened: students began reaching out to alumni, sharing their experiences and expressing gratitude for our support, thus extending a sense of connectivity and working together.

In general, isolation enables one to discover what's important, in part from seeing what's missing, to engage more with others even if electronically, and to give more as bonds develop. COVID became a unifier for a diversity of perspectives in pursuing a common cause.

My school's motto is *non sibi*, or not for oneself. It has served the institution and students well over a great many years and is particularly apt today. Students and others of the new generations seem to be favouring experiences, pursuing passions and serving others rather than the selfish pursuit of material gain, which only fosters a spirit of greed and consumption. COVID fosters a spirit of unselfishness by creating a new reality.

COVID was a curse that is being transformed into a positive unifier for good. It shows us how globally interconnected we are and illustrates the necessity of unifying and working together. COVID also provides an object lesson for how coming together can work and become a very positive experience, demonstrating how one's own actions can beget actions by others. The common causes and the institutions into which they can solidify become an obligation for all to sustain. My great hope is that we are entering a new era of compassion with a prevailing spirit for good.

It's OK to not be OK
Ruth Hawkins

I take off the headset and sigh. After seven hours of video sessions with clients, I really would like to have a glass of wine and just decompress. It is strange to feel so energized and present when working with a client and then so exhausted after. I don't remember it being this way when I saw clients in person instead of through a computer screen. I don't remember needing to take power naps during breaks between sessions. Life BC: before COVID... it seems an eon ago.

No wine. It would be a slippery slope. 'Self-care' for therapists doesn't include being an alcoholic. My concession to the long day is delivery of questionable nutrition. I sit alone on the couch in front of the TV and have my very late dinner, breaking several healthy eating rules all at once. I don't care. After a full day of supporting others through this pandemic experience, I need solitude and dissociation—no more listening, no more being fully present, no more empathy, no more feeling. Just sit. Reflect.

I feel numb, spent. Can I allow myself to feel *my* feelings while I'm overfull of the feelings of others? I struggle to find bits of empathy for my own family as they rail against the lockdown, new workplace demands, their loneliness, and busy signals on government phone lines. (Shut up, shut up, shut up). I don't say it and I don't tell them that I'm struggling. I barely admit *that* to myself. Time to cuddle the dog and press reset. Breathe.

I am supposed to be able to hold my own issues and triggers to the side while working with a client, and then take all my crap to my own therapist. This doesn't quite work during a shared pandemic experience; we have no blueprints or useful guidance to draw on. Most of the time, I feel like I'm winging it. I feel alone.

My own struggles are mirrored in what my clients bring to their sessions. This is what makes it hard: frustration and anger with family and friends who don't abide by 'the rules'; fear of catching COVID or, worse, fear giving it to people they love; and fear of not being able to make up 'lost time' spent in lockdown (for them, they worry that grandparents with dementia may not know them at the end of all this; for me, it's the sorrow of missing precious time with my new granddaughter). The aching loss in my clients resonates with my own. We are all in some form of mourning.

It can be a revelation when a client discovers that I too have a therapist. Maybe they think that, given my age, I would be 'done' with that. The fact is therapists need their own therapist. Especially now. A lot of the time we *are* OK, but not every day... not every week. Listening and supporting others going through this persistent, pervasive isolation and disconnection from others takes a toll.

Despite *having* a therapist, myself, I somehow thought I would be different and would be able to sail through these difficult times. Why did I think I was so different or special? Should my age and life experience have made it easier? It is true that I have more to draw from in understanding how life can take surprising shifts, both good and bad. Time gives the wisdom of lived experiences. It gives foundations upon which to understand the fears and challenges of others. But time is a double-edged sword for an elder: experience on one side, awareness of the lack of time remaining on the other.

For many months after lockdowns began, I was fine. And then, suddenly, I wasn't. For a while, I had this belief that others didn't see that I was struggling, and conversely grew resentful that they were not psychic enough to notice. I dropped hints, but my children and my partner seemed to shy away from noticing that the anchor in their lives was... what? Sad? Depressed? Not coping? Of course, when they ask how I am, I lie and say fine, hanging in there, blah, blah, blah. My adult children—having endured seven years of their father's slow death from Lewy Body Dementia—can't endure their mother not being hale and hearty (or so I suppose). I am their rock, their constant. And my partner? When I hint that I am not doing particularly well, I see the panic in his eyes. Or is it my own panic merely reflected? I do not do well with not doing well.

So, I keep my tears and deep sadness to myself until my next appointment with my own therapist. I muster the courage to tell her that I feel depressed and struggling. Simply admitting this, shifts something in me. I feel heard and seen. I am able to climb out of this COVID hole and move back into acceptance and flexibility, better equipped to endure this endless, touchless, distanced, and isolating world. Her acknowledgement that being 'not okay' is okay feels like permission to feel. It liberates me, and once again, I gain that vital awareness of *why* my clients need *me*, and I am able to carry on.

Prof with Parkinson's Zooms Her Way Through Pandemic
Betsy Hoffman and Jon Peirce

Learning how to teach virtually, through Zoom and other, similar platforms, would be difficult enough, one would think, for a fully-abled professor. For a professor over 70, and suffering from Parkinson's Disease, such a switch would surely be well-nigh impossible.

Not so, says Betsy Hoffman, an Iowa State University economics professor who has had Parkinson's for either nine or twelve years, depending on whether one starts with the date of her official diagnosis in 2012 or her earlier realization that her frequent falls and increasingly serious mobility issues were likely due to Parkinson's. If anything, Zoom has given her teaching career a new lease on life.

'I'm amazed at just how easy it is to communicate now, with Zoom,' Hoffman said in a recent interview, noting that in her lecture course, she can speak to the students and still read the slides. 'In fact, I read the slides better than before, because I no longer have to look behind, but can look right at the students.' The one issue she has had is with students turning their cameras off during class. After one request from her, the students in her grad class kept their cameras on during class. But she finally gave up asking her under-grad students, many of whom claimed they didn't have cameras in their computers.

During the period just prior to the COVID pandemic, Hoffman was having difficulty teaching her live courses. She required a four-wheeled walker to get to class and was forced to teach sitting down, as her Parkinson's and the aftermath of earlier back surgery made it difficult for her to stand while teaching. By the Spring of 2019, students were complaining that they couldn't hear her. For the first time in her long career, her teaching ratings slipped below the top level, though they still weren't bad.

A nearly fatal septic bladder infection in the fall of 2019 forced Hoffman to go virtual even before the start of the pandemic. 'The doctors didn't want me to go out, and for two weeks I didn't host my class at all,' Hoffman said. Going virtual at least gave her a way to complete the course.

'When the pandemic hit, I was relieved that I didn't have to go back to my office,' Hoffman continued. 'At that point, I would have retired—if I hadn't had Parkinson's.'

Under different circumstances, Hoffman and her husband, fellow economist Brian Binger, would have used retirement to do more travelling, something she'd already been doing a great deal of due to her involvement with many professional boards. But with travel next to impossible due to the pandemic, she needed some other source of intellectual and emotional stimulation. And teaching was it.

'Teaching keeps my brain active; it keeps me engaged at a time when there are so many things I used to do that I can't do anymore,' said Hoffman, who in addition to being a world traveler had previously been a passionate runner and downhill skier.

Not least of the challenges Hoffman faced was that of having to redesign her undergraduate public finance course. 'I couldn't use my previous textbook,' Hoffman explained, 'because it didn't have anything in it about the pandemic.' Fortunately, she found that the respected journal *Congressional Quarterly* had published a series of articles taking opposing viewpoints on various aspects of the pandemic.

Using the *CQ* articles as the new basis for her course, Hoffman launched what she called a 'threaded discussion' online. Each week she would pose a question; students would get credit either for initiating a discussion or for responding to an existing one. They were also expected to write a short paper each week. Perhaps as a result of these frequent assignments, Hoffman 'found that their writing improved dramatically through the term.'

The public finance course featured two 'high-stakes' assignments: a research paper, and a debate on a hot-button contemporary issue such as whether college should be free or COVID vaccination should be mandatory. While Hoffman had used debates in the course previously, she found that they worked better online than they had live. 'Online,' she explained, 'I could send them into discussion groups.'

How did Hoffman's students respond to learning in the brave new environment? 'They didn't like the different environment caused by the pandemic, but they've adjusted to it. Many students are desperate to get back together,' she said.

Certainly, the students in her courses appear to have adjusted well enough. At the end of the term, her evaluations were back up to the high levels they'd been prior to the pandemic.

Even through the pandemic, Hoffman has continued to serve on her departmental promotion and tenure committee. At the request of her chair, she has also been heading up an equity, diversity, and inclusion committee. To me, this seemed, frankly, beyond the call of duty. Why, at a time when she was already under significant stress, would she take on these extra duties? Her response was that the committee work 'allows me, as the only woman full professor in the department, to help shape the department's future.'

Amazingly, she has also managed to continue doing research during this stressful time. In addition to co-authoring several journal articles with colleagues, she prepared a detailed, massively-researched slide talk on the history of pandemics, delivering the talk (virtually) to, among others, her

Smith College class and a women's group in nearby Des Moines. (Parts of this talk appear in Section 1 of this almanac.) She plans to continue doing research, mainly in collaboration with her graduate students, for as long as she continues teaching.

What makes Hoffman's continuing to teach, do research, and serve on committees during the pandemic even more remarkable is that she did all of that while self-isolating. With Iowa one of the hardest-hit states in the country, the one-time world traveler didn't go out at all, except for medical appointments, for a full year, from March of 2020 through March of 2021, by which time she had been fully vaccinated. Essential errands were run by her husband.

But staying home did not, by any means, mean being inactive. Throughout her period of self-isolation, and even after it finally ended, she was part of a Parkinson's singing group, put together by a woman from the Iowa State kinesiology department who does therapy. In addition to choral singing, the group does chair boxing and chair yoga, and dancing—all activities requiring deep breathing to be performed effectively. With one class a week in each of the above activities, that means a lot of deep breathing!

Despite the long period of self-isolation, her new lifestyle appears to be working for Hoffman. When I talked with her in September of 2020, her voice was so soft that I had difficulty hearing her, and frequently had to ask her to repeat what she had said. This almost never happened during our two interviews for this piece, in April of 2021. Her voice was pretty much as I remembered it from our youth. (We've known each other since our college days.) Except for a certain huskiness, it gave no evidence of her disability.

What does the future hold for Hoffman? Does she plan to go on teaching despite the twin challenges posed by virtual technology and her own disability? On this point, she is quite determined.

'I intend to teach and to go to meetings—virtually—for as long as my mental stamina holds up,' said Hoffman, who as usual will be teaching a class this fall, and who has requested permission from her department chair and the university's human resources department to teach virtually even once live classes again become the norm at Iowa State—permission she thinks it likely that she'll receive. Far from being a barrier to her, the new Zoom technology has likely extended her teaching career beyond where she would have been able to take it 'live.'

'I think it [Zoom] is a boon to older people and people with disabilities, as well as to those who would prefer to save money, gas, and travel time,' Hoffman said. While others may have found that the new technology also has its drawbacks, there's no doubt that for her, it appears to have worked like a charm.

Volunteering During COVID
Lee Keener

In 2015, I retired, having completed a long career in academia at various universities, including Dalhousie University in Halifax, Indiana University in South Bend, the University of Alberta, and the University of Northern British Columbia in Prince George. My field was mathematics, but upon retirement I found I had little interest in doing any more math. It seemed like 43 years was enough.

Feeling a bit underemployed, I decided to expand my range of volunteer activities. Now, volunteer work was nothing new to me. Over my career I'd volunteered for several different organizations, among other things serving as a director of the Prince George Art Gallery and the Prince George Symphony Orchestra. And at the time of my retirement, I was the class secretary for the Amherst College Class of 1967, in which capacity I continue today.

This time, I thought I would try something a bit different. When I was much younger, I'd been a hosteling enthusiast, mostly using youth hostels (as they were then labeled) in Italy and the United Kingdom, one of my favourite hostels being the Borrowdale hostel in the English Lake District. Indeed, I had continued to hostel in my mature years.

With the extra time I had available after retiring, I thought I might give something back to hosteling, which I had enjoyed for so many years. One of my close friends had served as a director of the Canadian Pacific Mountain Region of Hosteling International (HIPMR). With his example in mind, I ran for a director position and was fortunate enough to be elected.

These positions are unpaid, but they offer a significant perk: free travel. The PMR region includes many of Canada's great national parks, such as Banff, Jasper and Yoho, as well as popular tourist destinations such as Whistler, Vancouver and Lake Louise. The organization has hostels in all these locations. Some are what are called 'wilderness hostels,' including a string of five hostels along the Icefields Parkway in Jasper and Banff Parks. We rotated our meetings through many of these venues and had great fun, while also tending to serious business. The people involved in the organization have been unfailingly pleasant and competent. I have made many lifetime friendships through my work with HIPMR.

Then came COVID! As we drove through a snowstorm on our return from a meeting in Tofino on the west coast of Vancouver Island in February 2020, none of us realized that we would not physically meet again for many months. Since then, it has been all Zoom. In September we elected three new

303

directors. None of them has met the older directors in person, or even each other, for that matter. Not only have our Annual General Meetings been online, so have our regular board and committee meeting. We even held a bit of a party online.

Having to operate online is of course a blow to social cohesion; some of the fun of working with the organization has been lost. Fortunately, for me, my commitment to PMR and my interest in its success have been compensation for other losses. For a new director, though, I expect that the situation has been harder and perhaps discouraging. For reasons that are not COVID-related, I will step down from my director position in September, after six years of service.

While others have had a more difficult time, I live in a comfortable home on a lake in a rural location. We have an immense home library, a large collection of films and music, and a grand piano, cello and clarinet (played by my wife, myself and my daughter respectively). We have a secure income and so are much luckier than most people. Indeed, I am luckier than the other members of my family (my wife and daughter). My wife continues to work online and is becoming very cyber-stressed. She is at her screen eight or 10 hours every day. Thankfully, she will retire at the end of June. My daughter is doing her first year of engineering at the University of Alberta at home and entirely online. By comparison, I am most fortunate.

The pandemic has adversely affected the hosteling organization, as it has affected every component of the hospitality industry. Most of our hostels are now closed. The few that are not are operating at significantly reduced capacity and are employing stringent safety measures. Government wage subsidies, hostel rentals, and an excellent CEO will allow us to survive the pandemic. But COVID has altered the lives of many of our employees who have been temporarily or permanently laid off. And the stress on our operations staff has been substantial.

My other volunteer position, as class secretary, has been much less affected by the pandemic. My work in that capacity has always been online, so COVID brought no changes. Even the nature of the correspondence with classmates has not much altered. Since practically all of them are retired, they have not by and large had to face financial problems. Only one or two have reported contracting the virus (with no apparent long-term effects).

Perhaps the biggest change to all of our lives has been the difficulty in travelling. Most of the members of the Class of '67 are still fairly healthy and in that time of life when health combined with retirement and an adequate income would normally mean heading to exotic places. Our family may be typical. We had to cancel a trip to Hawaii, a high school graduation trip to New York for our daughter (we had tickets to *Hadestown* and *Hamilton!*), and a school trip to London for our daughter. I also had to cancel a trip to Cambridge (U.K.) where I was to do a performance class on *Romeo and Juliet*.

Certainly 2020 was a challenging year. But it had its upside, too. I managed to read Proust's *Remembrance of Things Past* (all seven volumes). That's got to be worth something.

Easing the Final Slide:
Harder Since the COVID-19 Pandemic
Bill Newmann and *Jon Peirce*

For Olympia, Washington physician Bill Newmann, dying really hasn't been all that much fun since the start of the COVID-19 pandemic.

Come again? But lest you think Newmann some sort of bloody Frankenstein-type of figure, a bit of explanation may be in order. Since his retirement from general practice in 2009, Newmann has been an 'end-of-life' specialist. Preparing terminally ill patients for death and then attending at their deathbeds is what he does. With COVID and the substitution of Zoom and other forms of new technology for in-person contact with patients and their families, neither activity is even remotely like what it was prior to the pandemic.

Being there at the bedsides of dying patients to comfort them and their loved ones has been a source of deep and lasting satisfaction for Newmann, who reckons he's attended about 10 deaths since beginning his end-of-life work. 'The positive feelings I get when attending a death include the warmth and closeness of shared relief, peace and sadness, plus deep gratitude for the honor and privilege of being recognized as an important part of their lives, facilitating and supporting their loved ones' final request,' says Newmann.

From a longer-term perspective, Newmann views the experience of attending at patients' deaths as useful preparation for his own. 'Looking deeper, and lasting longer, I project, at some level, the image of my own death scene being as intimate, peaceful, comfortable and not lonely,' he says.

How has the pandemic changed Newmann's end-of-life work? 'Overall, I feel far less engaged,' he says, noting that COVID has made it hard for him to attend at deaths, although he did do so in one case where he had a close bond with the patient. Now, having been vaccinated, and with the end of the pandemic close at hand, he hopes to be able to start attending at deaths again before too long.

The other major component of Newmann's end-of-life work is serving as a consulting physician, helping terminally ill patients and their families prepare for death. Here, much of his attention has been focussed on documents known as 'living wills,' which provide guidance to patients' health care representatives as to the patients' wishes around dying and death. For example, when it's clear that the end is at hand, does the patient want to be taken off their ventilator immediately, so they can die immediately? Or would they prefer to be kept on their ventilator and given other medical treatment for a few more days or a week, to allow faraway loved ones to come and say goodbye?

Decisions such as these are complex and emotionally charged; it's critical that the consulting physician, as well as whoever the patient has chosen as their health care representative, understand the patient's values around end-of-life issues.

Newmann's work as a consulting end-of-life physician, work which has often involved his helping patients draw up their living wills, has provided a different but equally powerful source of satisfaction as his bedside work. Says Newmann: 'I get a different type of satisfaction when I do the consultation where I am actively engaged in finding out about the patient and his/her close family and/or friend(s). This is really what I enjoyed most as a family physician.'

Through the 40 to 50 end-of-life cases he has dealt with as a consulting physician, Newmann has found his greatest satisfaction in establishing bonds of trust with patients and their families, and in learning about the often-private details of their medical histories. Equally rewarding have been the insights he has gained into the 'social, emotional, occupational, avocational, intellectual and even spiritual contexts of their lives, including their sense of humour, and their physical surroundings.'

Further satisfaction has come in cases when he has been able to 'offer some useful ways of further exploring some of their medical concerns.' In such cases, Newmann has often been stimulated to learn more about his patients' medical picture by researching the medical literature and/or contacting their usual health care providers.

As in the case of his work attending dying patients, COVID has greatly diminished the satisfaction Newmann finds in his consulting work. With interviews almost entirely done over Zoom, he has 'missed the personal directness and the opportunity to get to meet and talk to the family members who are around. It's hard to establish any close relationships with people when everything's being done virtually.'

Is any special training required for doctors wishing to do end-of-life work? Perhaps surprisingly, no, although Newmann recommends a good background in pharmacology as 'important in understanding the impact of the various end-of-life drugs that we use.'

As for medical specialties that might lend themselves to a career switch to end-of-life work, Newmann suggests two: anesthesiology and pulmonary medicine. At the same time, he notes that many young doctors are opting to go into palliative care right out of residency. But most important of all, in his view, is experience—either personal or professional—with the process of dying. 'Being at the bedside of at least two or three dying patients is an invaluable experience,' he suggests.

'Beyond that,' he says, 'what's most important is how the person lives before dying. You have to be concerned (as an end-of-life physician) with how to help the person live their life to the maximum.'

Newmann's own interest in end-of-life work evolved more or less naturally, from seeing his patients age and, eventually, die, and from observing the struggles of two seriously ill family members: his brother and his mother. As a young man, Newmann had the experience of seeing his brother (John), just four years older than him, have his kidneys fail just after he got back from the Peace Corps. John became one of the first people to go on home dialysis for kidney failure. The experience led him to get a degree in public health and to become a consultant and an advocate for kidney patients. Among other things, he lobbied for federal legislation providing for home dialysis. John was a sort of role model for his younger brother.

Later, he started looking into medically-assisted dying when the Hemlock Society, dedicated to allowing terminally ill patients to die more humanely and on their own terms, had gotten started in Seattle. At about the same time, a similar organization called Compassionate Choices had started. He had one patient through Compassionate Choices.

All of this made Newmann seriously interested in the issue, and eventually he acquired on-the-job training through attending at a number of medically-assisted deaths. 'It became my way of keeping my hand in medicine after I had given up my regular practice,' Newmann says. His interest was further stimulated by a number of family tragedies, notably the experience of having his mother living with him and his wife for her last eight years, during the last four of which she was bedridden.

'I believe she suffered greatly in her last days,' says Newmann, adding that he believes that if end-of-life assistance had been available to her then, 'She would have taken that cocktail.'

Does Newmann (now 76 and with some health issues of his own) know how much longer he'll be carrying on with his end-of-life work? Despite his age and health concerns, he firmly insists that he has no plans to retire. 'As long as I can make myself available in this consulting role, I don't see it stopping until my physical and mental capacity decline much more than they have.' The work, he adds, is 'an important source of my involvement with the world.'

Meanwhile, Newmann has also been involved to a degree in mentoring and education around end-of-life issues, though he has no intention of making this his primary focus. 'I'm more interested in doing the work than in doing the advocacy,' he says.

That said, he *has* been reaching out to colleagues in the community and at conferences. While most comfortable talking to people individually, he will occasionally talk to a small group such as the local men's hiking club that recently asked him to talk to them about medically-assisted dying. 'I'm fine with talking to small groups but am not actively pursuing opportunities to do so,' Newmann adds.

As medically-assisted death becomes available in more and more North

American jurisdictions, and more and more widely accepted by society as a whole, it seems likely that more terminally ill people will choose to avail themselves of this option. One can only hope that those who do will have a physician as humane and as empathetic as Bill Newmann to accompany them on the final and in many ways most important journey of their lives.

Sudden Turns
Fran Ota

In my immediate past 'incarnation,' I was an ordained minister/musician, housewife, sometime artist, writer and gardener. In January 2020 I left a contract with a wonderful congregation, but one looking for full-time ministry. I knew that at 74 I didn't have the stamina to do that anymore.

You need to know a little history. Everything we do grows or emerges from something we've already done. In 1970, I went to Japan as a missionary with The United Church of Canada. I was a 'preacher's kid' and already used to moving around. Japan was a door opening into so much more: marriage to my language teacher, three years with education and refugees in Vietnam, then on to New Jersey, Australia, Michigan, and our current home, Toronto, and along the way in all those places, four children and more education. It was in Toronto that I shocked the entire family by signing up to go to seminary at the age of 45. That was the first 'sudden turn.' Several years into ministry, the next 'sudden turn' took me to Corner Brook in Newfoundland, leaving family and husband in Toronto for three years.

I am an inveterate traveler, and both Iceland and Norway have long figured in my wanderings, readings and followings. In January 2020, right when that ministry contract ended, Facebook mysteriously presented an ad: 'Study in Iceland—Master's Degree in Viking and Medieval Norse Studies.' It kept coming back; finally, I decided the Universe was sending a message. 'Check this out!' Luckily, I have a great family, all five of whom said, 'If you want to do that, do it!' I can hear my youngest, who at 44 finished an MBA, saying, 'Go for it, Ma!'

In January 2020, we were not really hearing much about COVID, and so the often-hilarious process of application began. I had to submit graduate and undergraduate transcripts and two references from people who had taught me at each level. The undergraduate degree had been 50 years earlier (50 already?!), and the references were from 25 years before! Transcripts were sent, and the two references were the last two professors still at the seminary who had actually taught me, both of whom were retiring in April. Talk about close timing! Still laughing, to be honest. And then there were immigration and an RCMP criminal records check, to be allowed to come to Iceland to study and live. So now I am a card-carrying legal resident of Iceland.

The program is an inter-disciplinary international degree in Viking and Medieval Norse Studies. It is free, and all taught in English. It is the brainchild of the University of Iceland, with one possible semester at Aarhus University and the University of Copenhagen, and the entire second year at the University of Oslo. (When I travel to Norway for second year it will be as a University of Iceland exchange student on the Erasmus Program, and I will be eligible for a grant.)

In April 2020 an acceptance letter arrived. Seriously? By then, COVID was much more real, but still not a big issue. Or so we thought. Now it was more paperwork, only this time it was immigration to Iceland complete with a full RCMP criminal records check, financial information, health information. I also had to buy health insurance for six months till Icelandic insurance kicked in, get an apartment in student housing, register for classes, and try to learn some language.

In August 2020, finally the time came. After two cancelled flights because of COVID and travel changes, I boarded a flight to Iceland via Frankfurt. Long but worth it. Iceland at that time had options for entering the country: a two-week quarantine in an approved location, or a test-five-day quarantine-test option. Now there is further testing added before travel, but that's a smart thing to do. Having an apartment meant it was possible to come straight here and fall into bed. I came with sheets, blanket, a mini-frypan and tiny pot, rice, Japanese dried food and tea, a couple of cups and bowls, and some cutlery. Having the apartment meant being able to quarantine without problem, start class, get acclimatized, and be relaxed.

I've been living here since August 19, 2020. My husband suggested a couple of times I could stay in Toronto and do classes from there. No, I couldn't! It's the *whole* of the experience, not just the safer bits. At 74, I made it here, set up living and started classes. I went into lockdown when COVID spiked but, even then, made friends and kept up with their lives. First semester I did four courses: Medieval Religion and Christianity, Old Icelandic 1, Old Norse/Icelandic Literary Corpus, and a Scandinavian history course. All of us were basket cases by the end of the semester, but we all got through. Now we are buried in Old Norse Religion, Medieval Archaeology, and Old Icelandic 2, reading medieval texts and leaning to transcribe them.

As I look back, the amount of learning—not just academic—has been incredible. Iceland took the long view on COVID, and as soon as things looked bad, a lockdown was instituted and enforced. And yet, although we could not go to class in person, we could shop and go for walks around the city. I have a lovely studio apartment in student housing, very close to the water. It's been a lifeline, and I've been extremely happy here. Much as I miss my husband's company, I would not have missed any of this, even the COVID bits. Iceland has provided free education and free health care. For those naysayers who insist it doesn't work; yes, it does. Here we are, 30 international students (there are many more in other programs) getting a free education, and covered for health insurance.

I've learned to navigate grocery store and restaurant websites, and to order groceries instead of going out to shop. I opened a bank account online, using Google translate. That's one of the things that has been so great here; banks and institutions were *ready* for COVID, and had everything up and running without a blink. The economy was affected but never shut down because the small business owners were treated as critical to the survival of the whole economy, without compromising safety.

Instead of driving, I'm back to busing, which I much prefer. I've made friends; within the current restrictions we can entertain so long as it's not more than 10. Easter dinner this weekend will be here, with three friends coming to eat.

The other piece is how much I have learned academically, of history, archaeology, religion, literature. There is so much, and it just gets better. Next August, for second year several of us will travel to Norway... hopefully. With COVID we never know, and that's another major lesson. We have to be able to adjust and carry on, and be hopeful that the conditions will improve.

Iceland is far enough north that the winters are very dark for a couple of months, and in Summer very light for a couple of months. In December, Reykjavik had four hours of daylight, but the nights were amazing, with Northern Lights putting on a show just often enough that even with city lights it was possible to get pictures. Now as we move toward Summer it's up to almost 13 hours of daylight. The temperatures vary much less than they do in North America, because Iceland gets the Gulf Stream which makes it a temperate climate in the south.

I have been here when a new volcano decided to form; a baby volcano, brand new. It hasn't been practical for me to get down to see it, but friends have, and the pictures are fabulous. It certainly would not have been the same watching from Canada. Over 50,000 earthquakes in a couple of weeks, and finally a very quiet and sedate extrusion of lava from the earth in the Gelding Valley, unnoticed until the red glow showed on the horizon at night. Here for history in the making!

I've been bemused by those people who insist that COVID and lockdowns have impacted their lives so severely that they cannot function. My generation lived with infectious disease, because there were no vaccines for many of those diseases, such as measles. So, we have a handle on what infectious disease means. Yet life indeed does go on; it's what we make of it while we're in it that's important. When I'm home in Toronto, there's a garden, painting, reading, writing, sewing; so many things right there to do, and there is never enough time, from my perspective. My husband and I have a home in Japan which his parents left and we are going there for five weeks in the Summer. Yes, we have to get tested and do quarantines, but we are quite happy with that. The pandemic has required adjustments, and it does require some flexibility, but life is still good and it is life!

This is only half the saga. On May 2, if the flights go, it's back to Toronto via Munich and Frankfurt—empty airports and short lines—and flying business class for both the comfort and a birthday treat, but mostly because of the extra weight allowance!

Second semester is almost over and it's been a blast all the way. In August the next part of the saga picks up in Oslo. Who knows where this will lead next? If I were to give advice, it would be that there is always something to do. Be open to those 'sudden turns' if you can, step out without knowing, tackle something new and different. Even mid-pandemic, learn as much as you can and have as many new experiences as you can.

Life is still good!

313

Un petit récit, pour se sortir des statistiques…
Camille Pellerin-Forget

Je suis physiothérapeute pédiatrique en réadaptation. Je me retrouve de façon volontaire dans la zone rouge d'une ressource intermédiaire pour personnes âgées. L'histoire est réelle, mais les noms, histoires et numéros de chambres ont été modifiés afin de n'y reconnaître personne, (mais de les entendre tous…).

Jour 1

Premier jour en zone rouge. J'y entre comme physiothérapeute, mais aussi comme préposée aux bénéficiaires, vers un inconnu considérable, un inconnu grisant. J'aime l'action, j'aime profondément les gens. Cela suffira.

Je vais *aux ordres*, la routine m'est encore nouvelle. On me dit « Ce pauvre homme, au 653, est mourant, tu lui fais sa toilette au lit et tu le rassures doucement. Il ne lui en reste plus pour longtemps… » Premier jour, première seconde dans mes souliers rouges.

J'entre au 653. Un sac poubelle fait office de rideau, la pièce est désordonnée quoique très propre. Des espadrilles, pantoufles, *loafers* jonchent le sol, deux fauteuils roulants encombrent l'espace. Des verres de styromousse trônent sur toutes les surfaces libres.

Je regarde *mon patient*. Il est couché, il semble dormir. À première vue, il ne présente pas de symptômes respiratoires ou de fièvre. Cette période du virus est terminée m'a-t-on dit. Je le réveille d'une caresse au bras, je lui explique ce que je suis venue faire. Au moment de changer sa culotte d'incontinence et de le laver, je lui pose quelques questions, courtoises et douces, sur le soin que je prodigue. J'ai déjà envie qu'il soit bien, qu'il me fasse confiance. Il me répond dans un râle expiré des mots inaudibles, ou pas de mots, peut-être.

Je m'essaie autrement, j'ai besoin qu'il existe au-delà du soin médical.

- Vous venez d'où, vous ?

J'espère qu'il entend ma sincérité, même drapée dans la bonhommie.

- Alma (dans un murmure).

- Ah… vous me comprenez, donc. Et vous pouvez parler. Alors on va parler un peu.

J'essaie de sourire avec mes yeux, ou même avec mon corps. Je ne maîtrise pas encore la façon d'offrir mon empathie en vêtements de protection, mais cela viendra. La danse de l'empathie se fait avec tout le corps, même s'il est masqué, ganté, et caché sous une visière et un vêtement jaune et informe. La douceur du geste devient notre seule façon de sourire,

314

les murmures de notre corps deviennent bienveillance.

J'observe le patient, il a l'air si jeune, trop jeune pour être un vrai *vieux*. Il en est à sa deuxième semaine de COVID, il bouge à peine.

- Vous êtes né en quelle année, monsieur Lavoie ?
- 1945, j'pense bien…

Et là, je l'entends, son accent d'Alma. Même soupiré, il chante, son accent. Ainsi, entre chaque silence, je lui arrache des morceaux de son histoire. J'ai envie de le connaître, ne serait-ce que pour mieux le rassurer.

- Bon, on a terminé. Que dites-vous de vous habiller maintenant ? Rester en culotte d'incontinence au lit toute la journée, je ne crois pas que cela soit bon pour le moral.
- Mmmh.

Il ferme les yeux, pour me congédier, probablement.

- Après je vous laisse tranquille, c'est promis.

J'ouvre les tiroirs.

- Vous avez de jolis vêtements, qui a choisi cela ?
- C'est ma femme.

Je lui fais une sélection de vêtements ; il hausse les épaules sans intérêt, mais ne ferme pas les yeux. Nous gardons la culotte d'incontinence, mais elle se dissimule sous des vêtements seyants. Une fois dignement—mais confort-ablement—habillé, semi assis dans un lit redressé, il n'a déjà plus l'air d'un mourant, monsieur Lavoie. Il n'a que 75 ans, après tout.

Jour 2

J'entre dans sa chambre pour le soin du matin : toilette partielle à la débarbouillette et changement de culotte. Je décide d'être un peu plus physiothérapeute qu'hier, aujourd'hui.

- Bonjour Monsieur Lavoie. C'est encore moi.

J'essaie de faire briller ma voix, d'en faire une mélodie agréable. Je dois faire attention, rassurer sans envahir. Et favoriser la lumière, pas la légèreté. Il ouvre à peine les yeux. Juste assez pour admettre ma présence. Je m'installe près de lui, le geste lent. Je ne veux pas le brusquer…

- Ce matin, j'aimerais vous asseoir sur le bord du lit pour vous habiller, d'accord ? C'est bon pour vos poumons, d'être un peu vertical. De bouger, aussi.

Il consent presque tacitement. Un petit hochement de tête, seulement. Je l'aide à s'asseoir au bord du lit, en utilisant la recette magique propre aux physiothérapeutes : il parvient à s'asseoir sans effort ni de ma part, ni de la sienne. Il semble surpris. Délicatement, je l'aide à se laver puis à se vêtir, en le laissant faire tout ce qu'il parvient à faire seul.

« J'veux me coucher maintenant », me dit-il, la voix faible. Il se laisse retomber dans le lit et s'endort aussitôt.

Nous recommencerons cet après-midi : s'asseoir au bord du lit pour boire de l'eau, discuter un peu.

Jour 3

-   Bonjour Monsieur Lavoie ! C'est moi !

Il me sourit en coin, ouvre un œil fourbu.

-   Vous êtes prêt à faire votre toilette ?
-   Non, trop fatigué.
-   D'accord, je vous laisse faire une grasse matinée de trente minutes et je reviens. Il n'est que huit heures après tout.

Je pose ma main sur sa joue, quelques secondes.

Il hoche la tête les yeux clos, et il me sourit encore. Notre complicité me rassure plus que je ne saurais l'admettre. À neuf heures pile, je retente le coup.

-   Voilà ! Je vous ai même apporté votre déjeuner. On fait la toilette et vous mangez après ?
-   Mmmmmm OK…

Comme la veille, je l'installe au bord du lit. Il le fait avec tant d'aise que je sens une petite vague d'excitation me submerger. Pour un professionnel de la réadaptation, un accomplissement, ça implique un nouveau défi. Ce qui est acquis ne sert qu'à créer de nouveaux objectifs. Préposée, d'accord. Mais physiothérapeute aussi.

-   Alors que diriez-vous d'aller à la toilette pour faire votre changement de culotte ? Je vous y emmène en fauteuil ! Vous en avez deux dans la chambre !
-   J'pas capable.
-   Mais oui, vous verrez, ça va se faire tout seul. Je sers à ça. Vous me faites confiance ?
-   Tu vas m'échapper. T'es trop p'tite.
-   Je vous promets que non. Je vous indique les étapes, et vous verrez…

En un instant, il parvient à s'asseoir dans le fauteuil roulant en mettant de la charge sur ses jambes, et en pivotant avec grâce. Il sourit encore, satisfait. En coin, au cas où je surprendrais son sourire.

-   Ah ben. Me v'là.
-   Maintenant, allons à la salle de bain. Vous pouvez avancer avec vos jambes ?
-   Mmmmmm.
-   Allez, je vous pousse pour vous aider.

(Je ne pousse pas le fauteuil roulant, je le laisse avancer des pieds, seul. Je sais. C'est de la triche. Mais il avance et bouge ses jambes.) Je suis si heureuse que je le prendrais dans mes bras. L'empathie se transforme doucement, je le sens. Comme tous les autres patients de l'étage, ils ne sont plus le 645 ou le 657, mais bien mes parents ou mes grands-parents, déjà.

- Monsieur Lavoie, ça me fait réellement plaisir cet effort que vous faites. Allons à la toilette maintenant.
- Hein ? Là-dessus ?

Il pointe la toilette, le regard incrédule. Je me demande depuis combien de temps il n'y a pas été. Je souris, à mon tour. Il ne le voit pas, mais il l'entend, je sais, mon sourire. Il l'entend.

- Oui ! On fait pareil comme au lit, mais ici.

Quelques minutes et un appel à un collègue plus tard (il s'endort sur la toilette, nous devons être deux pour le remettre au fauteuil ; j'y vois une stratégie de sa part pour avoir la paix) : je l'installe au lit. Épuisé, habillé, coiffé et propre, il s'installe sous la couverture.

- J'veux dormir maintenant.
- D'accord. C'est bien mérité monsieur Lavoie.

Je serre affectueusement son épaule, je veux qu'il sente la délicate familiarité. Ce lien tendre, il me permettra de demander l'effort quand il le faudra. De le rendre momentanément heureux, peut-être, aussi. On ne lésine pas avec le bonheur.

Cette histoire, cet homme, ces autres patients aussi, me font réfléchir. Je travaille habituellement en réadaptation pédiatrique. Avec les enfants handicapés, l'autonomie permet la liberté. Avec les personnes âgées, l'autonomie, elle, préserve la dignité. Je pose le déjeuner sur une table collée au lit, redresse le dossier à moitié et le laisse dormir, en me disant que le déjeuner, ça ira à 10 :00 h.

Lorsque je repasse plus tard, le déjeuner a été complètement englouti, le café bu. Il dort encore.

Jour 6

Sixième jour, le temps file, il me reste 4 semaines encore, je m'attache à ces patients, trop vite. Je les aime. Tous. L'empathie s'est muée en autre chose, de plus viscéral, de plus grand. Je n'ai jamais été bonne pour l'amour détaché, pour la douceur apprise… Je me lie aux patients, je n'y peux rien.

Monsieur Lavoie est assis au bord du lit à mon arrivée le matin. Sa nouvelle marchette siège près de lui, la chambre est libérée de ses fauteuils roulants. Les souliers sont toujours là, mais ils sont utilisés, maintenant.

- Bonjour vous !
- Hey salut toi ! De retour ce matin ?
- On prend une douche ce matin ?
- OK, mais pas trop longue, là ?

J'adore quand il s'impatiente doucement, quand il déteste que les choses traînent. Il se lève, tel qu'il l'a appris. Il marche jusqu'à la salle de bain, avec la marchette, aussi rapide que moi près de lui. Parfois, il oublie de la prendre.

C'est bon signe, dirait-t-on en réadaptation. En gériatrie, c'est différent. Oublier la marchette, c'est risqué. Une chute peut être le début de la fin. Et là, on ne peut pas gérer deux *fins de vie* en même temps, on en a assez avec la COVID…

- Je vous aide pour la barbe ou vous la faites seul ?
- Je vais le faire.

Je l'observe. Le geste lent, habitué, il mouille le visage, étend la mousse et entreprend de raser cette barbe qu'il a coupée des centaines de fois. Ce geste, il est rassurant. Ce geste, il lui permet de redevenir homme. Cette image est magnifique, j'en ai la gorge nouée.

- Ça ira comme ça ?

Il me regarde, l'air d'attendre l'approbation. Il a manqué des sections, c'est un peu irrégulier. Il est à croquer.

- C'est parfait. Vous avez de l'après-rasage ?
- Je ne sais pas.

Je trouve la petite bouteille, dissimulée derrière des murs de styromousse.

- Ah ! Vous êtes magnifique et vous sentez bon ! Monsieur Lavoie ?
- Oui ?
- Vous réalisez que ça fait 8 minutes que vous êtes debout sans appui ? Vous êtes prêt pour une petite marche dans le couloir, je pense. Après déjeuner ?
- OK, ma petite, tu viendras me chercher.

Jour 12

L'infirmière entre en trombe dans la zone rouge, elle brandit une feuille lignée remplie de noms : « Deuxième test négatif, monsieur Lavoie est *vert* ! Il redéménage demain ! »

Je me rends à peine compte que je cours vers sa chambre. Devant sa porte, j'enlève mes gants, lave mes mains, enlève mes vêtements de protection, lave mes mains et ma visière, remets un nouveau masque, lave mes mains, remets une nouvelle jaquette, ma visière propre. Lave mes mains encore. Je mets des gants. J'aimerais dire que j'entre en trombe, mais ce luxe n'existe pas en zone rouge.

- Monsieur Lavoie ?

Il est debout, dans les toilettes, à uriner. Ça aussi, c'est une façon de redevenir homme. Je ferme la porte et attends à l'extérieur. J'entends la fermeture éclair, j'entends le lavabo. Les filles ici avaient bien rigolé : « Tu travailles en pédiatrie, ça paraît, tu enlèves les couches des patients pour les remettre à l'entraînement à la toilette ». C'était pour rire, mais en même temps, c'était un peu triste comme constat.

- Quoi ? Ah c'est toi !
- Vous êtes guéri ! Vous n'avez plus la COVID !

318

- Le quoi ?
- Le coronavirus !
- Ah oui ! Bonne nouvelle.

Il ne partage pas mon enthousiasme, mais sa vigueur actuelle lui fait de toute évidence oublier d'où il vient. Il revient de *la fin de vie*, monsieur Lavoie. Il est tellement revenu vigoureux, de la mort, qu'il marche dans le couloir toute la journée, va au balcon, revient et en redemande. Il est tellement revenu fort de la mort que nous devons lui faire monter et descendre *l'escalier rouge* trois fois par jour pour le fatiguer un peu. Et il en redemande.

Mais plus maintenant. Il est *vert*. Il ne mourra pas de la covid. Il ne sera pas une statistique.

Oui, Monsieur Lavoie, il revient des morts. Monsieur Jacques, Monsieur Dufour, Madame Charrette et Madame La coursière ; ils reviennent tous de l'antichambre de la mort. Ils ne sont pas de cette histoire, mais ils ont la leur. Semblable, mais différente.

Ils sont revenus, eux aussi. À coup d'amour, à coup de petites bouchées « pour nous faire plaisir, s'il-vous-plait », à coup de *popsicle à l'Ensure*, ou de douches rafraichissantes. À coup de verticalisation, de marche quémandée (« juste une petite marche dans la chambre, ça me ferait tellement plaisir que vous disiez oui »), à coup de séances de musique, assis dans la chaise (« Vous, c'est Charles Aznavour, Mme Mertens, non ? »). Ils sont revenus des morts parce que « le lit, c'est pour dormir seulement, vous êtes d'accord ? ». L'antichambre de la mort ce n'est pas compliqué, en résidence de personnes âgées, elle se nomme souvent MPOC, insuffisance cardiaque ou Alzheimer. Ici, en zone rouge « hors hôpital », en CHLSD ou en ressource intermédiaire, ces maladies existent encore, mais l'antichambre de lamort, elle, se nomme simplement *le déconditionnement*.

Le déconditionnement physique, ou psychosocial, cette perte graduelle de nos acquis, cette difficulté à bouger après l'inactivité, qui mène à la crainte de faire quoique ce soit. Cette pente descendante vers la fin, qui empêche éventuellement de manger, de boire, de bouger.

Le virus, nous n'y pouvons rien. Mais ça, le déconditionnement, ça, nous y pouvons quelque chose.

La bientraitance au temps de la pandémie
Yves Rochon et Julie Fortin

Chez Logements de l'Outaouais, la bientraitance ça veut dire offrir à nos quelque 150 résidents et résidentes dont l'âge moyen est de 74 ans un milieu de vie accueillant, stimulant et sécuritaire où il fait bon vivre.

Le confinement rendu nécessaire en raison de la pandémie nous a posé de grands défis. Comment éviter que l'isolement forcé et l'anxiété ne causent de sérieux dommages à la santé physique et psychologique de nos résidents ? Afin de relever ce défi nous avons puisé dans notre bagage d'expériences et arrimé le soutien de vaillant-e-s bénévoles à notre personnel, constitué d'une petite équipe dévouée.

Dès le début du confinement, l'intervenante du milieu a entrepris d'appeler chaque résidente pour prendre de ses nouvelles, et au besoin répondre à ses questions ou tenter de calmer ses appréhensions. Le Club de loisirs des Joyeux Retraités a acheté des livres de jeux qui ont été distribués aux résident-e-s qui en ont fait la demande. Nous avons aussi constitué une équipe de résident-e-s bénévoles qui procédaient une ou deux fois par jour à la désinfection des rampes et poignées de porte des deux édifices, une façon concrète de participer activement à la lutte contre ce satané virus !

Bien que les salles à manger aient dû être fermées, l'animatrice communautaire du lieu qu'on appelle Le Bistro a rapidement mis en place un service de plats à emporter pour les deux repas qu'elle prépare en semaine. Passer chercher la nourriture devient l'occasion d'avoir un contact chaleureux avec cette animatrice bienveillante et à l'écoute. À l'édifice du 6 Lesage, où la moyenne d'âge frise les 80 ans, nous avons instauré la distribution des repas du midi à la porte des résident-e-s. Effectuée par des membres du personnel, cette livraison est l'occasion de prendre des nouvelles et de rassurer notre monde par nos sourires et notre bonne humeur.

L'intervenante du milieu s'est avérée une ressource précieuse pour recueillir les confidences et questions des résident-e-s qui ont fait appel à elle pour les aider à s'adapter à la nouvelle réalité.

Petites gâteries bien appréciées, une bénévole de l'extérieur a fourni à ce jour 12 douzaines de biscuits faits maison qui ont mis le sourire aux lèvres de bien des résident-e-s. Et ça continue !

Avec le retour du beau temps et la reprise de certaines activités de groupe —en respectant strictement les règles de distanciation physique !—espérons que le pire est derrière nous. La vigilance demeure de mise car la bataille n'est pas finie, mais on peut voir que la bientraitance, autour du mot d'ordre « nous

sommes tous responsables les uns des autres » a fait que « ça a bien été » …
et que ça va continuer de bien aller !

Julie Fortin et Yves Rochon
L'équipe de Logements de l'Outaouais
Gatineau (Québec)
mai 2020

Zooming Our Way into Oblivion
Denise Giroux

My friend and former colleague, Jon, is one of the editors of this almanac. Some time ago, he asked me to write a contribution as a 'worker;' an employee engaged in high-pressure, often adversarial union representation, forced to work from home fulltime because of the pandemic. I am a lawyer, employed until recently as an Employment Relations Officer (ERO) with a large union serving mostly scientific groups within the Canadian federal public service, in the national capital region of Ottawa/Gatineau.

The pandemic threw more than 300,000 federal employees—and their union advisors, like me—into unknown territory. Overnight, we moved from a nine to five commuter workday in an office setting and culture to full-time 'work from home.' This meant doing our best to carry on, in the midst of a generalized panic, some of us entirely alone in our homes, discouraged from contact and afraid, or forced to live and work with our spouses who were also often forced home full time, many of us with children forced home from school. The first few months can only be said to have been characterized by sheer panic and anxiety for the employees we represented and advocated for, as well as my own panic and anxiety.

Eight months in, as the second wave took hold, I found I had little energy left at the end of the workday to apply myself to writing about what I was experiencing. Each day rolled into the next, but I was never able to settle into any kind of satisfying routine; instead, I grew increasingly exhausted and tense.

Just a few short weeks ago, I 'retired' from that job after more than 15 years of service. Despite my desire to tell my story, I still could not sit myself down to do so. The simple truth is that in these early months of release from work obligations and stresses, I could not make myself think back upon it when all my body and soul wanted was rest, and, once rested, to relish the lightened load and begin to dream of what might be in the future. I can see that what I crave most is time to establish a new, healthier routine, a schedule set by me, for me, to ensure the variety of physical activity I need to try to make it for another 20-plus years, and to determine where my mental and political energy should be focused in the years to come. But I did, at last, sit and write this essay, to consider what the year had brought with it, and, above all, to document how I came to the decision to leave the job I was doing.

In early 2020, though news from Wuhan was reported daily and the deadly nature of the virus had been well-established, it still seemed to me an overreaction when, at my office, staff were called into an unplanned meeting to be told that Public Health had declared a state of pandemic and we were to take everything we would need to work from home with us, until further notice.

Some of my colleagues were already morbidly afraid of other people's germs—the world already a scary place for them—but non-germaphobes like me could not believe the pandemic would bring so drastic a change to our lives. I assumed at first that we would be back in the office in two or three weeks.

I already worked from home occasionally, when concentrated time was needed to do research or write up arguments in preparation for grievance hearings. I had a work-issued cell phone for calling members to advise them of their rights and obligations or to arrange meetings with their employers to try to resolve their workplace conflicts. Working from home, up to that point in time, still required pre-approval, and managers at the union generally had the same reactionary attitude of 'business,' preferring to see 'bums in seats' at the office. Even though the work required a significant degree of independence in setting my own schedule, the case load was unpredictable and member-driven. Support staff *had* to be in each day and *had* to take a one-hour lunch break, whether they wanted an hour or not; they just generally *had* to be seen as available.

I enjoyed the combined benefits of working both from the office and from home. I still benefited from weekly conversations with colleagues, conversations which could be about our work, exchanges on strategies and approaches, or our personal lives or even politics in the U.S.A. (yes, Trump and the insanity of his time in office and the election which finally saw him replaced with Biden). The office offered a well-established routine, the 'buzz' of common effort, a friendly overture from a colleague, empathy, and a place to store files. Going in required a near-daily effort to make myself present-able, to dress professionally. And, each day, on my way in to the office, I would listen to the news and analysis of current events on CBC or Radio-Canada. On my way out, I ran errands, got groceries, or dropped in on a friend before going home.

Working from home full-time, I re-captured more than two hours a day of commuter time, saved on gas, and reduced my carbon footprint. I was often *more* productive, and willing to work longer hours as I could do so and still recoup more personal time. I could make fresh food instead of packing a lunch, and throw in a load of laundry between tasks. I didn't have to dress up, and I might even be able to fit a dog walk in during daylight hours in the winter. It should have been the best of both worlds, but everything was tainted with the forced nature of the isolation and restrictions on normal social contact.

In this pandemic world, I felt immediately isolated; working from home did not seem particularly pleasant or convenient. With only the electronic media to listen to and no colleagues to commiserate with, I listened to the news and focused on my work Inbox as well as newsfeeds and tried to wrap my head around what this new reality might mean, in both the shorter and longer run. Because we were all in the same situation, unbelieving, attempting to adjust, none of us reached out to others those first few months. The Inbox kept us riveted to our computers, as it was chock full of government 'directives' and communications, guidelines and advisories, purporting to reassure their employees and union representatives that senior managers were at the same time ensuring continuing service to the public and showing concern for staff well-being.

Government workers were warned to stay off the VPN-secured, internal networks for the confidential work public servants often do, as the systems were crashing. Being told to stay off the network and standby might have come as some relief to those trying to support, nurture, and entertain their children even as they checked in with their managers, but the stay-at-home directives meant we were also unable to drop in on our parents, visit a grandmother in long-term care, be with a brother during his cancer treatment, or attend a dying relative. It meant working off the corners of our kitchen tables, unable for many months to access our stand-up desks, ergonomic chairs or special 'mice' along with the files needed to continue some of the work we aimed to do.

Each department, each deputy minister, and the Treasury Board which administers the public service generally issued countless updates on the pandemic: case numbers and deaths, directives on 'working from home,' access to the VPNs, delays in the usual grievance timelines, health and safety approaches, and work expectations. Labour relations representatives, our counterparts who advised management reps within the public service, were busy trying to respond to internal requests for support, with the result that our efforts to reach them were ignored for extended periods.

Consultation tables where union representatives and senior management were to discuss issues of common concern had been mandated by the Modernization Act of 2005, to promote participation by employees in consultation, collaboration, and co-development of policies affecting their working conditions. Fifteen years on, they were serving a much more limited purpose than originally intended, having largely been reduced to mere information-giving sessions, where managers updated the union on ongoing Phoenix (pay system) fiascos or announced changes to programs or HR services. As senior managers focused almost entirely on pandemic preparedness, defining essential workers and the safety measures in place for those employees required to attend at their workplaces (PPE and cleaning, etc.), consultation sessions became even narrower in scope, allowing for few if any submissions of agenda items from the unions. Too often, different departments' annual or quarterly meetings were just another 'meeting' amongst many others in a workday, meetings which all present were glad to see end as soon as possible with as little follow-up action required as possible; union representatives had become part of this rubber stamp approach. In short, the pandemic became merely one more reason for senior bureaucrats to limit the scope of consultation.

As an advisor to government workers dispersed throughout some 100 or so different agencies, departments, and commissions, I saw my inbox flooded with sometimes conflicting, sometimes subtly different guidelines from each of these departments; it was impossible to decipher a cohesive approach amidst the chaos. Still, I tried to keep the guidelines straight in order to be able to respond to the frenzied calls of members unable to keep up with all the changes themselves. My office manager did not make matters any simpler; clearly in an agitated state of his own, he seemed to be trying to carve out a useful role by forwarding to us the directives he had received from those same departments, as well as from within our own organization. He only succeeded in making matters worse, as he sent and re-sent communiqués we'd already received from the same sources. Inbox 'overload' was already a source of stress for EROs like myself, but his effort to try to act as some kind of central clearing house for the various communiqués did nothing to reassure staff that he understood that we, too, were dealing with the exact same pressures our members were experiencing. It didn't help that staff meetings were put on hold and team meetings did not resume for several months.

Like most people, I tuned in to the news for the latest numbers and facts about the pandemic in the first months, but the focus on cases and deaths and local restrictions became morbid and depressing, only adding to the general anxiety, so I tried to limit my intake. Eventually I spoke with some of my colleagues by phone, but it was a cold, late spring, and we felt holed up, isolated and unsure of what would come next, though we were still hoping that the pandemic would be short-lived!

The pattern of enquiries from our members took a clear turn, especially as the second wave began to take hold. Many of the calls reflected the stresses of parents—mothers especially—being harassed for needing to reduce their work hours to juggle parenting and new 'home teacher' roles, or feeling burned out because they had been making up lost daytime hours by working into the evenings, and now needed to rectify the balance to save their sanity, in the face of management expectations that they keep production up. Only in the fall did some of the departments begin to make arrangements to get special equipment to employees' homes, though in the national capital area, and at our union particularly, there was the assumption that we would all be returning to our offices very soon, leading to many employees, like myself, holding off getting their equipment sent home or replaced.

325

Many employees were required to share computer time or internet access with other members of a household, especially in regions where internet access was uneven. I live just half-an-hour from Ottawa, but the phone lines through which Bell provides the service are inadequate for the demand, and with everyone working from home, failures were frequent, putting me off one task towards another.

Our bread and butter as union representatives had always been holding face-to-face meetings with members and trying to broker settlements of conflict as it arose with their managers, but we had to adapt to replacing face-to-face meetings with one-on-one calls to managers—if a virtual 'meeting' could be arranged at all—over Zoom or MS Meets. I did not find the adaptation process at all easy. In a face-to-face meeting, I could appeal to reason and human compassion with oral argument, look someone in the eyes, and attempt to find common ground in discussion. For most of us, Zoom meetings were an entirely new way of 'talking,' as off-putting and impersonal as answering machines had been 40 years ago, creating a new awkwardness in communicating with our own face reflected back at us instead of that of the person we were trying to convince.

My strength as an advocate was in these meetings, laying out the facts and reasons for remedying a situation, and providing practical suggestions for doing so. The delays in reaching people and in getting those virtual meetings undermined my role. The format made it easier for managers to downplay conflicts which needed attention. No one was looking anyone in the eye, as all eyes were on a screen, and many simply removed their video image entirely even when they were speaking in order to save bandwidth. Even a full year from the onset of the pandemic and accompanying work-from-home reality, senior managers told us over and over again they needed more time to do anything requested. The pandemic became the excuse for ignoring or downplaying almost everything else. Even at the best of times, within the public service, the recourse mechanisms available to wronged employees are weak and slow, making accountability for bad decisions a long-term challenge. Without face-to-face meetings, in the virtual format, individual grievors, who would typically have preferred to resolve their issues through informal discussion, were forced to operate in a format most found unfamiliar and alien. The result was that members were frustrated, as was I, with both my role and my ability to be of service.

At this time, my cousin, an only child whose parents were long passed, was admitted to hospital in Hamilton, Ontario with advanced cancer in his stomach, spleen and liver. With the hospital in full lockdown, not a soul was permitted to visit him in person. He put on a brave face, and was willing to endure whatever treatment they could offer. I spoke to him by phone three days before he passed. He sounded scared, unprepared for what was coming, and angry that he would not be able to see anyone who mattered to him. I believe that, in the face of this reality, he effectively decided to let himself go quickly, and succeeded. Strangely, and inexplicably, for she had given me no advance notice of the possibility during a prior discussion, the social worker at the hospital called me within an hour of his death, as the next-of-kin, to tell me he was slipping away. *Now* I could visit him if I could make it to the hospital in a hurry. I could not get there—I live in Cantley, Québec—but his best friend Tony was in Hamilton, so he hurried over… too late. I have no doubt that Bradley could have benefited from a visit well before he was in the last stage of dying. I do believe that in most hospitals these inhumane restrictions have been relaxed, but Bradley's situation shook me up badly.

As his next of kin, I had to make arrangements for his body to be removed to a funeral home, and determine next steps. Even though Bradley had died a pauper, the decisions and coordination of funeral and related services and discussions with family demanded the same effort as they would have for a wealthy man, though the materials and ceremony were much different. This was an added challenge for me in the days immediately following his death. I couldn't shake the sense of horror and sadness I'd had at how he'd died, miserably, alone and scared. I still get upset when I think of him, and all those like him, who were forced to die alone in those early months of strict lockdown, with no caring presence by their side to help them through the ordeal. In September, some five months later, when restrictions were somewhat lifted before the second wave changed the rules again, we buried him. Even then, there were only 15 or so of us present, cousins and friends.

I also saw my mother's life severely circumscribed by the effect of lockdowns in her retirement residence. A contagion amongst staff and residents had all of them entirely isolated in their units for seven weeks in the late fall. Even prior to this quarantine and certainly after, she noted a visible deterioration in her fellow residents' wellbeing; not just overdue haircuts but a loss of interest in all things and increased physical impairment from forced inactivity. Social distancing requirements at mealtimes and masking, for people with hearing impairments (a common impairment for many elderly), are particularly limiting for them, as it is hard to hear one another at that distance without speaking loudly. And so, these restrictions keep their conversations short. If the 'stay-at-home' orders can be lifted, I hope to visit with her very soon, to take her out for day trips in some of our favourite little towns in the Niagara horseshoe area, or at least a lunch away from Sisco's pre-processed bland meal plans.

My father-in-law, in the meantime, was convinced to move into a retirement residence in the face of growing dementia, but the move coincided with total isolation within the residence, so that he went from living in his own home and visiting regularly with his girlfriend to eating and living totally alone in a tiny studio apartment. After just two months of this prison-like life, he insisted on moving back to his house—though his dementia and palsy are worsening—and he continues to live there. His two children worry, and being several hours away, they can't visit as often as they would like.

By November, eight months into the pandemic, calls from our members had increased significantly, as public service workers either started to get their heads above water and called us at last, or realized that the issues they were facing were not simply going to go away. And just as these additional calls increased demands on my time, the rollover of staff in our union office ramped up. Rollover was already a perpetual, unaddressed problem; now three maternity leaves and the departure of a senior staffer along with the manager—the latter much welcomed—was serious in an office of 20 employees. These departures always result in the transfer of caseloads from one officer to those who remain along with a search for experienced replacements to fill the vacancies. The lack of experienced applicants is another issue the union refuses to address. The burden inevitably increases on those who hang on.

As the most senior employee in my office, I'd observed and experienced the waning of all sense of team, in the face of and despite the organization's decision to 'restructure' the 20 employees into smaller teams of five to six members two years earlier. The pandemic was certainly a factor in the destruction of the last vestiges of collegiality or organization. Our own staff and team meetings were done virtually, just like the meetings with our members. Though some tried to lighten the mood when they had a chance to speak, the manager consumed three-quarters of the air-time with endless blah blah; there was less and less sense of common purpose, effectiveness, or solidarity.

Meanwhile, the union was saving thousands of dollars in reduced travel and in-person meetings of all kinds, including huge savings in taxi chits and mileage claims, committee work, meals and hospitality suites. None of these savings translated into meaningful support for the staff who carried on, to provide additional support to those servicing members in these difficult circumstances. On the contrary, our employer adopted two approaches that cut the wind from many of our sails. In August, our employer started preparations to press us all to return to the office, ignoring clear predictions of a second wave. They chose as the return date the first day of school in September; that is, the *same day* harried parents were to see their children return to school. Parents, my colleagues included, were naturally apprehensive about the safety of sending their children to live classes, and anxious for what it might mean for their extended families' well-being. The employer remained insensitive and obstinate on this for several weeks, before at last succumbing to pressures from the staff union (the union within the union that was my employer) urging them to delay. Soon case numbers started to rise in Ontario and Québec. By Christmas, those numbers had reached new heights, prompting the federal government to order even the 20% or fewer of government workers who had gone back to their offices to return to working from home full-time. In Québec, the high case numbers drove the provincial government to bring in a curfew—a curfew which remains in place more than four months later. (This piece is being written in April, 2021.)

Equally disconcerting was the employer's determination to exploit the situation with roll-back proposals at the negotiation table, where our union-within-the-union was meeting with them 'virtually' to discuss the terms of our next collective agreement. It was not the first time our employer adopted positions, vis-à-vis its own employees, that flagrantly contradict the values it claims to espouse when it negotiates agreements on behalf of its members (public service workers) with their employer (the Treasury Board). In this round of negotiations with its staff, the employer's near total lack of support and empathy for our circumstances, in the face of their significant costs savings, was particularly galling. A strong majority of employees supported a strike vote to counter the ugly proposals put forward by our employer, but in the end, the staff proved unprepared to take the necessary action to give effect to the strike mandate. The end result was the loss of seniority rights, some important health care benefits, and parental leave coverage. Worst of all, the employer repeated its 2014 refusal (in 2020!) to include a harassment policy in the agreement, or to revise its terms to ensure gender-neutral language, matters that would embarrass any responsible employer in 2020, given the existence of real cases of harassment made more harmful by poor handling at all levels of management.

The sad fact is that those of us who fight daily for respect of our members' rights, those familiar with labour history, labour laws, and the epidemic of harassment and discrimination, were outnumbered by other union staffers who are well-compensated for work which is generally more manageable, short on conflict or high pressure. The latter naively reasoned that we should not expect to make any gains at the table this round (ignoring the fact that we were being asked to give ground, not stand pat); they argued that we, unlike many other Canadians in the private sector who'd lost jobs and businesses, were still working, still being paid; we could 'aim to recoup the lost ground next time'(!). They did not seem to appreciate that our union was not negotiating with a mom-and-pop business forced to close down, our employer was itself financially secure, and in fact 'better off' than it had been pre-pandemic. For many of us, the collective agreement rammed down our throats by the employer was a bitter pill to swallow, reflecting the sad history of our own internal labour relations status. It reinforced what I had seen over several previous negotiations: the employer exploiting employees' naiveté exacerbated by pandemic-induced anxiety. This union benefits this way in large part because it has deliberately avoided training its own staff, over a 100-year history of existence, in labour history and principles, in contrast with almost all other organizations that call themselves a union.

I took some time off at Christmas. With all the added stress, it seemed appropriate to try to match my life for a couple of weeks to the slowdown of the earth's rhythms and shortening days, to try to rest. But the new year arrived, and with it, the third pandemic wave. That third wave is still raging in Ontario and Alberta, and, to a more limited extent, in Quebec, where I live. How long this full work-from-home scenario will continue, with all it means for the work union members do, is anyone's guess.

As for me, I simply ran out of steam: I no longer wanted to have to work in these conditions. The quality and appreciation of our members and the human interactions with my colleagues were what kept me going these many years. Though client/members still expressed appreciation for my work, and I was by this time having regular phone calls with some of my closest colleagues, the phone calls and e-mails were just not enough. In the virtual world, the frustrations of the work have little counterweight.

The pandemic heightens one's sense of vulnerability, and one's awareness of the fine line that exists between life and death, and of aging. In the time that remains to me—uncertain, of course, but without a doubt shorter than the time I have lived so far—I need to gain time for myself and those I want to be able to be with more readily, and to focus my energies on other projects.

When I started my career 32 years ago, I dictated my correspondence onto a mini-tape player, on my way out of a courtroom or in a taxi on the way back to the office. A secretary would transcribe the recording. Eventually each of us had computers on our desks; we learned MS-DOS to process word documents and accounting programs to handle the books. Fax machines were a miracle of timeliness. Answering machines came into existence somewhere in there. It was a strange thing to adapt to hearing our own voices recorded; it felt awkward talking to a machine. A significant technological milestone occurred in 2001, as I wound up my sole legal practice in Hamilton to move to Montreal. As the province of Ontario was turning to an entirely automated land registry system for property, lawyers still needed their own administrative assistants to complete forms. The internet was really just starting then to become a popular tool for e-mail and research, but we well know that things changed quickly enough that by 2005, union and legal representatives were expected to prepare all their documents independently. No assistants at all were available at the first large public sector union I worked for. All of these were technological changes I adapted to over time.

This last union I worked for tended to scrimp on resources and administrative support for the people doing representation, and our managers never managed to make inroads on the Directors' financial priorities to provide us with properly trained support for our work. PR (public relations) was gaining an increasing portion of the resource pie within the organization, and a whole new level of middle managers and team leads is being created; all of these are encouraged to see themselves as managers and avoid involvement with the staff union that they technically are still members of. Actual service provision—advice, organizing, negotiating, and representing members at every level—is under-resourced. The training section (i.e., the section designing courses for our members, not for training union staff) grew from one part-time person to three full-time people, but training sessions occur less often than before and in a much more limited number of areas, another casualty of the pandemic, perhaps. Yet the stewards we train are the eyes and ears of the union in the government departments' offices and laboratories and in the field; the quality and availability of their training make a difference. Sadly, training was already moving increasingly 'online' pre-pandemic, despite the fact that studies show how such training fails on every count to ensure sustained knowledge or the competence to actually apply principles in action, even in critical areas such health and safety enforcement. It is just another example of the union's hypocrisy in appearing to encourage engagement while at the same time undermining the measures needed to promote safer and happier workplaces.

Without trained support and resources, EROs like myself were being delegated increasing responsibility for carrying out arbitrations, on simple and complex matters, in my final three years with the organization. Prior to this, arbitration cases were generally contracted out to private law firms. Moreover, the procedural requirements of the Federal Public Service Employment Relations and Staffing Board were transformed, rivaling even the courts in the complexity of its disclosure rules, while it fails still to impose upon itself the usual types of requirements other administrative tribunals must comply with for timely issuance of decisions or scheduling hearings; wait times are unacceptably long. Despite these greater burdens, no law clerks or researchers are hired to support the EROs, though this would assist greatly in file management and trial preparation. Some of my younger colleagues seemed to take the lack of support in stride. Hired in the last three years with the downloading of this new responsibility, they are litigators, people who enjoy the complexities of litigation, formal hearings, and evidence. The strain of doing this while juggling a heavy set of demands and caseloads and increasing administrative responsibilities nevertheless takes its toll on them, especially if they are juggling new babies and small children too. The idea that we can continually do more, or do it all, without better support, raises, I think, reasonable doubts about the organization's priorities and whether it might be compromising competencies in the art of employment relations and effective informal advocacy.

I believe that these different responsibilities for Employment Relations Officers will ultimately have to be clarified and distinguished, as they are not entirely compatible. The public service is a huge organization with a 'wagons circled' approach to labour relations which fails for the most part to assess, value, and promote competencies in *humane* human resource management. Granted, there are some managers who *do* inherently have the skills to treat people fairly, but more effort is needed to priorize these skills along with the ability to deliver projects within budget.

In the remote working office, we were all expected to improve our own formatting skills. Mini-training sessions of an hour were offered, by Zoom of course, in Phantom/Foxit and Word programs to 'help' us in this, but my caseload never allowed me to put into practice what I might have learned from these sessions, as the numbers of enquiries and anxious calls from members increased in November and never let up until I retired.

This is the nature of work in 2020/21. As the third pandemic wave continues, I wonder: will things return to the way they were, or is this brave new technological world the way of the future? There is no doubt that colleagues who grew up with computers and gaming seem to have adapted with greater ease than I during this extra-challenging year. Do some human beings have an endless capacity to adapt to technology and change? Is it possible that most of us have a limited capacity to adapt to changes—only for so long, or so much in a lifetime—like a pre-determined number of heartbeats in a lifetime? Will my younger colleagues still be rolling with the changes 25 years from now, after seeing countless new technologies and applications change the way they work, as I did? Or will they too one day feel resistance, suffering benumbing fatigue at ever-increasing changes? How will this pandemic and their own isolation change their approach to living?

I am well aware that I remain one of the lucky ones after living through these 14-plus months of the pandemic. I was on the 'job' throughout, answering calls for assistance and support and providing practical advice ably and surely to professionals of the public service, based on real experience over 32 years. With the 'job' the paycheck continued… through the first, second and third waves. Though I, too, had adapted to the changed 'workplace' reality, I felt that the rewards no longer outweighed the costs.

Now, still in the earliest weeks of retirement, I am very glad to be free of the daily calls upon my energy and the hours focused on others' needs and requirements. I can sincerely say that the members I served are, on the whole, a very professional bunch of people, devoted to the work they do on behalf of Canadians. To work with the public service successfully, they have to be prepared to adapt to ever-changing policies, priorities and supervisors; governments, too, along with technological changes.

I'm very glad that I won't have to deal with the next 'recall' to the office, whenever that happens, and no longer need endure the endless strain of unreasonable expectations. For now, I have time to breathe, to redefine how my day is spent, to enjoy the Spring as it unfolds. I remain actively involved with the Nuclear Waste Watch coalition fighting to ensure responsible management of nuclear waste and protesting the insanity of investing in new nuclear reactors as a 'clean' solution to climate change. I am also president of the NDP riding association in the Pontiac, and all indications are that an election might be called in the coming months. I look forward to planning a little local travel, in Quebec and Ontario, and visiting with friends. Hopefully, after several months of rest, taking care of my own affairs: home repairs, support for my mother as a caregiver, my cousin's estate matters, some tennis and bike riding, I will find my energy renewed, so that I can focus on defining a next, new project, work that I can do on a part-time basis to supplement my small pension, and apply my skills in new ways. Hopefully, as well, the worst of this pandemic will soon be behind us. But even long after the pandemic ends, the ways in which it has changed how work is done will remain the subject of discussion and debate for many years to come.

SECTION 8

Technology

SECTION 8

Technology

I've been keenly interested in technology ever since I worked on the Labour Markets and Technological Change project at the Economic Council of Canada back in 1985. That doesn't in any way mean I'm an uncritical admirer of technology. Au contraire. But I don't think it any accident that technology has been the subject of a good deal of my writing, and particularly of my plays, over the years.

The pieces in this section offer three different takes on technology. Teresa Patterson's lighthearted short play 'BTW' puts a mainly positive spin on things like Smartphones and internet abbreviations—and how a senior might manage to adapt to such things. Harold Tausch's essay 'COVID, Technology and Me' provides a balanced appraisal of the advantages and drawbacks of new technologies such as Zoom for an actor and dancer seeking to continue performing during the pandemic. His having earned his living as a computer programmer for more than four decades adds a special richness to his piece. And my own short play 'The Virtual Apprentice' which, like the other plays in this almanac, was written in one of Colleen Naomi's online playwriting workshops, quite accurately illustrates my own deeply troubled relationship with new technology—a relationship perhaps best described as one of snarling détente.

335

BTW
A One-act Play
Teresa Patterson

CHARACTERS

RUBY BARNABY: 80-year-old grandmother, widowed.

FREDDIE BARNABY: 30-year-old grandson, single.

SETTING

The sitting/living room of an apartment of an 80-year-old woman. Two armchairs flank a side table. A telephone sits on the table. A sideboard sits against the wall to the left of the chairs. A teapot, a few cups and saucers and a cream and sugar set are on the sideboard. A small glass with teaspoons is situated near the cups. There is also a small decanter of spirits of some type. A basket of knitting sits in a basket beside one of the chairs.

TIME

Present day. Early afternoon.

As the lights come up, Ruby is seated in one of the chairs. She has a teacup on the table beside her and she is knitting.

A knock at the door is very loud and annoys Ruby.

RUBY

Come in! Come in!

FREDDIE

(Freddie enters from SR and makes his way toward the chairs, but stands by the sideboard) Good morning, BB.

RUBY

Hello Freddie. *(Jauntily)* And by the way, I'm not deaf, so there is no need to knock so loud.

FREDDIE

My apologies. Just wanted to be sure you'd hear me. You were expecting me though, am I right?

RUBY

Yes, you did tell me you were coming by. Please, sit down. Would you like some tea?

FREDDIE

No thanks, BB. I've already had coffee. (*He pecks her cheek*) Happy Birthday! (*He has a small package in his hand and it is very nicely wrapped*)

RUBY

Thank you. It's quite a milestone. Eighty years is a long time. (*She giggles*) And I still have all my faculties...including my hearing. (*He hands the package gently to Ruby. She puts down her knitting and takes a sip of tea*)

FREDDIE

Happy Birthday again BB. (*Freddie sits down in the extra chair*)

RUBY

(*Ruby puts her teacup on the table and accepts the gift box from Freddie*) Thank you, Freddie.

(*Ruby proceeds to unwrap the parcel and opens the inside box to find a brand-new cellphone*) Freddie, this is a surprise. I already have a phone. I did believe you would bring me a gift, (*Giggles again*) but this is really unexpected.

FREDDIE

This is a cellphone, BB. It's a Smart Phone and it will make a lot of difference in your life.

RUBY

Is it a cellphone or a Smart Phone?

FREDDIE

A Smart Phone is a style of cellphone. And it is very smart. You can make phone calls, send texts, look up articles on Google. It`s basically a computer that you use as a phone. I'll help you to learn some of the basics.

RUBY

Well, I hope so. (*She turns it over in her hand and looks at it a few more times*) I don`t think I could even turn it on.

FREDDIE

(*He shows her a few buttons on the sides of the cell phone and turns it on while very carefully showing her which button to push, then turns if off*) Here, you try to turn it on.

337

RUBY

(Ruby pushes one of the buttons and it does turn on) OK, done! Now what? *(Freddie takes the phone from her and plays with some buttons while Ruby picks up her knitting again. Freddie sets up the keypad so that he can show her how to text)*

FREDDIE

BB, I already set this phone up with phone numbers of family members and a few of your friends so you can text or call them even when you are out of the house. I also printed out this list of short forms that are used for texting. *(He hands it to her and she once again puts down the knitting, takes another sip of tea and tries to pay attention)*

RUBY

What does it mean to text?

FREDDIE

You can send a quick message without talking—kind of like leaving a note. That way if the person you want to speak with isn't available, they can check their phone later and see that you sent a message. It's really easy once you get the hang of it.

RUBY

(She is reviewing the list) What do all of these letters mean? LOL? IDK?

FREDDIE

LOL means Laugh Out Loud. What do you think some of the others mean? Like, IDK.

RUBY

(She shrugs) I don't know!

FREDDIE

That's right!

RUBY

How can that be right? I said, I don`t know. I don`t know means that I don`t know what IDK means. It looks like some medical procedure like an EKG, and I don't know what that means either. *(She has an air of frustration, so Freddie takes another stab at it)*

FREDDIE

Each letter stands for a word. The first one is I. It means I. The second one

338

is D meaning Don't. The last one is K meaning Know: I Don't Know. See if you can figure out some of the others.

RUBY

These are all single letters. Y! Does that mean Yes? I. Does that mean I? B. Does that mean Be, like to Be or not to Be?

FREDDIE

Y! means W- H -Y. I means E-Y-E. B does mean B-E. (*He spells out each word*) And O-M-G means Oh My God!

RUBY

Oh My God is right! If you use a short form to save time, then why use OMG? It's the same number of syllables to say OMG as it is to say Oh My God. And even if you type it, you still have to read it as three syllables. (*Her frustration is building*)

FREDDIE

It`s a form of shorthand, that's all. It's a bit like shortening names like we have done with yours. When I was a little kid, apparently I tried to say Grandma Barnaby to differentiate from my other gran, Grandma Rubin. I got them mixed up and it came out as BB. Everyone got used to hearing me call you BB and it stuck. So, you will get used to all of this once you get started. Would you like a fresh cup of tea? (*He goes toward the sideboard as if to take the teapot and head to the kitchen*) Shall I get some biscuits to go with the tea?

RUBY

No tea. If I hope to get used to these acronyms or short forms, I`ll need something a little more substantial. How about you grab yourself a tea cup, bring the bottle and we'll both have a go. (*Freddie obliges and brings the goods to the table. While he is pouring, Ruby continues*) With some fortification, I might just be able to figure all this out.

FREDDIE

First, let's drink a little toast to your birthday. Happy 80th birthday BB. (*They click tea cups and Freddie takes a sip. Ruby takes a gulp*)

RUBY

Here! Here! OK, let me look at this list again. (*She picks up the sheet and peruses it*) B-T-W. OK. That has a B in it. You said that means BE as in B-E, right? Looks more like a cryptoquote. At least that I could figure out.

339

FREDDIE

B-T-W means By The Way. (*Freddie takes the bottle back to the sideboard, then returns to the chair*)

RUBY

(*She gives him a look of disbelief*) So now the letter B means By?

FREDDIE

Well, it's not that one letter only means one particular word. It can stand for a different word in a different message. It is really just the combinations of letters that represent a full sentence or statement.

RUBY

I guess that makes a bit of sense. So, W-T-F? What does that represent?

FREDDIE

Whoops! I meant to delete that one.

RUBY

Well, now you must tell me, Freddie.

FREDDIE

Yes, I guess I should. W stands for What. T stands for The and F stands for F... (*Freddie looks directly at Ruby to gauge her response*)

RUBY

What the Fu... ohhhhhhhh...

FREDDIE

Yes, You're right.

RUBY

O-M-G! I think I need a fill up. (*She gets up and goes to the sideboard, pours a healthy dose of booze into her teacup and takes a gulp*)

FREDDIE

Are you OK BB?

RUBY

(*She sighs heavily*) Yes! I think I'm all right now. (*She pours one more shot and then heads back to the chair and picks up her knitting from the basket*)

340

FREDDIE

I have to go now, BB, and let you get on with your day. If you have any more questions about this list, let me know. Text me if you want. (*He pecks her cheek and leaves. He leaves and Ruby checks to see that he has gone*)

RUBY

(*Aside*) It used to be easy enough to connect with friends. You had a pen and paper and you wrote a letter to them. It took a bit more time, but there was always the anticipation of a response to be found in the mail. It was exciting to see an envelope with your own name on it. If something in the message startled you, you might respond to yourself Oh My Goodness, not OMG. These days they don't even teach cursive writing in school. But times have changed, technology has taken the world by storm and here I am with my very own cellphone. So, W-T-H. It's time to embrace the twenty-first century. Let's see who Freddie set up for me to text.

(*Ruby puts down the cellphone, picks up her landline and makes a call*)

Gladys. Oh, thank you. Yes, I'm having a good day. Freddie came by and gave me a cellphone for my birthday. Yes, I will give it a try. OK. Talk to you later.

(*Ruby puts the phone in its cradle, picks up the cellphone and exits SR. Lights fade to black to depict the passage of time*)

(*Ruby enters again in the dark and is on stage in her chair as lights come up slowly. Ruby has added a sweater to her outfit to indicate that this is a new time*)

(*Picking up the phone she holds it absolutely correctly, speaking to the audience as she types a message with both thumbs*)

RUBY

Gladys. I have been working on this texting for two weeks now. And B-T-W, U can say things like W-T-F or damn near anything you want to in a text. LMAO. H-B-2 me! TTYL.

(*She giggles loudly*)

CURTAIN

COVID, Technology and Me
Harold Tausch

Although I was a computer programmer for over 40 years, I've always been a bit of a Luddite—one of the last to adopt any new technology. There's nothing that will get me into a state of rage and frustration more readily than wrestling with technology when it is not working right or doing what I want it to do. The pandemic has forced me to use technology more than ever, and it has certainly prompted a fair bit of rage and many streams of profanity, but it has also at times been a godsend and a blessing.

We live in a time when we have access to an overwhelming amount of information and entertainment on the internet: 24-hour news, social media, podcasts, Netflix and its competitors, etc. So far during the pandemic, I've done a good job of resisting being sucked into the black hole of the internet. I seldom check my Facebook page, and I can't understand why anyone would use Twitter. Streaming services have resulted in an explosion of entertaining, well-written and acted series with wonderful production values, but I watch very few of them. Most of the time, I'd much rather be doing something than watching something.

The one thing that has been difficult to resist doing is reading the news on the internet. Particularly during the horror show of the American election and its aftermath. I found myself checking the news multiple times each day, reading about the same events on different sites, pursuing the endless internet trails. It was ultimately exhausting and depressing and led me to feel more and more pessimistic about the future of the planet and more and more cynical about the human race. Lately I've started to read the news just once a week (since I do want to have some idea of what's going on in the world), and I've noticed that I am more optimistic and there has been a considerable lightening of my mood.

A few years ago, I got back into acting after playing around with it in my 20s. 2020 felt like it was going to be a breakout year for me. I had parts lined up in two plays, a dance/theatre piece, a feature film and two short films. When the pandemic hit, all were cancelled or postponed except for one short film. One of the plays was for the Hamilton Fringe. When that was cancelled, they decided to have a festival of virtual plays instead. That was my first opportunity to wrestle with some new technology.

I was cast in a play called *Waiting for Mark*, which was about what happens if you die while on Facebook. It was performed live via Zoom and broadcast on YouTube three times. This was my first exposure to Zoom and, I suspect, one of the first attempts anywhere to perform a virtual play on this platform. I live in a rooming house and I discovered during the first couple of rehearsals that the WiFi signal in my room was not strong enough and all the other characters would suddenly freeze. Eventually I strung a 50-foot ethernet cable down to the modem on the ground floor, which solved that problem (although I periodically forgot to plug it into my computer after going to all that trouble, and a downstairs tenant tripped over the wire a couple of times).

One of the problems with Zoom is that each person has a different view, so there is no way of knowing where the other people are, and I found it quite distracting to have myself to look at as well. This was long before I discovered that you can hide your 'self-view' on Zoom, which has really improved my experience with it. I'm no longer checking out if I look all right every few seconds, and it feels much more like I'm interacting with the other people on the screen.

But the cast was terrific and I really enjoyed rehearsing and performing this funny little play. We probably didn't do that great a job, and we had some of the usual live theatre problems like incorrect or badly-timed sound cues. A good friend, whose judgement and honesty I trust, gave us a rather scathing review. I consoled myself with the notion that the first time we do anything we don't usually do it very well.

A few months later, I got my first ever voice acting job with some wonderful young people in Victoria. We were able to meet virtually via Zoom and rehearse and record together, although some of us were in Victoria, some in Toronto and some in Montreal. Technology was critical in making this project happen, especially during these pandemic times. It was a four-episode drama called *A Way Out*.[1] I played a man whose wife is slipping into dementia, who goes on a disastrous caving expedition with his daredevil grandson.

Of course, there were the inevitable technical problems. I bought a good microphone for the project, only to discover that I couldn't set the levels on the software we were to use for recording no matter what I tried. After many hours of research (and a good deal of profanity), consulting with the project's sound person, and messing around with various obscure settings, it still wasn't working. I started frantically downloading alternative recording software, none of which was any good, and managed in the process to get a virus on my computer that caused my screen to blank out briefly every once in a while. At that point, I remembered that I'd installed some software to filter out background noise on Zoom a month earlier. Without any great hope, I uninstalled it. Amazingly enough, after that the problem disappeared and I was able to adjust the levels on the recording software.

Shortly after *A Way Out*, I got another voice acting job in a horror podcast with a young writer/actor/producer named Adam in Vancouver, a project he created because there was so little acting work due to the pandemic. I played an evil immortal and his puppet. Great fun, again made possible by technology. We were using software designed for recording podcasts and, as usual, there were technical problems. If I plugged my headphones into my microphone and told the software that was what I had done, I could hear Adam perfectly but he could barely hear me. If I plugged my headphones into my computer and told the software that was what I had done, Adam could hear me perfectly but I could barely hear him. Somehow, I stumbled onto the solution: I plugged the headphones into the computer but told the software that I had plugged it into the headphones. Then we could both hear each other clearly. I had to lie to the software to make it work.

I am currently in rehearsals for another virtual play and I'm truly grateful that the technology exists to work with creative people all over the country, so that I can continue to gain experience and growth in my craft despite the pandemic and associated lockdowns. And the technical difficulties are allowing me to experience rage and frustration regularly, which will no doubt come in handy in some future acting roles!

One of the great pleasures of my life has been a variety of forms of social dancing—contact improvisation, freestyle dancing, and Biodanza—and I have missed that terribly since the pandemic started. As a single person, social dancing was my primary way to meet new people and to interact and have physical contact with others. I've tried a few times to dance virtually with some of my friends, but it just didn't work for me. I felt inhibited in my movement without the physical presence of the other dancers. Seeing little figures dancing in their living rooms just wasn't the same. Ultimately it left me feeling sad and lonely.

But there are aspects of virtual get-togethers that I'm really learning to appreciate. For almost 30 years, I've been a member of a men's group that meets every second Thursday evening. When the pandemic hit, we started meeting via Zoom. A few years ago, one of our members moved to Victoria; now he is once again able to take part in our meetings. We've decided to continue having a Zoom session open at our meetings even after we start to meet in person again so that he can continue to join us.

Recently, our oldest member died at the age of 85. We decided to hold a virtual wake for him via Zoom. Twenty-one people attended, including the members of the group, three of his children, his long-time girlfriend, his ex-wife and a few others to whom he had made a difference in his very rich life. We were scattered all over Canada and beyond: Victoria in the west, Sherbrooke in the east and Mexico in the south. It was a very moving and powerful celebration of the life of a wonderful man. And it could not have happened without technology.

I've started to prefer talking with my friends and family virtually rather than on the phone. It feels more like actually being with them. So much of our communication is non-verbal, and now I can see what their facial expressions and body language are telling me. During the first lockdown, I regularly met virtually with my younger son. I found our conversations often became deeper and more intimate than when we met in person.

It seems that any new technology has both good and bad aspects. Social media has allowed us to connect with people all over the world and to build new kinds of relationships. I've appreciated technology for allowing me to continue pursuing the acting adventure I am on and to stay connected with my loved ones. But I am longing at a very deep level to be in the physical presence of others, to sit in a lively restaurant, to walk down a busy street, to dance with my friends, to attend a theatre performance or a concert. We are social creatures and have a profound need for physical contact and community. The virtual world can give us only a pale imitation of that.

I can't wait for this pandemic to end!

The Virtual Apprentice:
A Socially-Distanced Modern Comedy
Jon Peirce

CHARACTERS

GEORGE BAKER: a bright but curmudgeonly guy who looks to be in his late 60s. A retired professor. Can be a bit of a show-off by times.

ELIZABETH WATERS: his neighbour from two apartments below his, bright with occasional tendencies toward didacticism. A high-level provincial civil servant. She's attractive and keeps herself well; she could be any age from about 40 to her late 50s—so long as she *looks* substantially younger than George.

SETTING

George's apartment, a large, comfortable, but fairly plain one on the third floor of a low-rise building in Metro Halifax. Furniture is adequate and functional—nothing more than that.

TIME

The present, early Spring.

SCENES

Scene 1: Mid-afternoon on a weekday

Scene 2: Mid-morning the next day

Scene 3: Mid-morning the day after that

As the play starts, George is sitting on his sofa, reading. He's dressed in typical pandemic attire, namely his L.L. Bean nightshirt, with slippers. He hasn't yet been outside and is feeling a bit stir-crazy, but would still like to get one particular piece of research in before he gets dressed and goes for his walk.

SCENE 1

GEORGE

(Thumbing through a very old dictionary) Virtual reality. Another one of those damned newfangled terms. Well, *(sighing)* maybe I can make some sense of it if I break it into its two component parts. Hm. 'Virtual. Being in essence or effect but not in fact.' Whatever the hell that means. Now for 'reality.' Oh, wow. 'The totality of real things and events. Something that is neither derivative nor dependent but exists necessarily.' Clear as mud. *(Stands up and*

flings dictionary onto the table) Screw it. Time to go get ready for my walk.
(Hears a timid knock at the door) Wonder who that could be. *(Breaks into song)*
Who's that knocking at my door; who's that knocking at my door? Who's
that knocking at my door—

ELIZABETH

*(Just as George opens door, UR. Like George, she's attired in pandemic gear—in her
case, a robe over her nightgown, and slippers)* Cried the fair young maiden![1]

GEORGE

(Whose jaw has by this time dropped several inches) Well, I'll be damned! Not just
any visitor, but a musically literate one. To what do I owe the honour of *this*
visit?

ELIZABETH

(Almost shyly) Actually, I was hoping I could borrow some yeast. I live in the
apartment two floors below yours, and I was just starting to make some
bread when I realized I was out of yeast. And I haven't been able to find
any anywhere—not at Sobey's, not at No-Frills, not even at Superstore.

GEORGE

(Amused) But how is it that you hit on me, of all people? Was it my *yeasty*
personality, or the fact that my last name just happens to be Baker?

ELIZABETH

(Laughing) Neither of those! You just happen to be the only one at home
today. Everyone else must be out working.

GEORGE

And you're not?

ELIZABETH

Actually, I'm working from home these days. Work for the provincial
government, and they give us flexible hours. Any eight between 7:00 a.m.
and 7:00 p.m. Things were going a bit slow, so I thought I'd fill in the time
by starting a batch of bread.

GEORGE

I see! Well, Ms—

ELIZABETH

Elizabeth. Elizabeth Waters.

GEORGE

And I'm George Baker. Pleased to meet you, Elizabeth. *You* just happen to be in luck. I have an unopened package of yeast in my fridge. My cleaning lady gave it to me the last time before she had to stop coming. Said if I started baking, it might help get my mind off the cleaning I would now have to do.

ELIZABETH

But won't you need it?

GEORGE

(Laughing) Not a chance. As you can see *(Striking a pose)*, I'm already a bit on the heavy side. Last thing I need is to make a whole bunch of bread and cakes and pies. If I did that, I'd be up to 320 in a flash. The yeast is yours!

ELIZABETH

Why, thank you! *(George goes off, DL, but quickly emerges with a packet of Fleischmann's yeast which he holds in a claw gripper and hands to her, very formally. The gripper is long enough that the two are close to six feet apart for the handover)*

GEORGE

See? Neighbourliness is possible, even with social distancing!

ELIZABETH

Thanks again. *(Puts the yeast into her purse, and then turns to look at the dictionary, which she regards in some amazement)* Say—what's that book you were looking at when I came in?

GEORGE

(Proudly) Webster's Collegiate Dictionary. Same one that got me through college and grad school. *(Pause)* I was trying to piece together a definition for virtual reality.

ELIZABETH

(Amused) Don't you think that dictionary's a bit out of date?

GEORGE *(Shrugging)*

And I'm not? What do you expect me to use—the *Hitchhiker's Guide to Lexicography?*

ELIZABETH

But I don't know *anybody* who still uses a hard-copy dictionary.

GEORGE

Guess you're not moving in the right circles, then. *(Pause)* What're we supposed to do when we play Scrabble—wait 10 minutes to crank up Big Bertha here? *(Pointing to his desktop)*

ELIZABETH

Leaving all that aside, was that dictionary working for you today?

GEORGE *(Unhappily)*

Well. . . no.

ELIZABETH

(Again, almost shyly) I could help you with some more modern tools. *(Pause)* That's if you want to, of course.

GEORGE

(Pause) Well, OK. Sure.

ELIZABETH

(Quite matter-of-factly) You would, of course, have to make certain adjustments in your attitude—

GEORGE

(Almost exploding—she has really hit a button here) Oh my God. Don't get me going on that! Back when I was in grade school, my teachers were always on at me about my attitude. That and group adjustment. *(Pause)* And when they were finished with all that, they'd haul out their Bonnie Prudden[2] books and quote her, telling us that our wimpishness had allowed the Commies to win in Korea, so we'd better do 200 push-ups and 50 chin-ups right away, or we'd all be speaking Chinese. *(Pause)* Now I'm not so sure I want to go through with this.

ELIZABETH

It's entirely up to you. I *could* always leave you to figure out virtual reality on your own.

GEORGE

(Aside) Fate worse than death! *(To Elizabeth)* Under normal circumstances, I'd tell you to take a hike. *(Pause)* But right now, you're the only game in town, so I guess I'll let you back in. Under protest. *(Pause)* Does 10:00 a.m. tomorrow work for you?

ELIZABETH

Works for me. See you then. In the meantime, start to think about that
attitude!

GEORGE

I'll try not to!

ELIZABETH

And thanks again for the yeast. *(She exits DL as he exits UR)*

SCENE 2

*Inside George's apartment, the next morning. George has removed the old dictionary, and
there's now a long, narrow table in front of the sofa, UR, but otherwise everything is the
same. Anticipating his visitor, George has spruced up a bit; he now wears good cords and
a cardigan over an Oxford-cloth shirt. Elizabeth wears a heavy tweed suit and 'sensible
Oxfords,' looking like a schoolmarm from George's youth. One more difference--she's
carrying a laptop. At precisely the appointed hour, there's a knock on the door.*

GEORGE

Come in!

ELIZABETH

I really shouldn't. But since you insist—

GEORGE

This table is well over six feet long. We can sit at opposite ends, just as if
we were a long-married couple watching TV on the sofa.

ELIZABETH

You're so cynical! I can tell right away I'm in for a challenge.

GEORGE *(Equably)*

We don't have to do this if you don't want to. We can talk about the
weather, the price of grain in Winnipeg, the price of tea in China, the
number of new cases in New Brunswick… Speaking of tea, I have some on
the go. Would you like some?

ELIZABETH

No thanks. Just had a big mug of coffee. I make it a rule never to mix my
stimulants.

GEORGE

Good plan! *(Pause)* Well—what *is* on today's agenda, then?

ELIZABETH

(Unfolding her laptop) You'll see. *(Boots up the machine)* Perhaps we'd best start with a definition of the term that was giving you so much trouble. *(Pause)* Well—here it is. Virtual reality for dummies—

GEORGE

Now, see here—

ELIZABETH

Sorry. That *was* a wee bit tactless. Here's a simple definition, intended for those with no special technical training. *(Reads in a school-marmish voice)* *Virtual reality* is an artificial environment that is created with software and presented to the user in such a way that the user suspends belief and accepts it as a real environment. On a computer, *virtual reality* is primarily experienced through two of the five senses: sight and sound. *(Long pause)* So, my friend, what do you think of that?

GEORGE

(After an even longer pause) Don't rightly know what I think of that. Got something to do with computers.

ELIZABETH

A step in the right direction, for sure. So, tell me George, why is virtual reality so important now?

GEORGE

Damned if I know. *(Pause)* Maybe it's because there's a whole lot of folks who'd normally be out working or playing golf or at least watching baseball on TV who've suddenly got nothing better to do, so they start reading these science-fiction books and talking about them?

ELIZABETH *(Cautiously)*

There is *something* to that. The term does appear in lots of science-fiction books, and yes, people are talking about it, and indeed working with it, much more than they were when we were still wide open. Could you take that just a little bit further?

GEORGE

Well, as I said, right now there's a whole lot of 'ordinary reality' that we

351

can't get into. So maybe this virtual reality is a kind of substitute. *(Pause)* But what's this got to do with my attitude?

ELIZABETH

I sense that you're not fully on board with virtual reality, George. You need to understand that it's here to stay. *(Rises, and strikes a pose, as if delivering a sermon from a lectern. She can even hold out an imaginary piece of paper if she wants)* Are you prepared to take it to your bosom? *(Looking down at his chest, George snickers)* Do you love it with all your heart and all your mind and all your soul? Have you accepted the Cyber God as your personal saviour? Are you prepared to love this new world of virtual reality better than the grimy reality we've left behind? Because that's what this means. Anything less than total surrender to the new dispensation means you will be left behind, abandoned to moulder on the scrap heap of history! *(Collapses back onto the sofa)*

GEORGE

(Emits a long, low retching sound, followed by a single, heartfelt word) Jesus! *(Pause)* I can't believe you actually believe this stuff yourself. You sound like Billy Graham and Billy Sunday and Jimmy Bakker all rolled into one. All I've ever seen converted around here are old farmhouses.

ELIZABETH

It's just that I felt so bad for you, using that dictionary from the Lester Pearson era in a mechanical attempt to figure out our world. You need to understand this *holistically.*

GEORGE

(Aside) Holistically, for God's sake! What next—a paradigm shift? *(To her)* You want to talk about attitude, Lizzie? I'll have you know that the Lester Pearson era, toward which *you've* displayed such a cavalier attitude, was a far more generous and humane era than our own! It gave us healthcare, collective bargaining in the public service, and much, much more. Now everyone seems hell-bent on taking away what the Pearson era gave us all freely. *(Pause)* Please don't take this personally. But the only missionary work I'm willing to be part of is done in the prone position.

ELIZABETH *(Reddening)*

Are you suggesting—

GEORGE

Not for a moment! *(Laughs)* Are you kidding me? *(Pause)* What I *am* suggesting is that my soul was lost ages ago, probably back in the

Pleistocene, and there's no point trying to retrieve it now. Ain't gonna happen.

ELIZABETH *(Almost desperate)*

But don't you see how much you're missing?

GEORGE

What am I missing? Do, please, tell me. Inquiring minds need to know. *(Pause)* But not today *(Wearily)* I've had all I can take today. Need *at least* three fingers of Glenlivet to wash that speech out of my ears. Tomorrow at 10:00?

ELIZABETH

I should just tell you to take a hike. But right now you're the only game in town. So, tomorrow at 10:00 it is. Under protest. *(Exeunt as before, she leaving DL slightly before he leaves UR, shaking his head as he goes)*

SCENE 3

George, dressed in jeans and a flannel shirt, sits on the couch nervously awaiting Elizabeth's arrival. She will turn out to be similarly attired. Although he doesn't let on, he finds her absolutely irresistible in jeans—which will only make the sparks fly faster in the following exchanges. This time, the knock at the door is firm and decisive. He lets her in and gestures her to the opposite end of the couch from the one he's been sitting on.

GEORGE

Well?

ELIZABETH

Look. I did go a wee bit overboard yesterday. Still, you need to understand—

GEORGE

Understand what? That I need to turn my soul into a machine to be able to function in this brave new world?

ELIZABETH

You'd be amazed at what the new robotic technology can do. It can give directions, organize your finances, check people out at stores, conduct a simple conversation—

353

GEORGE

(Striking a pose) Ven I hear a machine talking at me, I reach for my sledgehammer! *(Note:* 'Ven' is an attempt to recreate a German accent).

ELIZABETH

That's not very constructive.

GEORGE

Not very constructive, eh? How constructive is it to bring in new technology that destroys jobs by the thousands? You understand, don't you, that every time you use one of those self-serve machines at Shopper's or Sobey's, you're helping to put people out of work.

ELIZABETH

Progress, George. It's inevitable. No point in trying to fight it.

GEORGE

No? Well, I for one refuse to use any self-serve checkout machine. If enough of us think the same way, maybe the stores will take the machines out, and bring their clerks back. I understand some have already started doing that. And if not *(Mischievously)*, why, I can always come in at a slack time, and put a litre of molasses or a bag of nails through one of those brave new machines. That oughta learn it! *(Pause)* They just had a sale on molasses at No-Frills. I bought ten litres.

ELIZABETH

Did you now? I thought you said you didn't bake.

GEORGE *(Ominously)*

I don't. *(Pause)* Anyway—all those retail clerks who've been replaced by machines, what sorts of jobs are they supposed to get? Cleaning COVID rooms at the Infirmary, with a 2% raise and a promotion to hosing out dumpsters if they survive a year of that?

ELIZABETH

You're so cynical, George. I'm sure they'll find something, somewhere.

GEORGE

And I've got a bridge I can sell you, real cheap. What this world needs is… *(Stops abruptly)* But never mind. You won't listen to me. No one ever does.

ELIZABETH

Well?

GEORGE

(Wearily) Just tell me, please, what virtual reality can do for us in the here and now. I think we may have got a bit off-track here.

ELIZABETH

(Aside) If we were ever on track. *(To him)* You know all those things we used to do up until two months ago. Things like going to concerts, going to the theatre, having meetings, going to church services. Even singing in choirs.

GEORGE

(Still wearily) Yeah?

ELIZABETH

We can still do lots of those things—online. Ever hear of something called Zoom?

GEORGE

A friend of mine was making noises about it a while back. Didn't pay him any mind, because I didn't see how I could use it.

ELIZABETH

If you didn't need it then, you sure do now. It's amazing. You log in, push a button, and you're connected. You can see and hear everyone else who's connected and have real conversations. Almost as good as being there.

GEORGE

I don't know about that. Still, it might be a possibility. How do I get into that?

ELIZABETH

First, we have to make sure your computer is equipped for it. Then you have to download the program. That can take a while.

GEORGE

While I read *War and Peace*—

355

ELIZABETH *(Laughingly)*

No—just a novella will do. Maybe something about tennis and romance. Or a magazine.

GEORGE

Well, I'm game. Game because it's the only game in town. *(Laughs at his feeble pun)* What else is there?

ELIZABETH

You must have heard of Facebook—

GEORGE

Not only heard of it, but have it. *(Pause)* But I let my account go dormant in 2017. Got damn sick and tired of hearing about Trump all the time.

ELIZABETH

Can't blame you for that. But there's all kinds of good stuff there. Just like Zoom. Plays. Concerts. Even church services, if you're so inclined.

GEORGE

(Aside) Church services! God help us! *(To her)* How can you access these?

ELIZABETH

All you have to do is go onto the Facebook page of whoever's hosting the event, at the appropriate time, and press a button. Bingo. You're there.

GEORGE

(Has an 'Aha' moment) Oh, my God *(Very slowly)* Oh, my dear sweet everlovin' Jesus!

ELIZABETH *(Frightened)*

What? What's wrong? Are you OK, George?

GEORGE

It's like—it's like I just realized I've been speaking in prose. For my entire life.

ELIZABETH

I had that same recognition. About nine years ago. *(Briskly)* Well, shall I come tomorrow to help you set up Zoom?

356

GEORGE *(Still a bit dazed)*

If you like. Ten o'clock still work for you?

ELIZABETH

It does.

GEORGE

This is actually a great moment in my life. I think we need to toast it.

ELIZABETH

Well, if you insist. . .

George disappears, DL, but quickly re-emerges with two cups or mugs or glasses of something—what it is doesn't really matter. Hands one to Elizabeth, using the claw gripper, and keeps one for himself.

GEORGE

Cheers!

ELIZABETH

To virtual reality!

GEORGE

Virtual reality if necessary, but not necessarily virtuous reality! *(Pokes playfully at Elizabeth with the gripper as the lights dim. She responds in the same spirit, perhaps taking a dog leash or strap out of her purse to flick it at him)*

CURTAIN

Notes

---

[1] For those not in the know, the allusion is to the classic jazz song, 'Barnacle Bill the Sailor.' The best-known version is one recorded in 1930 by Bix Beiderbecke and Hoagy Carmichael.

[2] Well-known American writer from the 1950s on physical fitness, of the Marine Corps variety. A 1950s icon, alongside Admiral Hyman Rickover and Dr Norman Vincent Peale.

SECTION 9

Travel

Covid Travels to Family:
Into the Unknown
Sally Arsove

When will it be safe to travel again? To which countries will it be safe to travel? How can I prove that I've been fully vaccinated? What are the safest (and least safe) ways to travel? As the pandemic's third wave winds down and Canadians again start thinking about travelling to the U.S., to Europe, and to warm spots in the Caribbean, these and a host of other questions are on the tip of everyone's tongue. To say that the travel landscape is a fluid and rapidly-changing one is to understate. The situation, with regard both to travel within Canada and travel between Canada and other countries, has been changing on almost a daily basis. There are few signs that this is likely to change any time soon. Public health officials themselves have been disagreeing as to when it will be safe to resume travel, and where, and what precautions travellers should be taking.

The pieces in this section offer three quite distinct perspectives on travel. In 'COVID Travels to Family: Into the Unknown,' Sally Arsove describes the complicated planning needed to carry off a trip to family living in the U.S. at the height of the pandemic. The process she describes, often poignantly, is not one for the faint of heart. Next, Robert Barclay's amusing memoir lays out in dramatic detail what it was like to complete and then return from an around-the-world trip at the beginning of the pandemic. Finally, Jo-Anne Stead's memoir, 'Four Adults: One Pandemic,' describes what life is like when previously independent adult children move back in with Mom and Dad during the pandemic. Despite the inevitable frictions resulting from different ways of doing things, from housekeeping to taking walks, Stead comes away grateful for having had a 'unique opportunity' to spend time with her adult children and to live together as a four-adult family.

Covid Travels to Family:
Into the Unknown
Sally Arsove

Friends:
If you are thinking of travelling to visit family across a border—as we continue to limit our travels in the face of the great risks and uncertainties of COVID-19—below is my story, which could be your story, of travelling by air last December to January from Canada to the U.S.A. to visit family (I am a citizen of both countries), and some COVID Safe Travel Tips on getting through.

June 2020
Due to COVID risks, you cancelled your July trip to Seattle to visit your son and his wife and your 6-month-old granddaughter, who you have met only once just after her birth.

October 2020
After a Summer lull in COVID, you learn that a second grandchild is due in May 2021, and that with a new baby coming: you can visit again in either January 2021 or January 2022. So, you decide to first travel to Florida to visit you daughter over Christmas (she will be alone), and from there you will together to Seattle in January 2021.

You book your flight to Florida on Christmas Eve, directly from Ottawa to Fort Lauderdale. But wait: Ottawa is not on the list of cities from which one can fly directly from Canada to a foreign country! So, you fully expect notification from Air Canada of some flight changes, and finally in early December you get your first of several notifications stating 'your flight is cancelled and rebooked,' always for the same day. The changes were either to a different time to fill up flights, or to fly out on a smaller plane with a new flight number, hence a need to 'rebook.' While you understood that Air Canada is a business that needs to make money, the anxiety starts setting in: will your flight be full enough to actually take off?

Early December 2020
After many hours talking to Air Canada agents to figure out which flights tend to be full—time of day? Day of week?—then checking Air Canada Flight Status Information online to see what recent flights have been

canceled: you take the plunge and rebook to depart on Sunday December 20, on a flight that the Air Canada phone agent said was mostly full already. While you have heard a bit about some new COVID variants on the horizon elsewhere, there is nothing concrete, and while COVID has been increasing in Canada since the cold Fall weather moved people indoors, you decide to depart as scheduled on December 20. There is no lockdown/stay at home order in place in Ontario or Ottawa at that time.

How to stay safe in airport and airplane transit? Friends who have traveled advise you to wear a face shield as well as a mask. You have read that the air on the plane is as good as in a hospital, hence you should turn on your overhead air nozzle full blast. You pray that the person sitting next to you does not cough COVID directly upon you for the whole flight. And you decide that you will take the risk because you will be going to see *family*.

December 20, 2020

D(eparture)-Day arrives. You drive your car to the airport to avoid possible infection in an UBER. You have never done Long Term Parking, but you have been in Short Term and it has become Long Term for COVID, so you feel comfortable. You leave early, by two hours, and *arrive* at the airport.

You blot out all thoughts of catching COVID. By the grace of God, it's the Sunday before Christmas, and the Ottawa airport is empty, as is the Toronto airport, which is your connecting airport to the U.S.A. The water fountains had been operational in Ottawa, but you find them taped off in Toronto: good. And in Toronto every other seat in the waiting room is blocked off by a big red X. You feel safe in the airport. You feel safe!

On the flight, you sit next to a young man. You do not make eye contact and you do not talk. You turn on your overhead air vent full blast as advised and put a pashmina shawl over your head to keep germs off, in such a way though that you can still see around you. You hear no one coughing and you breathe a sigh of relief. You feel safe… you feel safe…

You land at Fort Lauderdale airport and you walk through a departure/arrivals area that is *crowded*. You wait for your checked bag at a carousel that is *crowded*. You try to distance from others. You hang around a pillar like a high school wallflower. You leap up when you finally see your bag that is identified with brightly-coloured ribbons. Are you still safe…

With your bag in hand, you rush to curbside and await pickup by your daughter. You wait away from others, distanced. Soon you hear a cheery voice and see the smiling face of your daughter. Nothing else matters, for now. But you are older, and must keep up your guard against COVID.

With family again! Still, your daughter drives you to a local Marriott extended-stay hotel where you have booked a room for your first four days as she lives in a one-bedroom apartment where it is hard to distance and neither of you has been tested for COVID. You feel very safe in the hotel: the room is not cleaned unless you ask, you bring your cold breakfast up to your room, and everyone wears a mask at the front desk and in the wide hotel corridors.

After those few days in the hotel, you take a chance with COVID and relocate to your daughter's apartment. You keep the patio door open all the time for ventilation. You do not wear a mask in her presence—a choice you make while you are staying with family—but you still distance yourself a lot, as you have been programed to do while living in Ottawa during COVID. You keep your activities outdoors with your daughter (who is not seeing her friends indoors) and you only see other people outdoors and distanced and you mask up when near to others outdoors. You avoid going into stores, and you buy most everything online.

Despite all the COVID-related complications, the time together is fun and precious and full of love. It restores a sense of mental well-being.

Your flight to Seattle is on January 6, so you and your daughter decide to get COVID tests on December 26 to reassure the family that you are not carrying COVID. The results come back negative; within 36 hours. From then until you board your flight to Seattle, you remain very careful about distancing and masking and limit contact with other people to the outdoors.

January 6, 2021

With great excitement—but also with some trepidation—you leave for the airport for your flight to Seattle. You had received a message saying that the flight was nearly full, so you upgraded to business class at a reasonable cost to be first off the flight at your destination and therefore less likely to get COVID.

You arrive in Seattle that night, and you stay in a Marriott Hotel at the airport as you feel very safe as their guest knowing that they follow COVID precautions. The next day, your son picks you up at the hotel with a smiling face and a big *hug*. You take a chance on that sorely needed human contact, putting your fears of COVID aside to enjoy that physical contact aspect of life.

You all drive to a spacious 'vacation rental by owner' house that you have rented in the mountains an hour from Seattle. You enjoy outdoor beers, the hot tub, the spectacular views of snow-capped mountains in the morning mist, walks with the dog Miss Tilly, family chatter and meals indoors, and your hilarious granddaughter… who admittedly is making strange with you!

New Development While Abroad

You are keeping up with the news and hear of scandal in Canada with Ontario politicians resigning after going to the Caribbean during COVID for a holiday. The Government scrambles to get tough on travel and imposes a requirement that you must have a negative PCR text within 72 hours of boarding your flight home, or you will not be let on the flight. You know that getting results of PCR tests can be quick or can be slow; there is no guarantee either way. A new level of stress is creeping in…

You begin to worry but try to hide it, so you can all continue to enjoy the pleasure of each other's company. You know you must quarantine two weeks when home, which is a good policy, but you begin to wonder if the government can shut borders even to citizens during a pandemic? You have no real answers. You had heard vaguely of new dangerous COVID variants before leaving Canada in December, and now in January they have appeared big time in the U.K. and all hell is breaking loose there, and Heathrow Airport is closed, as is their border. Once again you wonder if Canada could prevent you from coming back…

You had a flight booked from Seattle to Ottawa via Vancouver for January 14. Where should you get your PCR test, factoring in that the results could be delayed and you might have to delay your flight home? The tricky part is that your son is actually staying three hours from Seattle, so if you get stuck in Seattle and must take another PCR test and await test results again, you are facing heavy hotel costs… and no loving family to keep you company. What to do? What to do?

Decision taken. You fly back from Seattle to Fort Lauderdale with your daughter on January 14, so you can stay with her in case the PCR test results do not come back in time and you miss your flight home. Then you also buy *two* plane tickets from Fort Lauderdale home to Ottawa, in case you miss the first flight. This is adding some significant costs that not everyone can afford.

You Are on Your Way Home

It all works out. You get your negative PCR test results the day before leaving Seattle, and you fly back to Fort Lauderdale as booked where you make your first flight home to Canada. While waiting in line to board your flight home, you hear two young women talking about how much fun they had at the Hard Rock Café the night before! You know that even with their negative COVID test results needed to board the plane, they could well be carriers of the disease. And while they do board the plane, you decide to upgrade to Business Class, hoping that they will be in Economy. You are hungry and stressed and your guard is down, so with mask off you eat the 'free' hot meal provided to you… and you are finally on your way home.

Friends, you can see that while travelling during COVID is full of risks and uncertainties and stressors, if you need or want to travel to *family* and are doing so within the rules, here are some COVID Safe Travel Tips based on my travel experience last Christmas:

1. Be prepared for anything and everything to change: flights, travel restrictions, COVID testing rules, COVID passport requirements.
2. Be prepared for your travel costs to go up due to delays and unexpected events.
3. If you stay in hotels make sure they are following COVID precautions.
4. If you can afford it, upgrade to business class on airplanes so you are first off the plane.
5. Make sure your cellphone plan has enough roaming, and bring reliable IT devices and charge cords. A tablet is a good backup to a computer.
6. Always travel with carry-on luggage in case you need to change a flight at the last minute. You will not be let on a flight if you have a bag already checked onto another flight. Carry-on luggage also allows you to avoid waiting close to others at crowded luggage carousels.
7. On the plane, open the overhead air nozzle fully, as the air it blows on your face is very safe. It may be COVID-safer to choose a window seat over an aisle seat.
8. Take a shuttle to your airport hotel rather than a taxi or Uber, because shuttles tend to be small buses with few if any passengers, except you, and you are much farther away from a shuttle driver than from a taxi or Uber driver.
9. Wear a face shield at all times in transit and carry disinfectant spray and wipes.
10. Bring a shawl to put over your head on the plane in case the person next to you is coughing.
11. Bring enough healthy snack foods to get you through two days of travel, and an empty water bottle that, hopefully, you can fill with water once you are through security. Otherwise, you will need to buy water.
12. If you leave your car at long-term parking in an airport, be aware that animals can get into the engine and damage the wires, particularly if the airport is near open countryside.
13. Choose a purse that provides good organization and easy quick access to documents, etc.
14. If Air Canada cancels and rebooks you, find out how much time you have to request a different new flight without being charged a change fee or flight fare differential fee.
15. If you cancel and rebook a flight for COVID reasons, you may only get one free change.
16. Keep your cellphone topped up with lots of roaming data access in case you need to be on the internet, e-mail or the phone for long periods while not on free WiFi.

Physically Distanced from Home
Robert Barclay

How about finding yourself more than halfway round the world, 16 hours ahead of where the home hearth is, and with a pandemic looming over you like the tottering wall of a nearly demolished warehouse? How about that suggestion—so artlessly transmitted to us by our children back in Ottawa—that wherever you're staying at the moment, just get used to the idea of living there? Thank you very much for that. We were in Sydney, New South Wales in March of 2020 when our round-the-world holiday became terminal, but we had been brushed by the tendrils of the pandemic for some time before this. Nipping at our heels, it was. Twenty-twenty hindsight is a wonderful, but sadly quite mythical, human faculty. Just before we left Ottawa in December of 2019 a friend asked, regarding our global travel plans, 'Not going anywhere near Wuhan, are you?' The dragon of infection the Chinese were wrestling at the close of the year of the pig would escape its captors in the year of the rat, yet back then words like ominous, impending and dire were all easily ignorable. 'No, nowhere near.' Little did we know that we wouldn't have to go there; Wuhan would come to us.

The wisdom when we landed in London just before Christmas was that this virus the Chinese were wrestling with hadn't got out. So, in January, the worst bout of flu I had ever experienced in my life was just that, then—a nasty bout of flu? A planned visit to cousins in the West Country had to be cancelled. They had 'a nasty bout of flu.' Great to look back at it now and wonder if these were evidence that IT was already out and about, doing its very own round-the-world tour. So, maybe I've already had COVID-19, surely one of the most collectible of diseases? I use my bout of malaria at parties (remember when we used to have parties?) as a conversation stopper, although it's intended to be the opposite. While I don't collect illnesses as such, or don't go out of my way to incur strange injuries and medical conditions, I do have a good stock of medical party repartee, which I am sure always rivets my listeners.

But back to our travels. When we arrived in Kolkata from Singapore on the last day of January there were mobs at the immigration desk (there are always mobs at immigration desks in India) but on this occasion it was for a great form-filling *bandobast* because the Wuhan Corona Virus was on the rampage. The forms, hastily typed, photocopied on the slant with failing toner by someone with postural vertigo, and then realistically crumpled and stained, were distributed to all with accompanying cheap pens that had to be scribbled violently across said forms to coax their balls to issue ink. I don't want to know what the authorities did with people who wrote the word 'China' on their forms, but it probably wasn't pretty.

It was not until this round of tourism in Kolkata in early February that we first heard the term COVID-19. And where did we hear it? Not on the television, not on any of our newsfeeds, not in the free newspapers in the hotel foyer. Science City Kolkata has excellent technical displays that can rival many in the world's finest museums, and this was especially so of a spread of tall display panels flanked by two technicians in white lab coats. There were maps of the far east with graphics, colour-coded areas of infection spread; there were statistics, numbers, charts, tables and diagrams, and there was personal description by the technicians who updated their data daily. This was our first 'We haven't heard the last of this' moment.

In Thailand we were hosted by friends who met us in Chiang-Mai. Now, normally you would jump into a cab and visit the odd temple or two, or maybe an exotic market. Breathe in the oriental ethos... or something. Not this time. Our friends had flown in from Hong Kong, so the immediate mission was to ransack the drugstores for miles around for facemasks and bottles of hand cleaner. Hong Kong had long since run dry. Only when their supply of these life's necessities was assured could we do the tourist thing. By now the hotels were stopping guests at the door and aiming infrared thermometers at their—hopefully not—fevered brows. Hand washing was on the rise; globby dispensers were at every door that made your hands either sticky or slimy, but never feeling clean. The wearing of masks was already a cultural norm, a slap at urban pollution by those who sported them, although fully ninety-nine percent of the wearers had no clue how to put them on right, thus diminishing their efficacy to a mere token.

Back in Singapore in late February the social transformation from our last visit a few weeks before was profound. It's an executive luxury to sashay off the plane, be whisked through customs and immigration, and be led to your own, personal limousine in the span of minutes. When an airport is virtually empty, even the *hoi polloi* like us get this royal treatment by default. I'd swear the desk staff were delighted to see us; there's only so many Sudokus and crosswords you can do in the absence of clientele before you lose the will to live. Our taxi driver was equally delighted to see us, late in the evening and the first fares he'd had all day, poor bugger. People were seriously deciding that popping between countries might just have to be put on hold for the nonce. The strangeness of being in a twenty-percent occupied hotel was offset by the most effusive and attentive personal service. Before, that is, the layoffs began... What few denizens the hotel housed were waifs and strays and orphans of the great global tourism machine, cast off to sink or swim. We met jolly Australians without a cruise ship, dour English couples with no flights, retired Americans with grudges and loud shirts: all people marking time until 'they' did something.

We set off for Down Under, fingers crossed. When we arrived in Sydney, the pandemic clock was set back. All the angst and worry over viral Armageddon were hardly felt there. The wave may have been poised to come crashing down, but nobody in Sydney or the Outback, where we headed, was watching it crest. There were no worries at Alice Springs, mate. It was only on a wine-tasting trip near Melbourne that the hammer truly dropped. The Formula One race was cancelled! What? Get outta here! You don't simply fold up that multi-million-dollar international car racing celebrity circus just like that! Oh, yes, you do. And here was the news on the TV that Italy had closed its borders. What? You jest! You can't simply close up a densely populated, tourist-friendly nation of millions just like that! Oh, yes, you can.

It was clearly time to go home. A finger pointed right in our faces from halfway around the world: 'Your Country Needs You.'

Going home is great if you can book flights. The Air Canada and Aeroplan operatives must have wondered what had hit them. Their first reaction was to hang up on their customers; not even an automated message saying something like, 'Soo sahry, but all our lines are busy. Please try calling again in a month or two,' or 'Don't worry, at Aeroplan we've got you COVID.' You just got a busy signal, which is ironic because busy they were not, while not picking up the phones. Cut them some hindsight slack; it must have been a nightmare for them. Back to that kind advice our offspring gave us: 'Wherever you're staying at the moment, just get used to the idea of living there.' But, to give our kids credit, they took our case in hand and set all sorts of wheels, gears, pulleys and sprockets in motion to find a way to get us home. After a few days of panic, Aeroplan decided it wouldn't be a bad idea to let people talk to them again, so they opened the phone lines. However, half of the winter population of Canada was elsewhere, and all these elsewheres wanted to be in a very different elsewhere—indeed, a more homely elsewhere—than the one they were in at the moment, including us. Long-distance charges on a cellphone from Australia while waiting for an agent to pick up would hammer the piggy bank to shards. Long-distance charges on a hotel phone would have required a mortgage. As our eldest son was locked-down in Ottawa and working from home, it was easy for him to call the Aeroplan number, set the phone down beside his desk, and get on with his work. Three hours on hold, a sudden shock on hearing a human voice, then another hour finagling with the agent. We'd done the whole world around on Aeroplan points—business class all the way—and were contemplating the horror of steerage for those long, time-zone-reeling and thrombotic, knee-joint seizing hauls, but our progeny earned his inheritance (what was left of it after we'd been busy globe-trotting it away). Sydney to Tokyo, Tokyo to Chicago, Chicago to Toronto, Toronto to Montreal, all with blankets, legroom, reclinable seats and free booze. A mere 44 hours of transit.

Back we went to Sydney to wait a few days for our flights. The

367

transformation was as profound as the before-and-after view we'd had of Singapore. Circular Key was a wasteland of fluttering paper, shuttered cafes and a few pedestrians scurrying past. We ate at the last restaurant to stay open, bought some trinkets from the final souvenir shop to close, and returned to the self-imposed isolation of a hotel room that shrank progressively as the hours dragged on. There's no point in attempting to impose social distancing (as it was mis-termed from the very beginning) in the buffet of a near-empty hotel, so close it down and offer the few remaining guests room service. There were two long days of watching the world pulling up its tent pegs, sweeping its floor, and calling its citizens home like iron filings to a magnet. Two long days of walking the halls of our floor, three laps of the corridor every two hours, just to keep the legs and psyche from seizing up. Two long days of peering out of our window overlooking Sydney Harbour, and watching nothing much happening, and watching it happen over and over again.

The airport was madness. Flustered, bright red limeys with mountains of luggage and no flights to 'Eafrow jostled with blonde Swedish touring girls plying their cellphones in frantic appeals for Stockholm, Oslo, Copenhagen, or... daddy. Lines of desperate, sweaty humanity, displaced by touristic choice but now with the magic carpet of world travel whirled out from under them, stood in ovine order. A palpable miasma of misery hung above the hubbub. We absorbed a seething fear, half convincing ourselves that these tickets we held in electronic bondage in our phones would evaporate like faery dust and moonbeams, leaving us beached and castaway. There is an immense sense of relief to feel the double thump as the wheels are retracted, the plane climbs, and you know that there's no turning back. You wish there was a drug that would render time nonexistent, one that would zombie you through the travelling eons, only to wake you at your destination, fresh and amnesiac. The free booze in business class ought to help but, if anything, it makes time feel stretched, elastic seconds to minutes, minutes to hours, hours to days. Lo and behold, there does come a time when it's over and you're back on *terra firma*.

Canada was in lockdown when we stepped off the plane in Dorval, but our children had dealt with contingencies. A room was booked for us in the airport hotel, and on check-in we were presented with the car keys and a very detailed note. 'Wipe the entire car down with Lysol wipes provided... go straight home, do not pass Go, do not collect $200.00... Oh, and don't forget to wipe the stickshift...' They had left the car four days previously; the note said nothing about shelling out for the parking fee, which was considerably more than we could have earned passing Go anyway.

Home felt like the hotel in Sydney, although surrounded by all our stuff and with much more room for pacing. All in all, how privileged we feel to have travelled around the world in style, to have seen and experienced so much, and then, when the whole touristic edifice began to crumble, to find our way swiftly and safely home. In our travels we met so many folk not as lucky as us, and we must always think of them. How did the sunburned Londoners get back to Heathrow; what about the Swedish girls with their backpacks and broken dreams, and those stranded cruise ships and all their abandoned guests?

Yes… privileged, but conscious of it.

Four Adults, One Pandemic
Jo-Anne Stead

The pandemic brought a new reality to our world. I don't mean a new world order, or a different set of guidelines according to public health measures, but a new household order for our small world at home.

We started the pandemic by cohabitating with our grown children. This was a new working model for us. We'd been empty nesters for the past four years, with our oldest daughter, post university, launched on her own in Toronto, and our son at university. We'd become accustomed to a smaller two-person life, with simpler meals, and with the freedom to do what we want when we want. Nothing wild and crazy, but some nights we would just have breakfast for dinner. With both of us home in retirement mode, we often just shopped for groceries every day, buying whatever we fancied.

Then the pandemic hit. Our son, who'd just finished school and returned home in December, had luckily found a job in January. When the city, province and country started closing down around March 13, his office closed and he told us he would be working from home full time. No problem, we had enough space.

Then our 27-year-old daughter, who lives in Toronto and works in the television/movie industry, found out on March 16, a day before her new contract was to start, that it would be postponed indefinitely. She decided to come home to weather the quarantine here, since TO was in shutdown mode, and her small apartment was suddenly not so attractive. She thought her stay would be for only a few weeks.

So there we were, four adults, co-existing in our family home for an indefinite period of time. Usually, the only other times we are all home are for holidays like Christmas or Easter. During those times we generally pack in as much fun as we can into a short time period. The precious few holiday days are scheduled with the things we love to do: going out for dinner, visiting friends, going to movies, and making our favourite meals. Then before we know it, it's time to hug and kiss them good bye as they head out the door.

In the beginning, we treated our new arrangement like an extended holiday, doing things like deciding what favourite meals we wanted to make, ordering board games like Catan, or writing lists of the Netflix shows we wanted to watch. I developed a list of all the projects I'd been wanting to do but couldn't find the time for: organizing old photos, cleaning out junk drawers, writing more, and even cleaning out a basement still full of old toys. This was really going to be a productive 'time out' from the world.

Except that it wasn't, especially in the beginning, as I was glued to the TV and Twitter, listening to the news conferences and updates on the stats for the numbers in our corner of the world and beyond. There was a heightened sense of dread and foreboding about what was happening. Our daughter couldn't watch the news as it was too disturbing for her, and so I snuck in my own TV time when she wasn't around, or endlessly scrolled through my phone feeds. Somehow the atmosphere made me feel scattered and my to-do list didn't see much progress.

We soon settled into a routine. We all got up at different times and made our own way during the day, but then would meet up over dinner and usually spend some evening time together watching a movie or TV show.

I did bake more, which was great, except for my waistline, and it took our minds off the pandemic. I made bread, muffins and cookies during the first few weeks. The couple who wouldn't menu-plan and had sometimes shopped daily were now having to create detailed menu plans and grocery shopping lists for a week or two ahead. Our grocery bills, not to mention our liquor bills, were higher than ever.

The parent-child relationship is a long-established one. Theoretically, we had four adults living together, and everyone should have been taking on their fair share of the work. However, old habits die hard, and we soon slipped into the old parent-child dynamic. My partner and I ended up making the dinners most nights. It took some specific task-assigning and loud verbal reminders to ensure that those who hadn't cooked the dinner were taking care of the cleanup. I discovered that my daughter had become quite the gourmet cook, when she felt like it, and that my son liked foods he never had when he was growing up.

We also discovered some major differences in our generations. Our children are very attached to their phones, not just for communicating through texts and phone calls, but for entertainment. While I like to listen to CBC Radio when I am in the kitchen, they have their ear pods in and listen to their own podcast. This often led to the odd situation of two people in the same room listening to two different information and entertainment sources simultaneously.

Walks were also different. My children don't see a walk as I do. I love to walk and see it as an opportunity, often with my partner or friend, to chat and catch up and offer insights on the world. Often, I would see one of them heading out for a walk, and offer to join them. They would kindly decline my offer, saying they were looking forward to listening to their music or a podcast on their own.

Both children had been living on their own for a few years and with other young adults, so they knew the basics of how to cook and clean. However, home is home, and more relaxed. You could always tell where my son had been sitting since there was a collection of glasses and mugs around his chair, and a build-up of snack dishes.

A few weeks in, people started to get annoyed by the little things. Our daughter was the one to exclaim one day in the kitchen. 'Okay, whoever uses the last bit of butter in the dish should know to replace it with a new stick of butter!' before she stomped off to the fridge to get new butter. Okay.

We've never cooked so much. We've never done so many dishes. The dishwasher had never been run so often. With no company coming into our house in the foreseeable future, there is a new relaxed look to the place. Chairs have been moved around so it is comfier to watch TV. Books and magazines that were once in neat piles are now scattered around the house, picked up one day and never returned to their original location. And those old photos, junk drawers, and that overflowing basement? Well, we made a start, but somehow there never seemed to be enough time in the day to get to them. Too many other things—I can't remember what exactly—to do.

After three months at home our daughter returned to her apartment in Toronto, and we settled into a more relaxed pandemic routine at home. While those first few months might not have been the Brady Bunch bonding experience that we'd aspired to, it was a unique opportunity to spend time with our grown children and to live together as a four-adult family.

SECTION 10

Poetry

*T*he seven poets whose work is represented in this section cover a broad range of pandemic-related experience, and run the complete gamut of emotional expression.

In Valerie Buko's gently wistful 'Before,' a solitary walk through a local park occasions a somewhat melancholy reflection on how love used to be generally available there, pre-pandemic. In 'Pandemic Poems,' Elena Calvo, a photographer as well as a poet, takes a searchingly close look at seemingly ordinary things, such as an old man holding a baby's foot during a long flight, and emerges with a host of new insights into our brave new late-pandemic-to-post-pandemic world. Similarly, Kathy Figueroa's 'Five Pandemic Poems' invite us to take a new and closer look at everyday activities such as buying and eating snack foods. Figueroa is even able to find a few positives in the pandemic and its accompanying lockdown. If nothing else, as she points out in 'If a Silver Lining Has to Be Found,' there are far fewer germs around than there would normally be.

In 'Never Had I Ever,' Nova Scotia poet Cathy MacKenzie uses the title line as a structuring device in sorting out her many pandemic-era 'firsts,' most of them unwelcome 'firsts,' from long periods of self-isolation and public mask-wearing to being unable to hold family gatherings and hug close family members. For his part, Gatineau poet Yves Rochon starts out on a pessimistic note in his first wave poem, 'À l'abri de la tempête,' overwhelmed by all the new language of death and disease he's hearing every day. But then a look outside at nature, where trees and brooks and birds are 'recovering' nicely, thanks to the enforced lack of economic activity and reduction in driving, allows Rochon to end on a positive note.

Winding up our poetry section, Jagjeet Sharma, like Yves Rochon, finds inspiration and hope in nature. The sight of cardinals in a tree in the midst of a snowy landscape, as her poem 'Cardinals' tells us, not only reminds us that Spring, with its warm breezes and lilac-scented air, isn't too far away, but also suggests that like the Winter itself, pandemic-related lockdowns and shutdowns will soon be things of the past. Finally, Filipina-American poet Rowena Torrevillas' 'Because They Eat Bats' gives full voice to the loneliness, isolation, and disorientation resulting from the pandemic's first wave. The poem is a powerful description of what we have all been through with the pandemic.

Before
Valerie Buko

As I'm walking through my local park, safely distanced from the other
walkers, I'm feeling lonely.
I love the fresh air, moving gently through my hair,
But I'm still lonely...
Before this isolation,
before mask-covered faces and hidden hearts,
love seemed to be all around, waiting to be found;
if not certain, then surely at least probable, possible.
Before,
I'm thinking as I'm walking, love could be had by all,
if such luck upon you did fall,
and you could at least try it on for size;
if it didn't fit, you at least learned from the surprise...
I see a couple enter the park, walking closely, hand in hand, partners for
life,
who surely helped each other through this phenomenon,
and didn't have to endure this isolation, faces covered and hearts hidden...
Now,
I'm thinking that love seems to be only for the fortuitous, who found love,
had love
Before,
when love was all around,
just waiting to be found
and was more certain, probable and possible.

Pandemic Poems
Elena Calvo

flying back home
during the pandemic
an old hand
holds onto
the baby's feet[1]

fall 2020
my gynaecologist follows
a safe protocol
probing and touching
but no handshake[2]

behind branches
winter's bright moon
the fullness
of all the things
that hurt[3]

pandemic panic—
his head in my lap
reading haiku…
the long shadows
of Elche's palmeras[4]

harsh words
after months of absence
during pandemic…
his heart did not
grow fonder[5]

flying back to Canada
as the pandemic starts…
the icy geometry
of the landscape
chills an inflamed heart[6]

pandemic starts…
landing, exhausted
after a long trip
even the air pillow
collapses[7]

pandemic
life insurance
in my email
a welcome to my own
burial alert

emergency surgery
in a foreign hospital
during pandemic...
the orderly's eyes
behind the shield

trekking
the Acadian Fundy forest,
balsam firs and ocean...
on our backs
the weight of sorrow[8]

wind and hail
against the window
during lockdown
...
my restless mind

wind and hail
during lockdown
my mind[9]

Notes

[1] Haiku Society of America (HSA), 2020.
[2] *MoonBathing* (MB), Issue 23, 2020.
[3] *A Hundred Gourds* (AHG), online issue 19, 2016.
[4] Slightly modified version of poem published in *GUSTS*, No. 31, 2020.
[5] Slightly modified version of poem published in *GUSTS*, No. 23, 2016.
[6] Slightly modified version of poem published in *GUSTS*, No. 29, 2019.
[7] Slightly modified version of poem published in *GUSTS*, No. 20, 2014.
[8] *GUSTS*, No. 33, 2021.
[9] Haiku Canada Anthology (HCA), 2021.

Five Pandemic Poems
Kathy Figueroa

A Crimp in My Snacking Routine

Tasty barbeque chips, how I've craved you so!
But have had to do without, for to the store I rarely go
And honey-roasted peanuts are such a delight!
But these persistent yearnings, I've long had to fight

This pandemic has definitely put a crimp
In my daily snacking routine
And forced me to limit my munching
To what's at hand, and usually green

Though nutritious wild violet leaves
Are abundant out of doors
They don't pack the zip of a chip
Or other delicious stuff you get at the stores

Risking a brush with a coronavirus
That's mean and highly detrimental
Inspires a certain fear
That's primal and elemental

So, if to the supermarket,
I feel I must make a jaunt
Careful advance consideration
Is given to exactly what I want

A strategy is devised:
When will the least tourists likely be there?
Is hand sanitizer in my purse?
What sort of mask should I wear?

Shall I don the clear plastic face shield
That allows me to breathe free?
Or that paper surgical-type mask
Which fogs my glasses 'til I can barely see?

Yes, there are many details
To be given consideration and forethought
Before I head out shopping——so groceries,
Including snack food, can be safely bought.

If A Silver Lining Has to Be Found

No longer am I jostled in a crowd
Because large groups of people aren't allowed

Cashiers aren't able to cough in my face
For they're supposed to have a mask in place

In line-ups, no one can breathe down my neck
If they're closer than six feet they'll get heck

The pandemic's good side is hard to find
But improved public hygiene comes to mind

If a silver lining has to be found
It's that there are far fewer germs around.

Is This a Cold?

I've got the sniffles and 'the runs' too
Is this a cold, or maybe the flu?
I'm so tired… should I crawl back to bed
…Or drink more tea and take zinc, instead?

I'm feeling hot, my throat's getting sore,
Why can't I taste the food anymore?
Is this a COVID-19 attack?
…Or am I a hypochondriac?

I really don't know what's ailing me
And hope that it's just an allergy
But I'll still stay home and isolate
My regular life will have to wait

Safe Haven

The fragrance of baked apple fills the air
It's quick, tasty, and healthy lunchtime fare
Soup made from barley, lentils, beans, and rice
Will have a good flavour, with added spice

The kitchen's a safe haven these bleak days
As the virus mutates in scary ways
It's better to stay home, behind closed doors
When new strains emanate from distant shores

This Ecosphere

Bow to the might of the Pangolin and Bat
Leave them undisturbed in their wild habitat
Tremble before Creation in its glory
Know that Humans are but part of the story

Instead of plundering to ruination
Let Humans protect this wondrous creation -
This ecosphere, this world, this garden in space
This most marvelous home of the human race

Never Had I Ever
Cathy MacKenzie

Never had I ever
Expected to break my wrist—
Or any bone—
Is this the beginning of the end?

Perhaps it was, for:

Never had I ever
Heard such terms:
Physical-distancing, PPEs, flattening curves…
What the heck!

Never had I ever
Been imprisoned at home,
Allowed out once a week, alone, for essentials,
Though it's safer staying home!

Never had I ever
Experienced self-isolation,
Cruel and unusual punishment,
For no wrong of mine!

Never had I ever
Been afraid to grocery shop
Or enter a store—even step outdoors,
But the money I'm saving!

Never had I ever
Been yelled at
For walking down an aisle,
What's that? Floor arrows?

Never had I ever
Been treated like at leper at the ER
Because of my postal code,
Isn't that discrimination?

Never had I ever
Been forced to don a mask
Other than on Halloween,
But it hides my wrinkles!

Never had I ever
Imagined hugs and family gatherings
Would be forbidden,
Technological alternatives don't cut it!

Never had I ever...
Thought the world would change as it has.
Never had I envisioned a virus would—or could—
Shut down the world.
Oh, 2020, what have you done?
News was grim to watch,
Nova Scotia mourned and mourned:
Covid-19 deaths of many elderly,
Canada's worst massacre,
Six dead in a military helicopter crash,
The Snowbirds disaster,
Six fishers presumed dead,
Boots on porches for Dylan
With candles to guide him home,
A wee bit of hope that died.

So many 'never-had-I-evers'...

Alas, the world has changed
And not for the better,
But when our 'normal' returns
Perhaps people
Will change to better the world.
We can only hope and pray...
Oh, how I pray and hope.

À l'abri de la tempête
Yves Rochon

Cas, CHSLD, corona, confinement, contagion, COVID-19, décès, désinfection,
distanciation sociale, fermetures, hécatombe, maladie, mises à pied, morts…
Tout cela ne m'inspire rien de bon
Panne d'inspiration.

Expire… Inspire… Inspirer peut nous tuer
On retient son souffle, on fuit la moindre buée

Cependant qu'autour de nous, discrètement
La mère-terre pousse un soupir de soulagement.
Avions au sol, autos paralysées, usines muettes
Artères de toutes les grandes villes désertes :
Permission accordée à la nature de se faire de nouveau entendre
Les feuillages sont d'un vert plus tendre
Le ciel est plus bleu
Les oiseaux chantent, plus joyeux
Et les forêts renaissent de leurs cendres

Peut-être que ce petit virus agressif et sournois
En plus de broyer nos poumons jusqu'à ce qu'on en meure,
En plus d'ébranler les colonnes du temple ou l'humain se noie,
Nous aura-t-il atteint au cœur
Pour y faire germer une petite voix,
Le désir d'une vie plus en douceur?

30 avril, 2020

Cardinals
Jagjeet Sharma

I see
a cardinal or two
perched on naked
trees

their bright red coats
pleasing,
brighten up
my white backyard
squirrels make haste
over fresh, soft snow

soon it will all be over
lockdowns and shutdowns

soon we can smell
jasmine and lilac flowers
on warm evenings
in the twilight hours
when each creature
has gone to bed

and I seek solace
in the sinking sunset

Because They Eat Bats
Rowena Torrevillas

I have harbored racist thoughts
More than once.
I haven't hugged my grandchildren in months.
Grandson and I rode our bikes six feet apart,
Circling the college's empty parking lot, then
Even that wasn't safe, so we stopped.
I haven't been inside the grocery store or any
Enclosed space, in this silent town, though
I wear the N95 mask that gives me a headache.
The movie house is a distant memory, the streets
Are empty, the students all gone, their part-
Time jobs as well. Am I essential? we ask.
The governor hasn't ordered a lockdown;
Supposedly germs don't grow in Iowa's vast
Green landscape, untrammeled unto the horizon,
Which is where I feel safest, outside my room,
Where the maple tree outside this window has gone
From bare twigs to full leaf, overnight, it feels like
—Though in truth I have lost all sense of time:
Days and nights sleep upside down, as do
The bats, before they were eaten.

This poem was written for a forthcoming anthology of *Quarantine Poems*, coming out of Manila, which is in lockdown.

SECTION 11
COVID
and the Arts

Show and Sell
Taiya Barss

*A*s I noted earlier in the almanac, in my 'First Wave' pieces, the arts were among the hardest-hit of any sectors of the Canadian (or American) economies. As Peter Alexander says at the beginning of his masterful survey of the effects of COVID on the American classical music scene, the COVID pandemic 'struck a dagger to the heart of the performing arts,' with musicians, dancers and actors left either unable to ply their trades or forced to do so under extremely restrictive and occasionally even bizarre conditions. Neither Canada nor the U.S. provided the kind of comprehensive emergency relief for artists offered by Germany's enlightened government under Angela Merkel. (For more details about the German aid package for artists, see my earlier piece, 'Recovering from the First Wave: The Mid-Cycle Thaw.') Bassoonist Chris Millard's amusing piece gives some poignant examples of just how far classical musicians had to go to adapt their playing to the demands of COVID restrictions. At the other end of the musical spectrum, popular and folk guitarist Paul Lenarczyk describes how he maintained his performing chops while at the same time providing much-needed musical entertainment to Nova Scotians through his weekly virtual 'kitchen parties.'

Visual artists, whose work is typically done in solitude, did not face the same restrictions on doing their work as did performing artists. But they had many challenges of their own whenever they tried to exhibit their work publicly, as Taiya Barss' piece about mounting a painting retrospective during the pandemic well illustrates.

Of all the arts, theatre may have made the best adaptation to the pandemic. Colleen Naomi, who probably did as much as anyone to keep theatre alive in Nova Scotia during this difficult period, describes how she took her teaching online, offering numerous and varied theatre workshops through the new and sometimes alien medium of Zoom. My own piece, written from the perspective of a community theatre actor, describes some of the many ways I kept involved in theatre during this time—including taking several of Colleen's workshops. The later part of the pandemic's third wave saw me acting in a Zoom play—something that even a year ago, I couldn't have imagined myself doing. But then, I suspect a lot of artists in many different fields have found themselves doing all sorts of things they previously could not have imagined themselves doing. And that may not be such a bad thing.

389

Show and Sell
Taiya Barss

In the spring of 2019, I sold our house and moved to a one-bedroom apartment. In our house, my paintings had carpeted the walls, hanging in the hall, the living room, kitchen and bedroom.

Many paintings.

In my new, small space, I decided to be selective, hanging only the ones I wanted to keep, leaving some blank white areas of wall in between. My *Collection of the Artist*.

The remainder filled the closets or lived in boxes under the bed and bureau, or tucked behind the couch.

I needed space.

I needed to give these works a new home. Given my age, thoughts of a retrospective filled my head. Possible titles included *One More Kick at the Can*, *Last Gasp*, or perhaps *End of the Road*.

I mentioned my situation to my friend Dawn McNutt, who generously said 'I have a show scheduled for May, at the Craig Gallery. Why don't we show together?' I loved the idea. The Craig, a small gallery in the same building as Dartmouth's Alderney Landing Ferry Terminal, is my favourite gallery. It seemed just the right size, and her sculptures could inhabit the floor, while my work would fill the walls.

We amended her proposal to include me, and the gallery approved the idea. We were scheduled to have an opening night in early May and stay for that month. We are good friends, we have shown together in the past, and we were excited.

In March, however, our brightly coloured world turned a dull grey. The COVID plague was spreading over the earth, and our home, our city, our province, were closed, in lockdown.

The gallery contacted us, offering us the space, but told us that because of the virus, we couldn't show together and couldn't have an opening—that festive night full of strangers and friends. Only a virtual tour of our work would be available, online. The gallery would be filled with our work, but the door would be locked. The alternative was a show together in the Craig's first free month, August, 2022. Given that I was 77 and Dawn 82, we figured we had better proceed sooner rather than later. She chose May to exhibit her sculptures in the gallery. I chose June.

In early June, my son drove me and my boxes of paintings from Halifax to Dartmouth. He drove, I sat in the back, we both wore masks, and all the windows were wide open. I left the paintings in the gallery for director Lee

Cripps to hang. I went home, feeling dejected and forlorn.

Then I got a call from Lee, who said that restrictions had just been lifted a bit. The gallery was allowed to be open during my show. Just two distanced, masked people could enter at a time, but hallelujah!

I was jubilant.

My work is small and detailed, and people really need to stand in front of the paintings, looking at them closely to see all that is there. I started hustling, took pictures of my paintings and put them on Facebook, and was amazed at the enthusiastic and positive response. I took the harbour ferry across every day to visit my show, checking for the red stickers that would show a painting had been sold. I often invited friends to join me to tour the gallery, then picnic outside.

I was shameless. I needed space.

If the gallery had remained closed with my work only distantly peered at through a locked glass door, I would probably have brought home the whole lot, and been right back where I started.

I hung 50 paintings for my show, *Then and Now.*

I brought home twenty-five.

One closet, one box, and none under the bed.

A Dagger to the Heart of the
Performing Arts
Peter Alexander

The COVID pandemic struck a dagger in the heart of the performing arts. Both performers and institutions found themselves without performances to present, and therefore without income. Performers were adrift, with contracts cancelled and no performances to prepare. Performing arts organizations—orchestras, theaters, dance companies, opera companies and the vast industry we call Broadway—saw their income drop to zero overnight. And, of course, audiences found themselves without performances to attend.

Any summary at this date will be out of date before it appears, but here is one view of the past year and what it has meant for performers. Beyond the coming summer, which is just starting to take shape, we all are hoping for a return to whatever will pass for normal.

In my field, classical music, the response began in March 2020 with dismay and uncertainty, but over time organizations and artists have demonstrated resiliency and devotion to art. Creativity has opened doors leading to new avenues of performance, both virtual and real, that are likely to remain valid for the future. Everyone agrees that the shock of the pandemic has changed the arts forever, but in exactly what way no one can predict.

Among individual performers, the effect of the pandemic has generally been greater for freelancers than those with permanent fulltime positions. Many of the latter—members of symphonies, chamber organizations and choruses—have received reduced income and had some online performance opportunities.

Those who have full-time or part-time teaching positions have fared best. Most colleges, universities and conservatories have stayed open for online instruction, so their tenured faculty lost little income, even if their work became more complicated. Many have mastered the skills of teaching by Zoom and other online platforms, even though one lamented that she has students in Asia who she has never met in person.

Touring performances outside the academy, an important part of music faculties' professional lives, have disappeared. Solo appearances have to some extent been replaced by online recitals. Others have put together carefully distanced, streamed chamber performances, which at least serve to keep their performing senses sharpened.

It is the freelancers, including most opera singers in the United States, who have faced the greatest obstacles. With all gigs cancelled, they have turned to other sources of income. For example, I know an operatic bass who had just received his debut contract for three roles at the Metropolitan Opera for the fall of 2020. Needless to say, it was cancelled with no future prospect offered. This is more than the loss of a job; it is the disappearance of a major step in his career. He turned to delivery for Amazon around the holidays; others have found similar hourly work or retreated into living with family members. Many have patched together the occasional online performance.

Among freelancers, there has been widespread depression as musicians no longer have goals to work for. Last year, they may have been juggling three or more part-time connections, which always gave them music to learn, skills to keep sharp—then nothing. Left entirely to their own devices, some managed to create their own challenges, while others gave in to the realization that they had been rendered expendable by their employers.

Two particularly intriguing trends emerged among the more enterprising performers, and these are true regardless of any other jobs and income they may have. One is the mastering of new techniques—all the ways that material can be presented digitally.

Some have even created compilation performances playing all the parts themselves. String players, with wide ranges and cross-instrument skills available, have about the best opportunities. The most impressive of these, featuring Malin Broman, concertmaster of the Swedish Radio Symphony Orchestra, showing mad skills by playing all eight parts of the Mendelssohn *Octet*, Movement 4, can be found here:

https://www.youtube.com/watch?v=KWwLSsfdmNk

but many others, entirely home recorded and engineered, can also be found.

The other trend is exploring and performing new repertoire. With the pandemic coinciding with the rise of first the #MeToo movement and then Black Lives Matter, quite a bit of the repertoire has been music by women and composers of colour.

This trend toward performing new repertoire has also penetrated the institutions and larger organizations. Two orchestral works in particular have been just about ubiquitous: *Strum* by Jesse Montgomery and *Lyric for Strings* by George Walker. As worthy as these pieces are, they represent only a beginning, and it is a hopeful sign that both individual performers and institutions have pledged to explore more music by American composers who have been neglected, including Gabriela Lena Frank, Florence Price, William Grant Still, R. Nathaniel Dett, and many others.[1]

Orchestras, employers of so many classical players, have struggled. After an initial period of stunned silence and cancelled seasons, most orchestras have gone from raiding their endowments and urgent appeals to donors to give back the value of their cancelled tickets, to seeking creative ways to present content online. First, we saw compilation performances with players each performing from their own homes, but these require intense engineering to be successful. Some orchestras have archived material that they could present; for example, the Detroit Symphony, which has a long record of presenting online performances, was well positioned to move into digital concerts:

https://www.dso.org/events-and-tickets/your-visit/digital-concerts

Today, Detroit and many other orchestras are offering new performances, without audiences, with small and carefully distanced groups of players. Works for strings alone have dominated these programs, since the players can wear masks. In contrast, wind players have to be more isolated, and are often placed behind plastic shields. These types of performances, with performances distanced from one another, have been successful just about world-wide, and have allowed both the players and the orchestras to have income that keeps them afloat.

So many symphonies turned to small group performances, with players safely distanced in empty concert halls, on large stages or in unusual spaces, that 2020 became the year of the chamber orchestra. Works for strings were especially popular, since string players could all be masked while playing. Smaller wind sections were possible, especially if the players were placed at greater distances or seated behind plastic shields.

This was not left to experimentation. There were several scientific studies of the spread of aerosols by wind players, most prominently one that was undertaken by the University of Colorado and jointly funded by the NAMM Foundation, National Federation of State High School Associations, D'addario Foundation and College Band Directors National Association:

https://sharpsandflatirons.com/2020/11/01/keeping-instrument-rehearsals-safe-during-covid-19/

This and other studies provided firm guidelines for rehearsals with wind instruments.

Coincidentally, one of the most successful orchestra seasons was staged in Boulder, Colorado, where the Boulder Philharmonic recorded a series of five concerts over 10 days in a local airplane hangar. The hangar provided all the space needed for safe distancing—and unusual background settings—plus professional video recording equipment and operators. The programs:

https://boulderphil.org/reimagined

featured guest soloists with members of the orchestra, and included solo works—pieces written for chamber ensemble or small orchestra—as well as string arrangements of larger works, including Schumann's Cello Concerto and a Mozart piano concerto. Each program was produced for video in two days—three rehearsals and a recording session—and the concerts were broadcast through the year, allowing the Boulder Philharmonic to maintain something like their usual concert series.

Opera poses greater challenges, since the singers cannot be masked while performing. Nonetheless, opera companies have found ways to keep performing, offering some of the most creative solutions posed by the pandemic. There have been performances for drive-in audiences, an opera performed in a baseball stadium, and taped performances that maintain safe distancing among the cast members. (For singers, that means more than six feet; 12 feet is the usual standard for wind instruments and singers, because of their ability to spread aerosols.) At the University of Colorado, rehearsals of *Hansel und Gretel:*

https://cupresents.org/performance/11799/cu-opera/hansel-and-gretel/#top

were interrupted every hour to sanitize and air out the working space. In spite of these hurdles, full performances by two casts were safely recorded and streamed.

Benjamin Britten's *Turn of the Screw*—an opera well suited for safely distanced performances due to its small cast and orchestra and ghostly subject—received an especially intriguing production by OperaGlass Works when planned live performances were replaced by a filmed performance staged in an abandoned theater (available through Marquee TV:

https://www.marquee.tv/videos/operaglassworks-turnofthescrew

Other companies produced pieces customized to the pandemic, adapted scenes, or presented arias by individual singers.

Most opera singers in the U.S. work entirely freelance, with no long-term contracts. This is somewhat different from Europe, where opera houses hire singers below the very top stars on multi-opera contracts. In most cases those singers have been paid a reduced salary through the year, as is true of orchestras and choruses in Europe. This is why the creativity of the opera companies around the U.S. is so important; without streamed and drive-in performances, the singers would have no work and the companies would have no income beyond their donors' generosity.

Not all organizations have made their musicians a priority. Some included them in their recovery efforts, but others cut them loose. In other words, the experiences of freelance musicians—at least in the United States—varies from being stranded with a complete loss of income, to partial support that has enabled them to survive. In Europe, with extensive government support, it is more common for institutions to support their musicians to a greater or lesser extent.

One extreme has sadly been represented by the Metropolitan Opera in New York, which furloughed all employees at the outbreak of the pandemic, without pay. At this writing, first the Met chorus—one of three full-time professional opera choruses in the country—and the orchestra have received limited pay for returning to the bargaining table after nearly a year, while management tries to negotiate a permanent pay cut. Met stagehands remain under lockout by the Met management.

The pandemic has been devastating for the Met's renowned orchestra, of whose members 10% have retired early and another 40% have been forced to leave New York altogether. Some have even been forced to sell valuable instruments to cover rent or mortgages; others have moved to Europe for work.

Whether a comparable orchestra can ever be reassembled is an open question. The hardline stance taken by Met management and general director Peter Gelb is seen by the players as union-busting; Gelb is known as a staunch enemy of New York's strong unions. Meanwhile, Gelb has a deputy and six assistants still on the payroll, and the Met administration has continued to raise funds for the company—but not the musicians—by streaming performances by star performers, mostly from Europe. In a step undermining the locked-out stagehands' unions, they have also contracted the building of sets for the 2021-22 season outside the United States.

For the record, the St Paul Chamber Orchestra recently signed a two-year contract with its musicians with no cut in pay, the opposite end of the spectrum from the Met. Most other orchestras are somewhere between these two extremes.

Looking to the short-term future, summer festivals are moving toward re-opening. Many are presented outdoors, or will incorporate outdoor elements. Ravinia, summer home of the Chicago Symphony, has announced a summer season to take place entirely outside, with limited admissions. Aspen has announced an 'in-person… summer season, making use of out-door spaces.' Something similar is expected at Tanglewood, summer home of the Boston Symphony, although no announcement has been made at this date.[2]

The Santa Fe Opera, which performs in an open-air theater, has announced a season with anywhere from 30 to 80% capacity, depending on the recommendations of health officials. Central City Opera has moved its 2021 season—a re-scheduling of productions originally slated for 2020—from its intimate theater in Central City to an outdoor performance venue in the Denver suburb of Littleton. Glimmerglass in Cooperstown, New York has built a new outdoor stage for the 2021 festival.

Internationally, the Glyndebourne Festival has announced a 2021 season. Salzburg has postponed its summer season into the Fall. All this represents a tentative return to live performance… even if not quite 'normal.'

But no one knows what 'normal' will be next year or after. With musicians having developed new skills for streaming content, a lot of classical music will probably continue to be presented online. It is clear to the orchestras, players, singers and opera companies that audiences can be reached in this way who may not come into the concert hall. When you add the fact that no one knows when and how audiences will be willing to gather in large numbers, seat-to-seat with strangers, it becomes evident that 'normal' will look different in 2022 than it did in 2019.

It seems unlikely that all institutions will survive. Surely some regional orchestras and opera companies that have been surviving marginally will disappear; others, having found new skills and new audiences, will probably thrive. It may be evidence of the post-pandemic sea change that one of the most eminent institutions, Columbia Artists Management, Inc. (CAMI) closed its doors in 2020 after 90 years in business, due to the 'prolonged pandemic environment.' CAMI's demise shocked the business end of the music world. Today, no one is willing to guess who is next.

Notes

---

[1] I am pleased to report that this trend toward playing more music by previously neglected composers can be observed in Canada, as well. Composers such as Florence Price and William Grant Still are now frequently heard on CBC Music's classical programs, as are many previously rarely-played female composers from Europe, Canada, and the U.S.

[2] Hollywood Bowl and Red Rocks Amphitheatre outside Denver were at full capacity for the summer of 2021, and most summer festivals were open to limited audiences. By the beginning of 2022, most organizations are forecasting a return to full attendance.

The Kitchen Party Piece
Paul R.J. Lenarczyk

Almost exactly one year ago, the global pandemic was declared. Here in Nova Scotia, for one high school teacher this declaration meant that his prediction to his students, made on the day before March Break started, was coming true. When students had asked me 'Do you think we'll be back in a week?' I'd answered with a confident shake of the head. I could tell something was brewing, though I had no idea how bad a cup of tea it would be.

The lockdown, for my family, meant that my wife and I and our four-year-old kid were home alone all day every day, in the last weeks of Winter and through the Spring and almost into Summer. We are not outdoorsy people at the best of times, but in the Winter we hate the outside. So, we were cooped up in our little house, and our poor little kid was stuck with just us. Sure, there were Zoom play dates with her daycare classmates, but that just wasn't the same as seeing them in person.

Now it was St Patrick's Day. I've always been a big fan of that particular holiday, since Irish music had long been a favourite of mine, even before I first became a 'Roving Minstrel' at King's Landing Historical Settlement in New Brunswick in the summer of 1991. Ever since then, the folk songs so rooted in Irish Celtic culture and transported to the new world by the earliest European settlers had been my go-to tunes to play on my guitar and sing.

And so, the idea came to me. There was this thing called Facebook Live which I'd been long meaning to try. And I had a guitar, though I hadn't played it for some time. My last year at King's Landing had been 2009. I'd played a bit here and there since. Probably at least as much Van Morrison as Irish Rovers, but he was Irish too, and so were U2, another favourite group of mine. The idea was that I would do a loosely-Irish themed St Paddy's Day show on Facebook Live just for my family: the two girls locked down with me in Halifax, and my widely dispersed family around the world.

I have no idea how many people tuned into that first show, but it was popular enough that someone suggested I should do it regularly. It was an excuse to pick up an old abandoned hobby—playing guitar and singing—and practice both again. Some people make bread, others make music. I was never much of a chef or baker, so I chose the music. And for a while it became a regular thing. First it was three times a week, but that was way too hard. So, then it was twice, and I think later just once a week, on Saturday afternoon, when I'd sit down in front of the webcam, guitar in one hand, beer in the other, and play some favourite tunes or new ones I'd learned that week. Almost every episode had some common features. There was always at least one Polish song, because I'm Polish and some of my audience is Polish too, and always a Celtic or Maritime tune from my King's Landing days as well. There was usually a tune from a musical, because I'm a musical theatre nerd. And there was usually a dance number from my kid, who loved seeing herself on the screen as well. I wonder where she got that...

The 'kitchen parties' connected people and brought me in touch with Facebook friends with whom I hadn't really exchanged more than a 'like' or 'heart' in years. I'm an only child, so I have no natural siblings. But I have cousins who are as close as siblings, and I also have many siblings by choice, most of whom live in different parts of the globe. Somehow, they would tune in, whether live or by watching the stream after it was finished, and they'd write comments and choose songs for the next show, and we would bond. I found an old teacher of my mother's, or rather she found me, and we reconnected. I renewed friendships with friends' parents who started commenting on the shows. The siblings by choice and by blood also encouraged me in the endeavour.

Were my 'kitchen parties' life-changing for anyone? I don't know. They were certainly very meaningful for me. They helped get me through those darkest days of uncertainty early on in the pandemic, and they then got us through the challenging time after the Portapique mass-shootings. I think they helped the family keep going. And they allowed me to rediscover the joy of playing music, while getting me back in touch with people from all around the world. They also became a much more pleasant venue in which to consume that cup of strangely brewed tea, or perhaps something a little stronger. And of course, those connections which are so hard to make in a pandemic became stronger instead of fading away, and music, that universal language, helped us all to make those connections. And that can never be a bad thing.

The Next Breath You Take…
Christopher Millard

Basing a life on the bassoon is at best a fragile proposition. We make a living blowing into a curious and oddly expensive wind instrument. I've been working in symphony orchestras for 47 years, so a lot of hot air has passed through my instrument. Rarely strenuous, the act of bassoon playing is more about collaboration than virtuosity. Composers have understood for three hundred years that it's a friendly instrument operated by sympathetic people; we generally play well with others. But playing the bassoon in The Time of COVID has not been for the faint of heart.

As symphony orchestras slowly re-emerged, we looked for ways to animate our lifeless concert halls while respecting the need for safety protocols. We've had to meet some auditory challenges: spaced-out seating, massive Plexiglas panels, and all of us black-masked like the Lone Ranger. Without audiences, our perspectives on projection and sonority were shaken up while we tried our best to project our music-making into fields of empty red seats—all under the cloud of the coronavirus.

While safety measures offered some consolation, 60 people gathered together on an indoor stage remained an unnerving proposition, and we quickly became focused on several 'elephants in the room.' We were all lounging on the upstage risers, disguised as wind and brass players, with buzzing lips, vibrating reeds, and torrents of expelled air and spit. Violinists, violists, and cellists were all sharing the same stage with us and had little trust that their flimsy masks would provide protection from superspreading trumpets or oboes.

Orchestras everywhere started out by limiting programming to strings-only repertoire. It was not enough. Though Bruckner symphonies seemed to be temporarily lethal, was Beethoven possible? Even Haydn and Mozart required some wind players. With trepidation, we started to creep onto the stage, though with every note we sounded our poor colleagues imagined trillions of marauding coronavirus particles. For months we desperately followed the emerging science. Which instruments allowed the greatest amounts of aerosol particles to propagate? Flutes? Trombones? Every study suggested different protocols. We ran fog machines on our empty stages, trying to make sense of the flow of air. Downstage, upstage or just *up*? Were there clear patterns or just chaos in the potential aerosol pathways? Was two metres safe or did we need 20?

We calculated stage dimensions and theatre volumes and investigated air exchange rates. If a hall had three full exchanges of air per hour, could we say that was safe? Or was it simply less menacing? Was our viola section at risk from that innocent clarinetist five metres upstage? Could we ever control the potential spread from an asymptomatic brass player whose child had brought COVID home from school, the conductor fresh off a trans-Atlantic flight or perhaps a bassoonist exposed while shopping for vegetables? We surrounded our wind sections with glass panels, only to learn that these might actually *increase* danger by blocking efficient air flow.

So as the Fall 2020 orchestra seasons gasped for air—to create *something* —we began to ask if our exhaling wind and brass delinquents could actually wear masks. Sure, but if you *can* produce a sound by inserting a mouthpiece into a slitted mask the AIR was still going through the instruments and happily propagating *everywhere*. So, let's mask the instruments as well!

We then started looking for fabrics that would cover the bells of a tuba or an oboe and might filter some critical portion of those creeping COVID cooties. Too dense a fabric and the tone became too dull and the instrument's response unpredictable. Too thin a fabric and perhaps there was no meaning-ful mitigation of danger. Would the result of all this be high trumpet notes suddenly less certain, horn players navigating massive sleeves over their bells, low notes on oboes refusing to come out. And what about the woodwinds and all the open tone holes? Well, thank goodness we had a study for each instrument, except... the conclusions were so variable and uncertain. Was there any true value or was it just illusion? In the high schools, we saw saxophones safely hidden in pillowcases and the proliferation of dozens of cumbersome body bags. Good for malaria but a challenge for Mahler. We had to draw the line somewhere.

So, we covered our faces at every reasonable moment, raising our face masks when there were sufficient measures of rests in our parts. As the months progressed, our non-wind colleagues began to appreciate that tight masking with good filtration was likely giving them significant protection as they shared the air with us. But in a Brahms symphony, wind and brass players have to take in air a thousand times, and every unfiltered breath might be our express ticket to an ICU.

Ultimately, all of these somewhat uncertain ways of dealing with an insidious enemy will be abandoned as vaccines are administered and im-munity builds among performers and audiences. But there's a very bumpy road ahead. Symphony orchestras were already enormously challenged before the pandemic, with aging audiences, deteriorating music education, and a Eurocentric culture in a rapidly diversifying population. With almost two seasons of avoiding concert halls, will our patrons return? For sure, programming will never be as it was.

It will come as no surprise that many performers of a certain age have found COVID a time of great personal clarity. For me personally, after years of constant concert preparation and practice and above all a sense of continued discipline, I've found the past year has brightly illuminated my own imminent path to retirement. As I ponder the challenges facing my energetic younger colleagues, I've come to recognize that it's time for a younger bassoonist to take my chair. Many of my similarly aged cohort are coming to the same realization.

I'm confident that the very act of breathing—vital to our music making —will quickly become unencumbered by any fear of disease, but the re-engagement of audiences and the continued cultivation of classical music will always remain a fragile proposition. As I leave my own career behind and enroll in the ranks of listeners, I will be content to simply breathe along with each familiar phrase.

Theatre in a COVID World
Colleen Naomi

On March 15, 2020, I received a phone call from CentreStage Theatre in Kentville. When I hung up, I cried. For the first time in 11 years, I would not be teaching a youth theatre camp at CentreStage during March Break.

I'd been heavily involved in all aspects of theatre since my own youth. When I was seven years old, I wrote a script on our Atari, gathered a few friends for rehearsals, and performed the ten-minute play in my front yard for friends and neighbours. I even printed programs on our dot matrix printer. This was the first of several similar projects.

At the age of 10, I became involved in community theatre, starting in the tech booth running a follow spot light. I never left. Well, to be clear, I did leave the tech booth. But the theatre had captured me, heart and soul.

Over the years, the performing arts increasingly became an anchor in my life. My theatre community has seen me through marriage and divorce, parenting, illness, injury, family moves and many other ups and downs.

As Artistic Director for South Shore Players in Nova Scotia, I know that The Show Must Go On! Theatre, by nature, is creative, so even in the face of a pandemic I needed to find a way to stay true to that motto.

Those involved in theatre are of all ages and stages of life. I was especially aware of those who were retired, most of whom live alone or with only one other person. Even as I was absorbed in my own large blended-family life, I was aware that there were those who were not surrounded by loved ones. I realized that for many, the closures would result in a much greater sense of isolation, which could be devastating for people's mental and emotional well-being.

I firmly believe that theatre is not only a fun, artistic learning experience, but also beneficial to our health. Like other art forms, theatre is an incredible form of therapy. We are continually called upon to look inward at ourselves, while exploring the motivations and intentions of others, all in a supportive group environment.

Knowing that people were isolated from friends and family, as well as disconnected from their theatre community, was heartbreaking for me. But what could I really offer? How could I tell people that theatre was continuing, even as we were announcing the cancellation of our spring production? Well, I know that theatre depends on stepping out of our comfort zones, trying new things, and putting ourselves out there, and I was not going to let my community down.

My first step was to reach out to our theatre community through monthly newsletters, giving a sense of connection, hope, and perhaps even excitement! But as the pandemic continued, I realized that I would need to look beyond the conventional 'live theatre' box, and this would mean developing new skills in technology. I've never been one to grab hold of the latest trends and gadgets. When people ask me for my cell phone number, I'm forced to admit that I don't have one. I rely on my children to show me photos on Instagram, and I really want to believe that Twitter is just something birds do. But my initial reluctance notwithstanding, in a spirit of innovation, I learned Zoom, honed my use of Google forms, and started developing online theatre opportunities.

During May of 2020, I offered my first two online acting workshops. When these filled up quickly, with waiting lists, I planned more for June, July, and August. I used the experience of my years teaching youth theatre programs, as well as my upgraded computer skills, to design enjoyable and informative workshops. These were mainly attended by seniors, with some joining from outside our local area and even outside our province. While a few of the participants were already comfortable with Zoom, for many it was their first time attending an online workshop. Everyone embraced the learning curve, appreciating the miracle of technology that allowed us to join together while being apart. With the world feeling shut down and people increasingly isolated, I knew that at the end of each workshop participants were looking forward to the next one. I received continual positive feedback, with the main message being 'Do more!'

In the Spring and Fall, I offered two four-part scriptwriting series online. The participants were primarily retired and included people who had never written before, as well as those looking to enhance their skills in a collaborative group setting. Each person who attended wrote and refined a 10- to 20-minute play in a month. Three of those plays are included in this almanac.

By the end of the year, I had taught 24 online theatre workshops. And they are still going strong.

Without performances going on, I also wanted to reach our audiences and those members who aren't drawn to workshops. From August to October 2020, I hosted a series of 12 weekly *Conversations with Cast and Crew*. These videos featured interviews with 24 local people of all ages who had been involved with South Shore Players. We had more than 5000 views! It was a tremendous response, demonstrating how many people were missing the familiar faces of local theatre.

By the Fall of 2020, I was itching for a production. Things here in Nova Scotia were going well as far as our pandemic numbers were concerned, and although it was not possible to offer a typical show, we were able to gather in groups of ten, with social distancing.

Rehearsals for *Christmas Spirits* included six actors, three musicians, and myself as director; over half of those involved were over the age of 60. All performers remained six feet apart throughout the production, with the exception of a real-life couple who was in the cast. Once we were ready to perform our show, we moved into a bigger hall, where our lighting technician and videographer were able to join us. At that point, restrictions allowed us to have audiences of 10 people to view the filming: masked and seated in household bubbles, twelve feet from our performers. We had two performances which were filmed, edited, and presented on YouTube for two weeks in December. We learned a lot and laughed a lot, though I won't pretend that there weren't moments when I asked myself 'what was I thinking?' But in the end, we had a show ready to present, and again the audience response was heartwarming.

One of the most wonderful things about directing *Christmas Spirits* was hearing those involved talk about how fortunate they were to be able to be in a show, at a time when so many were unable to do so. That reaffirmed how to me the importance of the work that we were doing.

When I reflect on the journey of the past year, from that first phone call to my current schedule of theatre workshops, I can't help but feel incredible gratitude. My theatre family has been crucial to helping me stay mentally, emotionally and creatively healthy over the past year, and I know that is true for others as well. I reached out to many people and they reached out to me.

I'm proud of our theatre community. I'm amazed at the way people have stepped up and stepped into different ways of exploring theatre. I'm excited about the eleven new short plays now in the world that were developed at scriptwriting workshops that I led. And I'm thankful for those who have called me to check in or sent me notes of appreciation.

I hope in the future I will return to my work with youth, but I'm also committed to continuing my work with older adults, because really, who couldn't use a bit more theatre in their life?

Theatre During the Pandemic:
A Community Theatre Actor's Perspective
Jon Peirce

During the second half of my nearly eleven-year stint in Nova Scotia, from 2009 through 2020, theatre was an extremely important part of my life. I appeared in ten different plays, taking on roles as varied as those of Judge Omar Gaffney in *Harvey* and crime writer Edgar Chambers in *Anybody for Murder.* I was also assistant director for a Monk Ferris farce at Dartmouth Players and served on two community theatre boards, those of Bedford Players and Dartmouth Players, and on the playreading (script selection) committee of the latter. I even taught a Seniors' College course in Truro that entailed putting on a short play. In the end, none of my students were able to memorize their lines, but we did manage to pull off two quite creditable staged readings. Beyond all of that, in a continuing effort to hone my skills as an actor and aspiring director, I also took a number of workshops, on subjects as varied as doing comic scenes for film and dealing with physical intimacy on stage. Except during the summers, when community theatres were usually 'dark,' there was scarcely a time between 2014 and early 2020 when I wasn't doing something or other directly connected to theatre.

It was perhaps not surprising, then, that Saturday, March 14, 2020, the next-to-last day before widespread pandemic lockdown measures began to take effect in Nova Scotia, was a full and joyous day of theatre-related activities for me. In the afternoon, I went to a cast party for *A Tribute to Broadway,* the Passage Players musical in which I had just appeared in Cow Bay. The 30 or so of us in attendance sang, danced, ate pizza and a wide array of decadent sweets, laughed, hugged, and generally had a great time. The only sign of the impending pandemic was the reluctance of one or two of my fellow players to shake hands. Curiously, no one seemed to mind being hugged.

That evening, I went to a performance of David French's comedy *Jitters* at Bedford Players, the theatre where I've done more acting than anywhere else. I laughed and exchanged sly, witty whispered remarks with those seated next to me; at this point we were still able to sit close enough to each other that our whispers could be heard. At intermission, I drank coffee and chatted with several long-time theatre acquaintances, one of whom was directing *Jitters,* another of whom had directed a play I'd been in three years earlier. By this time, shaking hands was starting to seem a bit awkward, but I went ahead with it anyway, figuring that with no cases officially reported yet in the province, we would probably be safe enough. Little did I know that it would be another three months before I would even *see* my next handshake, let alone engage in one myself. Even now, nearly 14 months later,[1] I can count the number of hands I've shaken since that night on one of mine.

I have still yet to attend a live theatrical performance since *Jitters,* let alone appear in one, let alone make it through to a cast party. But does this mean I've abandoned theatre? By no means! As this is being written, I am involved in twice-weekly rehearsals for a Zoom play being put on by Rural Root Theatre, one of a surprising number of small theatre companies within striking distance of Gatineau, Quebec, to which I moved at the end of last summer (2020). And I'm also participating in weekly Zoom workshops in improvisational theatre being put on by Perth Studio Theatre. Other comparatively recent activities have included reading parts—also over Zoom—for two short plays being workshopped by Kanata Theatre, participating in online play reads held by Bedford Players, and auditioning for a part in a radio play being put on by yet another nearby theatre, Theatre Wakefield right here in West Quebec. And, yes, you guessed it; that audition was also conducted over Zoom. Up until this point, I've thought of myself as a Boomer. Now, it might be more appropriate to call myself a Zoomer. This isn't to say I'm by any means expert at using this strange new technology. After ten months of working with it, I can perform perhaps half a dozen relatively simple operations. If my level of knowledge were to be translated into the hierarchy of military ranks, I'd be a corporal. But there are now, believe it or not, people less adept with Zoom than I am. And I've certainly come a long way for a man who, a year ago, had yet to make his first electronic Internet bank transfer.

The longest I've gone without taking part in any organized theatre activity since the start of the pandemic has been seven weeks. The only reason I went that long was that during the period right before my move, I was totally engaged with packing and other move preparations and actually had to pass on one or two workshops I'd otherwise have been delighted to take.

To a great extent, the person responsible for keeping theatre going for me during the pandemic is Colleen Naomi, the artistic director of South Shore Players, yet another of the Nova Scotia theatres whose boards I trod during my time in the province. Colleen had been offering occasional workshops for years before COVID hit. I remember taking one on directing. But once the pandemic hit and she could no longer do her usual work with South Shore Players and youth theatre, the workshops started coming fast and furious.[2] Her Spring and Summer offerings included a playwriting workshop (*Scriptease*), a directing workshop (*Director's Chair*), and at least four workshops on various aspects of acting, including script analysis and character development. I wound up taking all of them. She also offered (and continues to offer) a bi-weekly Tuesday night improvisation workshop. The fall saw a second *Scriptease* scriptwriting workshop, as well as two on vocal training and accents offered by an outside expert, Sherry Smith. And the

winter and early spring saw her offering a workshop on preparing mono-
logues for audition and one on stage management, taught by fellow South
Shore Players member Teresa Patterson. I managed to work in all of them
except for the one on stage management.

Taken together, this broad range of workshops kept me and quite a few
other people, many but not all from the Lunenburg area served by South
Shore Players, happily and productively engaged in theatre through the
pandemic's first year. Some of the workshops worked better for me than
others. For me, the most useful ones were the two *Scripteases* where each
participant wrote a short play over a four-week period. I don't think the
virtual format cost us anything; indeed, it made the whole thing possible, at
a time when out-of-town travel was still problematic and distinctly frowned
upon by provincial authorities, and when in any event it wouldn't have been
possible to gather half a dozen people indoors. And the virtual format also
allowed me to continue to participate even after my move to Gatineau,
Quebec at the end of August.

It is a measure of just how successful those online playwriting workshops
were that the three plays in this almanac were all written in one or other of
them.[3] Even should the authorities in Ontario and Quebec open up those
provinces to in-person theatre performances and workshops, I would probably
continue to take Colleen's online scriptwriting workshops for as long as she
cared to offer them. The weekly format facilitates the sort of intensive
thinking and writing one needs to do to turn out a play, while the involvement of other like-minded people provides a further stimulus to creation.
And the informal workshopping that occurs when the completed plays are
read out loud at the final class is invaluable. I only hope that Colleen will still
be able to find the time to offer *Scriptease* online once the theatres open up
again in Nova Scotia.

During my first few months in my new home, I didn't try to reach out
and see what was going on in the theatre world of Ottawa or West Quebec.
Quite frankly, I had neither the time nor the energy to take on new theatre
challenges, occupied as I was with setting up my new place and first preparing
for, then recovering from, inguinal hernia surgery in early November.
Through the fall, Colleen's workshops and an occasional play-reading night
with Bedford Players were more than enough. But as fall turned into winter,
and I began to recover my strength after the hernia surgery, I became curious
to see what the local community theatre world looked like. My first Internet
foray connected me with Theatre Wakefield, a group I'd heard about before.
As one who has written a radio play or two himself, I was pleased to discover
that they were auditioning for one. Even though I wound up not being cast,
just going through the process and having the chance to talk, however briefly
and remotely, to theatre people was itself a rewarding experience. I came
away from the audition feeling that in the fairly near future, I might just be

able to find a home for myself somewhere in this brave new world of online theatre.

And my hunch was right. By February, largely through a chance encounter with a fellow author and playwright at an Ottawa Independent Writers meeting, I'd connected with Kanata Theatre. There, I was given the chance to read parts in two plays that the company was workshopping. And through Kanata Players' newsletter and various notices about things going on at other theatres, I learned of the two online activities that are providing me theatrical sustenance at the moment: a weekly Perth Studio Theatre workshop on improvisational theatre, and a Rural Root theatre play, for which the company was holding auditions. I did indeed audition and to my surprise and delight wound up being cast as a cab driver in *Fishing for Fate.* I'm greatly enjoying being part of this play, even if it does of necessity entail learning a lot more about Zoom than I wish I knew. (This part of rehearsals will go better once I am 'off book' and can concentrate on my actions without having to hold a script in one hand).

It would be possible to write an entire essay, indeed an entire book on how Zoom acting differs from traditional stage acting. But such a task must await other, more gifted hands than mine. For now, suffice it to say that working on Zoom demands a rethinking of one's entire movement vocabulary and manner of delivering lines. I suspect that what we'll be emerging with will be some sort of hybrid form, part way between traditional stage acting and traditional film acting. If my present experience winds up being the first step of a transition into film acting, then so be it. I must say that the thought of acting in front of a camera does appear at least marginally less terrifying than it would have a year ago. Who knows what the future might hold?

At the moment, as was the case during the Fall, I find myself too busy, between my 'day job' (putting together this almanac) and my two ongoing theatre ventures, to seek out new theatre opportunities against the time when my current gigs come to an end. Given what I know now, however, I feel fairly confident that there will be a number of those opportunities—and in the fairly near future. Meanwhile, it's hard to believe that our four-night run is less than a month away; to me, it seems as if we've just barely started with rehearsals.

What have I learned from this year of doing theatre offstage? What I've discovered, first, is the surprising resilience of Canada's theatre community. Thanks to an almost universal 'can-do' attitude and a surprisingly innovative use of technology that most of us hadn't even heard of 18 months ago, we've continued to do theatre, albeit in different ways than in the past.

Secondly, especially as we become more conversant with the new technology, we'll need to find new ways of reaching out to the broader community, so as both to maintain our old audiences and to attract new ones.

Jon Peirce

Here I see a myriad of possibilities for all kinds of outreach activities, from doing plays outdoors 'in the round' on the grounds of hospitals and long-term care homes to facilitating online play reads and play discussion groups for people physically unable to attend live performances. Nor should we forget about the potential offered by the schools. A writers' group I belonged to in Nova Scotia, the Writers' Federation of Nova Scotia, used to conduct (and as far as I know is still conducting) *Writers in the Schools* workshops in primary, middle, and high schools. Why can't we do the same with theatre (*Actors in the Schools*), doing our workshops live when possible and otherwise virtually? Such workshops could 'kill two birds with one stone,' giving members of the theatre community an opportunity to practice their craft, while at the same time introducing young people to theatre and encouraging them to become the theatre audience of the future. If we went about it right, it might even be possible to make a little money in the process.

Finally, I've learned, or at least am beginning to learn, that theatre has a universality that transcends the particular form or forms it may take. This I am learning particularly through my Perth Studio Theatre workshop with Carolee Mason. As we come to fully appreciate that universality, our ability to reach new audiences increases, while our ability to communicate with existing audiences is deepened and strengthened. Such an appreciation adds both breadth and power to our acting, and provides all sorts of new possibilities for creating theatre, whether through traditional scripts or in other ways. Right about now, it would be really neat if we could link up with community theatre people in other countries and see what *they've* been doing to adapt their art to the changed circumstances demanded by the pandemic. What a rich learning experience that would be!

Meanwhile… if I could just get into that goddamn Zoom one more time.

Gatineau, Quebec
May, 2021

Notes

[1] This piece is being written at the end of the first week of May, 2021.
[2] Colleen has written a piece for this almanac about her theatre experiences during the pandemic. It's entitled *Theatre in a COVID World*.
[3] In addition to the play by yours truly—*Virtual Apprentice*—the almanac plays were written by Teresa Patterson and Paul Pickering.

SECTION 12

Milestones
and
Ceremonies

*W*ith the pandemic, all sorts of activities, from moving and travel to celebrating birthdays and weddings, suddenly became far more challenging, if not impossible. Moving, particularly for elders who have been accumulating possessions over most of their lifetimes, is difficult at the best of times, rating as one of the most stressful activities a person can undertake. Given the many restrictions on travel and personal contact imposed during the pandemic, even moves like mine, from Nova Scotia to Quebec, that might otherwise have been relatively straightforward turned into major adventures. A great many of us seeking to move during the pandemic were forced to delay our moves for a significant length of time. Some, like Marcia Brumit Kropf and her husband, were forced to jump through a series of hoops that seemed almost to have been crafted by Franz Kafka himself.

This section contains pieces describing two different types of move. Kropf's was made entirely within New York City and involved significant property transactions. Mine, though much longer (about 1500 kilometres), was conceptually simpler, as it involved no property transactions at all. Still, I was faced with the logistical challenge of incorporating interprovincial travel restrictions into my planning process, and then, later, with the physical challenges entailed in making a major move while encumbered by a major hernia. Fortunately, both our stories have a happy ending. Both Kropf (and her husband) and I landed on our feet after our big moves, and all of us are happy we made those moves.

Family weddings during the pandemic have also posed significant challenges for elders. While we all want to be there to help celebrate our relatives' special day, the dangers of COVID arising from such events are very real, as the saga of the superspreader wedding reception in Millinocket, Maine in August 2020 clearly demonstrated. My cousin Don Peirce's piece about his niece's wedding offers a mostly lighthearted take on just such a wedding; it describes his attempt to work out a compromise solution which would allow him and his wife Joyce to be there for the wedding without subjecting themselves to undue risks of contracting COVID.

The section's remaining piece is about my being 'Poutined In' at a Gatineau pub late in the winter of 2021, during a period of comparative relaxation of pandemic restrictions. Thanks to some very supportive friends, this show did indeed go on, though in much more muted fashion and with many fewer friends in attendance than would normally have been the case. Will I have another, noisier celebration of my new status as a Quebecker once all restrictions are lifted and we can again gather by the dozens in pubs? Most likely I will, providing folks can tolerate my version of a French accent as I recite some piece or other of French literature. . .

413

Farewell to Nova Scotia:
Mr Chips Leaves God's Country
During the Pandemic
Jon Peirce

This was it—finally. After years of partial preparations and false starts, after dozens of calls to movers and U-Haul companies and hundreds of searches of apartments in places as scattered as West Quebec and Victoria, British Columbia moving day was at hand. Or the first part of it, at least. At around 2:00 p.m. on August 26, 2020, I opened my Dartmouth, Nova Scotia apartment door to two men from Campbell Movers. Though they never seemed to hurry, they worked with surprising efficiency in loading my furniture, books, clothing, and non-fragile dishes and cooking gear onto the truck, sometimes toting two or even three big boxes at a time down the back stairs. By 3:45, their work was completed. I signed the loading papers and sat for a moment in my one remaining chair, a rickety piece destined for the recycle bin two days later, contemplating a now nearly-empty apartment. I then walked to the nearby hotel where I would, perforce, be staying for the next two nights, no longer having a bed to sleep on. After leaving my overnight bag there, I walked home, and from there drove down to the *Ship Victory*, my 'go-to' pub throughout my eight years in Dartmouth, for a last feed of fried haddock, washed down by a draft Guinness. As I enjoyed the tasty fish dinner, I wondered if I would find a pub I liked as much in my new home, Gatineau, Quebec.

While unfailingly courteous and friendly, the movers didn't wear masks. Under different circumstances, this might have bothered me. At the time, though, there were practically no active COVID cases in the entire province of Nova Scotia. Given this fact, and given that it was a warm, muggy August afternoon, to have asked the two to wear masks would have seemed a cruel and unusual punishment. More selfishly, I also figured it would not have improved their attitude toward me or the job at hand.

Two days later, also at around 2:00 p.m., I began the second part of my move, driving my fully-laden Toyota Camry out of Dartmouth and onto Route 118 and then Route 102, the Trans-Canada Highway. My destination was Fredericton, New Brunswick, where I had a dinner date with a dear friend of mine from the theatre world, Lita Llewellyn, who had been my director in Joanne Miller's comic murder mystery *Habit of Murder* the year before. I hadn't planned to leave so late. My initial plan had been to leave at around 10:00 a.m., which would have allowed plenty of time for a nap in my Fredericton hotel room before dining with Lita. But due to some electrical malfunctioning in my car, which fortunately turned out to be quite minor, my departure almost didn't happen that day at all. I'd only just turned out of the parking lot and started up Boland Road toward the Trans-Canada when the car emitted the sort of agitated beeping that normally indicates one is out of oil, or that something else is seriously wrong. Alarmed, I pulled over and tried again five minutes later, only to hear more beeping within the first 100 metres. Not wanting to take any chances with a seriously malfunctioning vehicle on such a long and important drive as this, I called CAA and asked them to tow the car to O'Regan's, the dealer from whom I'd bought the car and where I'd always had it serviced. After CAA had come and hitched up the car, I took a cab to O'Regan's, in North End Halifax.

Initially, the man at O'Regan's said they were very busy just then, and I would have to wait my turn in the queue. It might, he said, be 5:00 or 6:00 o'clock before they could look at the Camry. I then pleaded, cajoled, and did a bit of a drama king act, saying it was absolutely imperative that I be in Fredericton before dark, whereupon they relented to a degree, saying they would do the best they could to work me in. Not wishing to hang around, which I didn't think would do anyone any good, I took another cab back to the Dartmouth hotel, figuring I could at least sit and wait there and at worst would have a place to stay if I needed to delay my trip until the next day. As it happened, that worst case scenario never materialized. Within the hour, O'Regan's had called me on my cell phone and said one of their mechanics had driven the car himself and found nothing wrong. I asked if the beeper had gone off; they said it hadn't. Still concerned, I asked if the mechanic could look at the car. The service rep said she would see if she could get him to do that.

Half an hour later, I had another call on my cell. It was the service rep again. The mechanic had not only driven the car but had looked it over. Again, he'd found nothing wrong. But he did have a possible explanation for why the beeper had been going off. Evidently some boxes in the front seat of the fully loaded (possibly even overloaded) car had been setting off an alarm connected to the front seat air bags. While annoying, this was in his view nothing to worry about. Once I'd picked up enough speed, the beeping alarm should stop. Still more than a little apprehensive, I decided to take the risk, and took yet another cab back to O'Regan's, where I paid my repair bill, thanked the staff profusely, and finally, just before 2:00 p.m., set out on my journey.

It turned out that the mechanic had been absolutely right. Though the beeping alarm, true to form, did go off two blocks away from O'Regan's, it stopped once I'd picked up a bit of speed. The drive to the New Brunswick border was the proverbial piece of cake. With surprisingly light traffic, I made that border in about two hours, and was delighted to see only a handful of cars ahead of me in line.

The border stop was something I'd been dreading for months. Not only was I expecting a long wait, given the many Internet stories I'd seen about the long lines there; I was fearful that something (such as a sudden cough) might come up that would jeopardize my chances of being able to cross at all. Indeed, so afraid was I of developing a sudden cough, that I'd completely stopped smoking weed in July and August, relying instead on THC oil when I wanted to relax. To my immense relief, none of the awful things I'd been prepared for actually transpired. Within mere minutes of my joining the queue, I was showing my carefully arranged letter of permission to enter and drive across the province from the New Brunswick Department of Public Safety. The young woman checking papers did little more than glance at my letter before waving me through. 'Take good care, dear!' she said as I started to drive away.

My one remaining fear was that the beeper would go off again while the border guards were within earshot. Once again, I was in luck. Perhaps because the car had been running for so long and was thoroughly warmed, the beeper would not go off again at all until the next day, when I was leaving Fredericton. Meanwhile, the remainder of the day's drive proved totally uneventful. By 6:30, I'd arrived at the beautiful Crowne Plaza Hotel, where I'd be staying, and had checked in and taken my luggage upstairs. Half an hour after that, I was enjoying a delicious patio dinner with Lita and her rescue dog, Rosie. It was really great to catch up with her.

Due to the outbreak of the pandemic, we'd been forced to cancel two previous attempts to get together, made while she was still living in Bedford, Nova Scotia.

The rest of the three-day drive to Gatineau was also quite uneventful, though I did find it passing strange that the motel in Rivière-du-Loup, Quebec, where I stayed on Saturday night, had no blankets for the bed and only a child-sized toilet in the bathroom. Given that the temperature in Rivière-du-Loup was only plus 8° at the time of my arrival, blankets (plural) would have seemed appropriate. But if that was the way it was going to be, that was the way it was going to be. So, after making two calls to the office to request blankets and not getting any reply, I cranked up the thermostat to around plus 25°—no doubt costing the strange motel owner as much in excess heat as he would have spent for a proper blanket—and managed to get a fairly decent night's sleep despite it all.

Did the lack of blankets for my bed have anything to do with the COVID pandemic? This was a hypothesis advanced by one of the friends to whom I told my bizarre story later on. But that was (and is) a hypothesis I find hard to credit. If sheets and pillow cases can be safely laundered, so can blankets, providing they are of the right material. Thus, the reason for the lack of blankets for my bed seems likely to remain forever a mystery.

By 4:00 the next afternoon, having completed the longest leg of the three-day drive virtually without incident, I'd arrived at my new home in Gatineau. My lady friend, Ann McMillan, was already there, waiting outside in her car for my arrival. Ann was a huge help to me in unloading the car, something I couldn't do all by myself owing to my hernia (about which more later). Later, my long-time friend and old union colleague Denise Giroux would arrive, to help with the early stages of setting up the house. The weather having in the meantime returned to the mild and sunny conditions I'd experienced in Halifax and Fredericton, the three of us joined Joe Michel, my new landlord, and his girlfriend, Sylvie, for a tasty patio supper at a nearby sports pub called *Forum*, where Ann and I would enjoy several more meals before the return of the pandemic forced its closure after Thanksgiving weekend. (I'm pleased to be able to report that *Forum* is now again open and doing a booming business). I was well and truly ensconced in a lovely half-duplex in Gatineau, only about 100 metres from the Gatineau River and within a short distance of several excellent walking and biking paths.

Setting up my new home took a good deal longer than it would normally have done, due to the now-overgrown hernia, which made it impossible for me to lift anything weighing more than about 20 pounds. But I had help from Ann shoving boxes around, and help from Denise hanging my collection of artwork on the walls. By late September, I was pretty well set up at 11 Rue Marengere. All the boxes had been unpacked, and all the clothing had been suitably stowed away in dressers or closets. Was I fully settled? No, not quite. There would be dealings with healthcare staff and Motor Vehicle Registry staff before I could say I was *fully* settled. But I had a place to call home, a place I really liked, a place to which I would be proud to bring friends. Here in my new house, I could start a new life for myself at long last.

As some of you may already have deduced from this piece's opening paragraph, the move from Nova Scotia to Quebec was one that almost didn't happen. In a way, the drama of my final day in Nova Scotia was a fitting end to my stay in that province.

I'd actually been thinking about moving out of Nova Scotia as early as the fall of 2016, when, frustrated by my seeming inability to crack the literary and theatre communities, as well as by my continuing lack of a relationship, I first recognized that I probably didn't have much of a future in the province. One place that quickly caught my eye was Victoria, British Columbia, which in addition to its equable climate, offered a strong theatre community and an equally strong literary community. But the city's high rents and the huge costs of moving there made such a move an economic non-starter. So, I reluctantly crossed Victoria off my list of possible relocation destinations.

My second possible destination was West Quebec, just outside of Ottawa. There I would be close to the two children I had who were still speaking to me. Equally to the point, there I had two very dear friends: my old workmate Denise Giroux, who lived in Cantley, and my old literary friend Elena Calvo, who lived in Hull. Having such good friends close at hand would be a big help when it came time to actually relocate. And Ottawa had a strong literary community featuring Ottawa Independent Writers (OIW), which had been such a big part

417

of my life when I'd lived there, and a vibrant theatre community as well, of which I had been a tangential part as an understudy for an Ottawa Little Theatre production. West Quebec had a vibrant theatre community as well. The rents appeared manageable, and the moving costs, while significant, were far less than those entailed in moving to Victoria. And so, early in the fall of 2016, I began to explore both drive-it-yourself and commercial moving options.

I'd just begun packing when U.S. Election Day came. Against all the odds and all the polls, Hillary Clinton lost to Donald Trump. Trump's election sent me into a deep depression from which it took months to recover. Any thoughts of moving were put on indefinite hold, as I once again hunkered down in Nova Scotia for security.

Financial constraints and a continuing need for security driven by Trump's increasingly demented antics kept me from seriously considering a move again until the spring of 2019, even though I'd long since realized I had next to no chance to grow so long as I remained in Nova Scotia. On the relationship front, with the exception of a fairly brief (three-month) fling with a Halifax woman about my age, I continued to strike out completely with the dating services and in personal encounters with possibly eligible women. And things were going little better in the theatre and literary worlds. Despite the fact that I was far stronger physically than I'd been four or five years earlier, at the start of my theatre career, and had acquired significant acting experience in a variety of roles, I was garnering at least half a dozen rejections for every successful audition; a far worse record than I'd had with a seriously gimpy hip as a raw beginner. In the literary community, I was effectively a non-person, picking up a single 'Writers in the School Workshop' in the Fall of 2018, after seven years of unsuccessful applications to that program. Though I found doing the workshop extremely rewarding, the fee I received for it didn't even come close to paying my Writers' Federation dues for my time in the province.

In the spring of 2019, shortly after the closing of *Habit of Murder,* I fell into a deep depression. While a stretch of 'post-partum' blues is perfectly normal at the end of a play's run, this was something else again. This was a depression that went deep to my core, leaving me all but paralyzed emotionally. Meditation, deep breathing, therapy with two different counsellors, vigorous exercise—none of these helped. Finally, in desperation, I re-read A.H. Maslow's *Toward a Psychology of Being,* which had been my beacon through college and early adulthood, and his classic 'hierarchy of needs.' The specific question I needed to answer for myself was why Nova Scotia, which had worked so well for me when I'd first come to the province in 1970 as a graduate student, had worked so poorly for me during my return stay, starting at the end of 2009. Maslow's hierarchy of needs provided a ready answer.

In 1970, when I'd been unemployed and with few job prospects in the offing, my needs had been the primary ones of economic and physical security. Dalhousie met those needs amazingly well, even giving me a place I could call home for a few years, which met some of the 'belongingness' needs we'll be talking about in more detail shortly. In 2019, my situation was quite different. As a pensioner, I had enough to live on, and a bit to spare, my previous financial problems having finally been solved. Materially, I wanted for nothing. But I was bitterly lonely: lonely for friends, lonely for a family that scarcely existed for me anymore, and lonely for a close, physically affectionate relationship with a significant other, of the sort I hadn't had for many years, as well as for connection with fellow writers and theatre people. In short, what I was missing was a sense of connection. None of the plays I'd been in, board meetings and church services I'd attended, and hours I'd spent at the tennis club had managed to provide me with that. I was striking out completely on Maslow's Level 3, his 'belongingness' level. To all intents and purposes, I was alone in the world in Nova Scotia, beautiful though the province was (and is). Recognizing this was a key factor in solidifying my resolve to move, as it demonstrated the futility of attempting to do anything more about the situation where I was. In June of 2019, I decided that unless some huge event took place, more or less compelling me to stay, I would leave the province in the fairly near future. Nine-plus years seemed to me more than a fair try.

I formalized my decision to leave Nova Scotia during a meeting with my three old literary friends, Elena Calvo, Adele Graf and Ralph Smith, with whom I'd been meeting once a year or so since leaving Ottawa at the end of 2009, at an outdoor café in Centretown in late July of 2019. 'Why should I be leaving, when you're the people I want to be with?' I asked them. Over the iced tea and lattes, I pledged to move back to the area within one year (it was then late July).

Having announced my decision out loud in front of three witnesses, I felt the kind of commitment to it that I might not have felt had I not verbalized it. Though my resolve would waver a bit during the middle of the pandemic's first wave, it would never falter. The pandemic would delay my arrival only three months beyond the date initially planned for it.

But how exactly did the COVID pandemic affect my move? I'd finished packing most of my books and was confidently looking forward to giving my notice at the end of March and proceeding with the move at the end of May, when the first COVID case was diagnosed in the province, just before the middle of the month. At that point, neither I nor anyone else had any idea how long the pandemic would last or what effect it would have on one's ability to move from one province to another. For a time, I wasn't even sure that I and my possessions would be allowed to enter New Brunswick. In the face of so many unknowns, I decided to put the move on hold for one month and await further developments. At the end of April, with Canadian cases mounting into the thousands and still no clear sense of whether the move would even be physically possible in two months' time, I put it on hold for another month.

An important issue was what to do with the boxes of books which were sitting, packed, on the floor waiting to be moved to Ottawa. Given that it seemed likely to be some months before I could actually make the move, I recognized that I couldn't go on living with them taking up half my floor space. Either I would need to unpack the books, put them back on the shelves, and then repack them later, or I would need to find some other place to put the boxes. I opted for the latter, figuring that unpacking and reshelving would be entirely the wrong message to send to myself. With a bit of rearranging, I was able to get all the boxes onto the now nearly-empty bookcases. I was even able to put two small suitcases containing high-end books destined for sale in Ottawa on a shelf. And the big suitcase also containing high-end books went into my bedroom closet, which had plenty of room available. All in all, it was a good short-to-medium term solution.

I came closest to calling off the move near the end of May. The COVID statistics coming out of Quebec were extremely worrisome. As of May 13, despite having less than a quarter of Canada's population, Quebec had about 55% of the country's total cases and around 60% of its COVID deaths. Its recovery rate, as a percentage of non-fatal cases, was an anemic 28%, compared to over 50% for Canada as a whole, and around 80% for neighbouring Ontario. I also wasn't sure whether I would even be able to cross over the border into New Brunswick, let alone Quebec. And even if I could get in, did I really want to drive straight into a pest house?

Now I began to feel paralyzed with fear and indecision, as I had so often in the past when contemplating the move. And as I had so often done in the past, I thought about security first. Nova Scotia, when all was said and done, really hadn't been a bad place to spend the pandemic. Maybe it wouldn't be so bad to go on living there. It seemed likely that Nova Scotia, along with the other Atlantic provinces, would be among the first Canadian provinces to 'recover' from the first wave, and thus to be able to allow its citizens to resume something approaching a normal life. Did I really want to take the risk of moving? Maybe I should try one more time to make a go of the theatre and dating scenes.

Fortunately, at this critical juncture, instead of remaining wrapped up within myself spinning wheels, I decided to reach out to my friends for advice. First, I called Denise who, without positively insisting that I should make the move, provided strong encouragement in that direction. She then called my prospective landlord, Joe Michel, who painted a glowing picture of life in Gatineau—one that contrasted sharply with the exceptionally boring life I was then living in Nova Scotia. At the rent he would be charging me, the half-duplex in Gatineau would be practically a steal! During our conversation, Joe also let it be known that while he could hold the place an extra month for me, he couldn't hold it indefinitely. Finally, I called my lady friend, Ann McMillan. After a good talk, I asked Ann if my staying in Nova Scotia would be a barrier to her continuing the relationship. She allowed as how it would.

Knowing that I had a great deal on an apartment and a wonderful girlfriend waiting for me 'on the other side,' but could well lose both if I shilly-shallied too long, proved a spur to my flagging will. At that point, I was able to step back from my immediate situation, and recognize that the same things that had bothered me about Metro Halifax for many years would continue to bother me once the pandemic had ended. Despite superficial appearances, nothing had really changed. I would continue to be a misfit, not even comfortable in my own apartment, into which I was for some strange reason ashamed to invite guests. There seemed no reason to delay the move any longer. I called Joe and told him I would take the half-duplex, starting no later than the first of October, but probably the first of September, and resolved to give notice on my Dartmouth apartment sometime in June.

There remained, to be sure, the problem of New Brunswick, which had for some time been turning away visitors at its borders. I didn't want to go to be among those turned away—especially not after having given up my apartment and thus having nowhere to stay if I had to go back to Nova Scotia. But a call to New Brunswick's Public Safety Department confirmed that that need not be the case. People driving across New Brunswick to move to another province were permitted to do so, providing they had a letter attesting to their new residence in their new province, and providing they drove straight through, without stopping for the night. (Stops for meals, gas, and the calls of nature were permitted.) Though I wasn't happy with this rule, which meant I would need to stop the first night in Amherst, Nova Scotia, in order to make it across the province of New Brunswick in one day, I figured I could live with it. Furthermore, there was always the possibility of an easing of restrictions by the time I actually came to make my move.

As things transpired, those restrictions did ease. At the beginning of July, the four Atlantic provinces established an interprovincial 'bubble,' by means of which a resident of any Atlantic province who had not travelled outside the region or been exposed to the virus could freely enter any other. This meant that I would be able to drive through New Brunswick in civilized, even leisurely fashion, stopping in Fredericton to spend the night and then moving on to Rivière-du-Loup, Quebec, for my final night on the road.

The one remaining obstacle to my move was my hernia. I'd had it for over a year, but had thought it only a minor nuisance and occasional inconvenience, as through the beginning of July it had rarely caused even minor pain. But then, late in July, just as I was beginning to get into some serious packing, the hernia had suddenly flared up, after two probably inadvisable tennis sessions in the same week. All of a sudden, this thing that had been the size of an extra-large egg had swollen into something the size of half a football! Unable to bear the pain, or to push the hernia back into its proper place, I sought help at Halifax Infirmary's emergency room, and within three and a half hours had received it.

Unfortunately, I was not able to obtain the surgery I obviously needed. But the highly-skilled emergency room doctor was able to massage the giant lump back into a safe place, using a technique that she showed me and which I would use, quite successfully, myself, until I was finally able to have my operation. I called that technique 'wrestling the turtle.' She also managed to convince me that I could probably get by without surgery for a couple more months, until I arrived in Quebec and could have the hernia seen to there. While far from reassured about my longer-term medical situation, given what I'd already heard about Quebec's health care system, I figured I could still get on with my move as scheduled, providing I got help with the heavy physical parts of the job, such as packing my dishes and loading my car. Thankfully there were people around who could give me that help, allowing me to proceed with the move more or less without a hitch.

I could not, finally, be myself and continue to live in Nova Scotia. This recognition, along with the likely loss of an excellent rental deal and a great girlfriend, was what confirmed to me the wisdom of my decision to leave, despite the far higher COVID risks in Quebec, despite the move's significant financial cost, and despite the obstacles thrown in the way by my suddenly recalcitrant hernia (which I would manage to have repaired at Ontario's Shouldice Clinic in early November). Only time will tell if I did in fact make the right decision in opting for growth over security. At the moment, some five months into my new life as a Quebecker, all the evidence suggests I did. Even at the worst of the second round of lockdowns, I have a far richer interpersonal life here in Quebec than I did in Nova Scotia before COVID. Despite all the difficulties, ranging from my occasional struggles with French to my frequent difficulties in dealing with the motor vehicle registry and healthcare system, I feel that the move has freed me for my best shot at a successful closing chapter of my life.

Gatineau, Quebec
February, 2021

Yes, I Really Did Move During a Pandemic!
Marcia Brumit Kropf

The year 2020 was the year of the COVID-19 pandemic... and the year we moved to a new apartment in Manhattan.

I am quite experienced at moving. My family, with my airline-executive father, moved every five or six years as I was growing up. As an adult, married, I have moved eight times, living outside the U.S. and in three states within the U.S. In 1985, I moved to New York City with my husband and two-year-old, recognizing the importance of my Brooklyn-born husband's tenure offer. I never expected to stay. Thirty-five years later, New York is home and I think of myself as a New Yorker. The 2020 move, though, was different than any other I'd ever experienced.

First, let me say that this move was a privileged move. We moved voluntarily to a place we took a long time to find, and we had the financial resources to make the move safely. Many, many New Yorkers suffered economically and emotionally during this pandemic and had much more difficult experiences. My family faced a long, hard year with some difficult setbacks, but is safe and surviving.

So why did we choose to move? In February 2010, my husband Roger and I had purchased a small one-bedroom apartment on the east side of Manhattan. We downsized. Our two children were in their mid-20s and no longer living with us. We were nearing retirement and planning a lot of travel. And New York was just coming out of the 2008/2009 recession, so apartments were slightly more affordable, making it feasible to give up renting. Ten years later, our two children were married and had given us four grandchildren. The apartment was no longer a place where we could host a family dinner or a grandchild sleepover (well, we did but it meant using an air mattress on the floor of our bedroom).

In 2019, my husband met a real-estate friend who convinced him that this would be a good time to look at Manhattan real estate. We had some difficult demands for an apartment. It had to be below a certain financial threshold. It had to have two bedrooms but, unusual for NYC apartments, we wanted a quite large bedroom for us and a smaller bedroom for guests (rather than two equally-sized bedrooms). We wanted to stay on the east side of Manhattan, near my son's family in Manhattan and my daughter's family in another borough. In addition, I was committed to finding and buying a place before we sold the current apartment. I didn't want to have to move to a hotel or a sublet for months, which would mean moving twice. That required financing to allow us to buy before selling. My theory was: When would you ever not be able to sell a Manhattan apartment?

In December of 2019, we put down a deposit on a lovely two-bedroom apartment in the mid-town east area of Manhattan. It was exactly what we were looking for: just spacious enough, with a large bedroom for us, a small bedroom for guests, and large windows overlooking a small park with beautiful trees. But co-op building real estate transactions in New York are not fast. The next steps were finalizing the financing and going through the co-op board approval process. Note that the co-op application itself was 76 pages long, not including all the required attachments, among them three professional and three personal letters of reference for each of us. The financial part was actually simpler! We focused on the Winter holidays and family gatherings, looking forward to 2020 with a lot of excitement.

And then, on my 74th birthday, January 9, 2020, the World Health Organization (WHO) announced a mysterious coronavirus-related pneumonia had appeared in Wuhan, China. See below for a brief chronology of the early stages of the pandemic in the U.S. and in New York state:

- January 31: WHO declared an international emergency.
- February 3: The U.S. declared a public health emergency.
- March 7: The Governor of New York declared a state-wide emergency.

Despite the various emergency declarations, we were fairly calm and comfortable. We started being very careful about being in crowds and washing our hands. We bought hand sanitizer. We kept scheduled appointments, thinking at the time that the pandemic would be a short-lived, well-contained problem.

The co-op board application was submitted in early February. Our interview with members of the co-op board was conducted in the evening of March 12. We felt it went well and went out to dinner at a near-by Persian restaurant highly recommended by a good friend. Little did we know that this would be our last restaurant meal for months. We talked about how excited we were to begin exploring this new-to-us neighborhood. We then took the bus home (and that was my last ride on public transportation for months). On Friday, March 13, we were informed that the board had approved our application. We started discussing a possible closing date with the sellers, the lawyers, and the banks.

Sunday March 15

The Mayor of New York City announced density rules, closing bars and restaurants for all but take-out and delivery. My seven-year-old grandson's school closed, as did my three-year-old granddaughter's nursery. We were told that the schools would stay closed for the next four weeks, expecting them to reopen after the Spring break in April. The jobs of both my children and their spouses were affected, as organizations closed, sending some employees home to work and furloughing others. As working parents, they were providing child care and remote schooling on their own while working fulltime; and we couldn't help. We began to realize that the situation was more serious than we had first thought. On March 22, 2020, the New York State PAUSE Plan went into effect. All non-essential businesses were closed and all non-essential gatherings were banned. We were asked to socially distance from others and we began to wear masks. Discussion of the apartment closing went nowhere because no one knew what to do. The management company for the co-op and the lawyers had only done closings in-person with everyone present and signing documents. On April 9, we learned that the co-op would no longer allow anyone to move into the building. We then asked that the closing be postponed until a time when we could move in.

We stayed isolated in our current apartment from March through the summer. I didn't want to pack because there was very little room in the apartment and we needed to live there comfortably until we could move. I tried to sort out things that we wanted to donate, but even that was difficult, as organizations in the city had stopped accepting donations. During that time, the city was at the height of the first wave. Our apartment was near several of the big hospitals, and we continually heard the sirens of ambulances taking people there.

In late May, there were signs of the virus ebbing, and the Governor began a four-stage plan to reopen across the state. On May 26, we learned that the co-op would now allow new people to move in. The closing was scheduled for June 29, our 52nd wedding anniversary. We began to pack.

Everyone involved was now improvising, trying to figure out how to hold a real estate closing in the city, especially one that involves the transfer of shares from one person to another, during this time of limited gatherings and concerns about transmission. The closing became a multi-day affair and reinforced how lucky we were to have a car.

Friday, June 26

By 11:00 a.m., we were receiving electronically documents to review, documents to notarize, and documents to deliver. All had to be printed and pored through by us and our lawyer. At 1:30 p.m. we drove down to the financial district to the building where the co-op management company has offices. We parked at a corner and alerted their representative that we were there. She came down, took our driver's licenses upstairs to copy, came down, watched us sign documents on the hood of the car, and accepted the six personal checks we had written for different things. So much for virtual transactions! At 3:00 p.m. we drove up to the new apartment and did the walk through. Thankfully, we were still very happy with the apartment. In order to do the final walk-through, we were asked to follow RESBNY (Real Estate Board of New York) guidelines by the new co-op. That meant 1) signing and returning a health questionnaire about exposure to COVID-19 before arriving; 2) signing and returning a release from liability re: COVID before arriving; 3) having our temperature taken upon arrival; and 4) wearing masks and gloves during the walk through (we would have worn masks anyway but disposable gloves in a months-long empty apartment seemed a bit much).

Monday, June 29

Roger began the morning by trying to make a wire transfer of the dollars left that we were contributing to the purchase of the apartment. He found that he could not do the transfer remotely because the amount was larger than the bank allows you to debit daily. He tried calling and learned that he could not do it over the phone either. He had to walk into a branch office. He went over and clearly this was the first wire transfer that the person at the bank had done, but eventually he was told it had gone through and came home. A bit later he got a call from the bank saying that they had forgotten to have him sign a specific form with the reference number on it. So, he had to walk back again and sign the form in order for the transfer to go through.

At 2:00 p.m., we had a GoToMeeting with our lawyer and the mortgage bank's lawyer. We went through a huge pile of papers while they watched us sign. Every time we signed a document, we had to move the computer camera so they could see our hands making the signatures. We then scanned documents and sent them to the lawyers. This was slow going, as we have a small home printer with no fax function. Scanned documents were sent to my computer, which I forwarded via e-mail to the lawyers. I sent the very large document files in nine e-mails, as the file sizes were too large to be sent in one e-mail. The bank's lawyer's assistant then printed them on their end for her to review. I had suggested some other much more secure and streamlined options regularly used in business such as Dropbox, but the bank's lawyer was committed to the e-mail approach.

After the one-and-a-half-hour meeting, Roger walked to Federal Express to drop the paper copies in the mail so that the bank would have the originals. The bank's lawyer now had to send the papers to the bank for final approval and then the bank had to send the funds to the sellers (who were to have a similar meeting where they signed their documents). Once that was done, then the co-op would send our shares to the bank to hold and we would own the apartment. Happy Anniversary!

Wednesday, July 1

Our lawyer informed us that we now owned the new apartment and could pick up the keys. Our 'virtual' closing had taken four business days and required several in-person interactions.

Wednesday, July 8

We selected paint colors for the apartment and finalized the painting contract with a contractor who worked regularly in the building. He agreed to begin the work on July 14. We were finding that, with restrictions loosened, people were focusing on upgrading their homes and workmen were very busy.

We were also hearing that many New Yorkers were moving, either out of the city now that they could work remotely or to larger places within the city. Roger began to spend quite a bit of time looking for a mover. The first company recommended to us was not available due to high demand. Roger then read online reviews to identify some options and completed the online request forms for three companies, asking about the week of July 26. None were available. He then went back and requested the week of August 3. One came back to us: the quote was reasonable. Now we had to get both buildings to finalize a date that worked for the movers. And the movers had to agree to the more stringent building requirements related to the COVID-19 situation, as follows:

- The shareholder/unit owners or their subtenant is responsible for informing the moving company that they must supply their employees with proper Personal Protective Equipment (PPE) consisting of a nose and mouth face-covering/mask, gloves, and shoe coverings, *which must be worn at all times in the building*. Additionally, they must be informed that there are no public restroom facilities available to them in the building. The Co-operative/Condominium reserves the right to deny building access to the moving company's employee(s), or suspend or cancel the move, if proper PPE is not worn at all times while in the building.

- The moving company will only be allowed into the building through the basement via the service entrance. The moving company will be provided a dedicated elevator to transport between the basement and the apartment floor only. A building staff member will be positioned in the basement and on the apartment floor in full PPE.

- All personal items to be moved into or out of the apartment must be placed on the sidewalk and/or inside the apartment. No items are to be kept in the basement corridor or in the hallway floors.

- The building staff will perform a cleaning of all touched surfaces on the apartment floor, the elevator, and the basement when the move is complete.

- All residents on the same floor as the apartment which is moving will be notified in advance of the move. *REMINDER*: Residents should be wearing a face covering (nose and mouth) when in the hallways, elevators, lobby, basement and other common areas of the building.

427

Tuesday, August 4

The *Move*. I hadn't slept at all the night before because I was so worried about Hurricane Isaiah. It's difficult enough moving with the additional safety precautions related to COVID-19, but now, a hurricane? When I went to bed on Monday night, the forecast was for rains to start at 6:00 a.m. I spent the night worried that; 1) the movers would have to postpone the move, leaving us to manage on our own with everything we needed packed; or 2) the move would go forward in heavy rain, adding water and mud to everything. The good news was that somehow there were windows of time during the day when there was no rain.

The four men from the moving company arrived at the apartment at 9:00 a.m. Everyone was masked, gloved, and careful. They did a wonderful job of assessing the work, covering all the furniture, and packing the truck. The heavy rain held off until close to noon, so almost everything was in the truck. The truck got to the new apartment close to 2:00 p.m. By then, the heavy rain had stopped, but there were terrible winds. However, the crew were able to quickly bring everything into the building. They took great care, setting up the bed and unwrapping everything. We were very impressed. My 'open me first' box with towels, sheets, two plates, and two sets of flatware was fabulous. It was the only box we opened, and it got us through the night. Roger cleaned the bathroom and I set it up and got the bed made. We ordered dinner from the nearby Persian restaurant and then went to bed exhausted.

The next few weeks were spent unpacking and carting stuff from one place to another. This was in part because we had decided to move the art ourselves, leaving it on the walls in the old apartment until the new apartment was set up. In addition, in a strange turn of events, my son's family and my daughter's family had also moved as well, illustrating the trend described earlier. They each moved to places that were more conducive to working from home and had private outdoor spaces for the children to play. These were moves they had been considering anyway; the COVID-19 situation simply sped up the decisions. In the end, all three of our families moved within a month of each other. We weren't just moving things from our old apartment to the new apartment; we were also moving things among the three families.

By September, we all felt settled. It had taken about eight months from the signing of the initial contract to the actual move into our apartment. We were very glad we were both retired and could spend the time required to handle all the complexities of the situation. And we are very happy in the new apartment and glad to have more space, as the pandemic lingers through the beginning of the new year. We are also enjoying living closer to and visiting Central Park. Unfortunately, we can't really show off our new place, host family gatherings, visit with nearby friends, try out the restaurants in our new neighborhood, or visit our favorite now-closer museums.

Perhaps in the coming year we'll again be able to do these things.

Meanwhile, is anyone interested in a lovely one-bedroom apartment in a wonderful Manhattan neighborhood? It is January, 2021 and the old apartment is still for sale...

My Niece's Wedding
Donald Oluf Peirce

'Uncle Don, I want you to walk me down the aisle.'

My niece, Diana, had just shown my wife Joyce and me her engagement ring though my front door screen. She was ecstatic. She had called me earlier to say she had a surprise and wanted to drop by. She was showing off her ring through the front door screen since she could not enter our house due to the world-wide COVID pandemic. She seemed so happy.

She wanted me to walk her down the aisle because her father, my twin, had died six years earlier and, since we were identical and she considered me her 'Second Daddy,' she thought it would be wonderful if I did that for her.

Diana had had problems with dating relationships due to her parents' controlling who she could date. Now that she was 43 years old and had finally found someone her mother approved of, she couldn't wait.

We had never met her fiancé, Barry Zimmerman II, so it was a total shock to my wife and me that a man we didn't know had proposed to her. We hadn't even known she was dating.

It was the end of August 2020, and the world was in the middle of a COVID pandemic. To get married at such a risky time seemed absurd to me.

'Diana,' I tried to explain, 'having a wedding is a dangerous thing to do at a time like this, when thousands of people are getting sick and dying. Everyone, including the minister, would have to wear a mask. The guests would have to mask and social distance. It will not be matrimony as usual and it could become a super-spreader. I suggest you wait until a vaccine is developed and the world is safe. After all, Aunt Joyce and I waited 14 months to get married because *her* dad was in the hospital at the time and she wanted him to walk *her* down the aisle.'

'I can't wait that long,' she said. 'I'm 43 years old.'

She didn't say, but I assumed she wanted to get pregnant and her biological clock was ticking away. To wait would be unthinkable.

The day of the wedding arrived, November 14, 2020 at 11:00 a.m. The wedding party consisted of the groom's parents and my twin brother's widow. There was a matron and maid of honor, one bridesmaid, her brother Daniel's wife, Rebecca, a best man and two groomsmen: Daniel and someone I'd never met. There were also a junior bridesmaid and two ring bearers—Daniel's boys—Micah, 10 years old, and Liam age five. All told, there were 14 in the wedding party and about 60 guests. Diana's brother Daniel took my place, and walked her down the aisle.

I have to confess that I didn't see a lot of masking in the wedding pictures, which I viewed on Facebook, but I was limited to what was in my field of vision. Fortunately, I haven't heard of anyone getting sick. Since I wasn't there, I can't vouch for people following COVID protocols.

The day of the wedding, Joyce and I drove up to the church, timing our visit so we would arrive at the end of the ceremony. As I drove into the parking lot behind the church, I saw her minister standing near where I was parking. He came right over to our car and introduced himself. I asked him if he would please send word to Diana that Joyce and I were there, waiting to see her and her new husband. I had told her we would be there.

When Diana came out from the church, all were masked, but as Diana approached the car, I noticed her mask was below her nose. Half-masking is no masking, so I asked her nicely to 'Please cover your nose.' She started to lift her mask up and then got peeved.

'I don't have COVID!' she said, in an irritated voice. 'I have no symptoms.' Then she added, 'I won't have you ruining my wedding.' And with that she spun on her heel and headed back into the church.

So much for meeting her new husband. Joyce and I were shocked, but her minister came right over and started talking to us, and that bit of friendliness took some of the sting out of Diana's reaction.

Much later, she talked to us on the phone, and I made an effort not to rile her up, but I was very much concerned with her earlier rudeness and wanted to tell her so. I never did get the chance to admonish her, but she came over to our house a week later, and she and Barry stood outside our screen door while we talked to him in an effort to get to know him. In addition, she gave us a very nice eight-by-ten wedding photo, good for framing.

A few weeks later, Diana called to ask me to check out the wedding video she had just posted on Facebook. I have to confess, I didn't see a lot of masking in the wedding video, but I haven't heard that anyone got sick, either. Apparently, you can have a wedding in the middle of a pandemic, disregarding all the protocols, and everything will come out all right.

As I mentioned earlier, Diana had always considered me her second Daddy, since I was identical to her father. In the end, her love for her Aunt Joyce and me shone through and all was forgotten as well as forgiven.

See, among many others, Anon., 'How a Small Wedding in Maine Became a Deadly COVID-19 Superspreader,' *Healthline*, November 17, 2020 (Downloaded June 18, 2021.)

Being Poutined-In:
Ceremony In a Time of COVID

Jon Peirce

Moving from Nova Scotia to Quebec has been a profound life change for me. A change that deserves to be marked by something other than three-month battles with the motor vehicle registry over transfer of my car registration, or a two-month search for a healthcare clinic. But how to do this? Eventually, taking my cue from Newfoundlanders' 'Screeching-In' ceremony, which involves, among other things, kissing a codfish, I decided that, as I had never before eaten a poutine, Quebec's national dish, I should be 'Poutined-In,' with as much pomp and ceremony as it would be possible to muster in the circumstances. Why should Newfoundlanders have all the fun?

Ideally, the ceremony should have taken place within my first two months of residence in the province. Two things made this impossible: first, an immense hernia, that would have rendered the consumption of large quantities of fatty food most inadvisable; and, second, the closing of Quebec's restaurants and pubs for a period of nearly four-and-a-half months, starting on Thanks-giving weekend.

Being 'Poutined-In' is no more something one does at home than being Screeched-In. A cardboard container of the stuff from Pierre's Palais de Patates, accompanied by a can of beer—or worse, Pepsi—simply won't cut it. But in November, I'd had the hernia seen to, and in mid-February, Gatineau's restaurants and pubs finally reopened. Once the restaurants had reopened, and we could again enjoy draft beer with our food in a social setting, I knew there was no time to waste. If I waited much longer, I wouldn't really qualify as a new Quebecker. There was also the distinct possibility that the restaurants, which had so recently reopened, could be shut down again owing to another COVID resurgence: the dreaded 'Third Wave.'

And so it was that on a Saturday night in early March, accompanied by my lady friend Ann and dear friends Denise and Greg, I hied myself to the *Bon Vivant* pub in downtown Hull, where Denise had had her election night party after running for Parliament in 2019.

On first entering the *Bon Vivant*, we were greeted by amorphously atonal music at a volume that would have more suitable at a rave, and frigid temp-eratures that would have been more appropriate inside a meat locker. The music did little to enhance conversation between the two tables (yours truly and Ann at one, Denise and Greg at the other), which in accordance with COVID regulations were six feet apart. But after a couple of requests to our server to please 'Turn the heat up and the music down!' I stopped shivering, and we were able to conduct a conversation of sorts with Denise and Greg over our draft Guinness and white wine.

You may find it hard to believe that a Canadian citizen had reached the age of 76 without ever having ordered a poutine, but it's the God's truth. I was not exactly looking forward to the experience. Some of the poutines I'd seen, whether in the flesh or in a picture, looked like a rough draft for a Jackson Pollock painting, while others looked like something the dog might have brought up on the living room floor after a rough night with the neighbours' garbage cans. I thought, briefly, about wearing a blindfold while eating the poutine, but quickly discarded the idea as not really sporting, and more important, something liable to leave my *shirt* looking like the rough draft of a Jackson Pollock painting. If there is, indeed, 'many a slip 'twixt the cup and the lip,' how many more there would likely be between a dish full of dripping, greasy potatoes and one's lip when one was blindfolded!

Having operated without a gall bladder for the past 32 years, I have a rather limited ability to digest fat. I knew that I would need to have plenty of greenery inside me before diving into the poutine, in order to 'grease its skid,' so to speak, through to the nether regions. With this in mind, I ordered a large green salad, which Ann and I shared, along with a very tasty calamari starter.

There were various options for different kinds of poutine. After some thought, I decided on the plain one, consisting solely of French fries, cheese curds and beef gravy. Initially my plan had been to order a poutine and a burger separately. But when the server told me I could, for a small extra charge, have the poutine as a side for the burger, I pounced. What a great idea! I'm sure I wound up getting a smaller poutine this way than I would have had with a separate order, though the one I got, which filled two-thirds of a good-sized soup bowl, was definitely plenty big enough!

When the poutine finally arrived, about a third of the way through my second Guinness, I was pleased to see that it did *not* look in any way gross or disgusting. Indeed, the dish seemed quite austere in its plainness; it might almost have graced a monk's table, providing he were a Quebec monk! Noting that some of the things on top had a bit of a greenish hue to them, I asked if those might be some other vegetable, such as green peppers. But one of my companions laughed and said that was just what the potatoes looked like when swimming in the gravy—a bowl of gravy that seemed quite endless, as I set myself to the task of actually eating the dish. If this was a side poutine, I could only imagine what the main dish one might have been like!

Slowly, even methodically, I worked my way through the poutine, having long since finished the burger. I seem to recall alternating between a fork and a spoon. By the time I reached its bottom layer, it was little more than lukewarm. Under different circumstances, I'd have sent what was left back to be reheated in the microwave. But I didn't want to drag the ceremony out any longer than absolutely necessary. While the reheating would undoubtedly have made the last part of the dish taste better, the delay might well have killed what was left of my appetite for it, resulting in the unforgivable sin of my *not finishing every bite in my dish.* Besides, we were all up against an absolute deadline: the nightly 9:30 curfew, which was fast approaching. I live only 10 minutes' drive from the *Bon Vivant,* but Denise and Greg, who were dropping me off since Ann was headed in another direction, had a full half-hour to go after that. At such moments, gastronomic elegance must give way to the exigencies of *la loi.* As much fun as all this was, it wouldn't have been worth a $1,000.00 fine for breaking curfew.

With the poutine finally finished, I sat for a moment, drinking it all in… and waiting to see if I needed to belch before moving on to the ceremony's next and final phase. Thankfully, I didn't; indeed, I'm happy to report that at no time during the entire evening did I belch, or for that matter secrete acid reflux. What a relief!

And now the moment was at hand—the moment when I would complete the 'Poutining-In' ceremony, and thus qualify for adoption as a Quebecker, by reciting something in French. After taking a deep breath and requesting silence from my companions, I plunged right into La Fontaine's classic fable about 'Le Renard et le Corbeil' (The Fox and the Crow), which I'd had to memorize for French 2 back in my sophomore year at boarding school. What I remembered went effortlessly, and while some slight improvisation was necessary to fill in a missing part of the ending, that went off without a hitch as well. Best of all, the whole thing took less than a minute. I don't think I could have gone on much longer than that. Not enough in the tank because there was too much in the tank, if you know what I mean.

And then it was time to give each other borderline illegal hugs and make our various ways home. Even with all the COVID restrictions, there'd been enough of a ceremony to qualify me for adoption as a Quebecker. We'd certainly all done the best we could, and I was glad the thing had happened. At the same time, like others I've read about who'd carried out other ceremonies such as weddings during the pandemic, I couldn't help feeling that something was missing. What was missing was the joyful noise that under normal circumstances would have been raised by the dozen or more additional friends in attendance; the laughter, the drinking songs, the clink of glasses, the added recitations and performances. And so, like the newly-married couple planning to repeat their vows in a second, far more public ceremony, I plan to do the same, when the pandemic has been licked to a sufficient extent to allow me to do so safely. Being adopted into a new province is a significant enough milestone in one's life that it deserves to be celebrated by *all* of one's family and close friends. And now that I know, I'll order a poutine with something other than that deadly brown gravy as a sauce. *A bientôt, mes amis!*

Gatineau, Quebec
March, 2021

SECTION 13

A Glimpse
of the
Future

SECTION 13

A Glimpse of the Future

What kind of future can we expect when the current COVID pandemic is finally behind us? The pieces in this section offer two quite different perspectives. In her short story, 'It's the Old World After All,' Ann McMillan paints a gloomy picture of a dystopian society dominated by sterile architecture and in which citizens are under near-constant surveillance. Then, in her short but intensely powerful poem, 'Quarantine 1,' Betsy Hoffman declines to commit to any particular vision of the future, ending the piece with a series of question marks which neatly sum up the uncertainty felt by so many of us as the third wave finally starts to recede.

It's the Old World After All
Ann McMillan

The squat grey building didn't resemble my mental image of a love nest at all, but perhaps that was for the best. As I strode purposefully through the shiny, metallic lobby and took the immaculate, mirrored elevator to the 6th floor, I felt, as always, the strum of the surfacing sexual excitement that had been bottled up inside of me. I'd always fought my sense of rebellion and suppressed my needs for physical contact, but it was a losing battle from the beginning, and like many ill-fated heroines before me I needed to live until I died.

The trip from the airport had been slow, but uneventful. The promises of intelligent, self-driving cars had taken decades longer than anticipated to be implemented; and although those cars were safe, they were pathetically slow. But at least one could relax inside and pay attention to a computer or phone without being on the alert for the approach of careening vehicles or squishy pedestrians. If there were delays, the pervasive drone system made sure that they were minimized by directing repair workers quickly to the points of congestion. Still, after my trip I was feeling my 60 years and more than ready for a few hours of more complete withdrawal from the pressures of 23rd century life.

Canada's big cities of the early 2200s appreciated high-rise, high-density living in a way that seemed incongruous given the national character, so long based on wide-open spaces and appreciation of nature. Nature, in this building, consisted of a few minute white spiders that scurried away, pale as ghosts, if they sensed a movement; they had probably fallen off the flowers in the lobby, the only other 'natural' presence in the space. Heaven knew what the spiders lived on in this barren, ultra-clean environment. The building was surrounded on three sides by towering behemoths of buildings topping 200 stories, and as a consequence, except in the middle of the day when sun seeped in from the south, which faced over the street, was perpetually in a state of twilight.

I opened Room 632 and entered, appreciating the wisps of sunlight that came in through the wide glass balcony door from the south. As I had done many times before, I quickly unpacked the basics, used the washroom, and scrubbed my hands before tapping lightly on the door interconnecting into Room 634. There was no answer, so I checked my phone, found no new messages, and sat back on the ultra-modern, uncomfortable sofa to wait, giving a small sigh of disappointment. After a few moments I got up, made myself a cup of disgusting coffee from the ultra-clean machine perched beside the TV and reached into my bag to pull out my latest old-fashioned book to read. Margaret Atwood from the 21st century had certainly had a vivid imagination, even if she had gotten it all so wrong. George Orwell had chronicled the subtle changes that infect a world that lives in fear. Aldous Huxley, ironically the first writer of the three, from the early 1900s, seemed to have a much better sense of where the world was really going to go in *Brave New World.* I was fascinated by the future, as seen from the past.

Some time went by as I quickly settled into my happy place to read. Suddenly, in horror, I realized that the light was waning and leapt up to tap on the interconnecting door again. Again, no answer. A wave of worry passed over me, and I began to analyze my situation. As a senior researcher with the government, I was exactly where I should be, when I should be. That was reassuring. After all, even with all the gigantic technological advances since the great C-19 depression, they couldn't read my mind. This was a government hotel and thus regularly swept for bugs of the electronic kind. Here, safely in my hotel room, the drone reconnaissance network could not video my doings as they were rumoured to be doing more or less constantly now. It was rumoured that the drones were being equipped with real-time equipment not only to record sounds from those within, but also to see through 'soft-sided' buildings, only kept from reconnaissance by steel and concrete. The young technocrats were beginning to flex their muscles in society by demonstrating what their modern technology could accomplish, and feeding rivers of streaming data into every vein of the bureaucracy.

The changes were pervasive. With the failure to assure immunity from the rapidly mutating virus, everyone had to be hypervigilant all the time to avoid catching the latest version of it. The shocked scientists had discovered that without the ability to develop effective antibodies by surviving a first attack or to stimulate the immune system with new immunizations, people always remained at risk of contacting the latest version of the virus. And it was a very smart virus, which now killed about 20% of the people it infected.

Isolation had ceased to be a short-term accommodation, necessary to prevent initial spread of the deadly disease, and had become a life sentence. Most young and healthy people could survive one attack, or even two, but the virus loadings in their bodies increased with each attack, and by the third or fourth attack the body's immune system collapsed and they drowned in their own leaking and bleeding lungs, with or without a respirator, often alone, save for health professionals completely swathed in protective clothing.

At first, while the search for a means of prevention, treatment or cure was new, there had been a sense of suppressed optimism as in 'We'll beat this thing.' Over decades that optimism had faded. The second baby boom, a product of those who had stayed at home for months in 2020 and lived to tell the tale, surpassed the prior generation of boomers in both numbers and sense of entitlement. Many of them died in childhood from the rapidly mutating virus. Those who lived risked their lives to meet, marry and procreate. The elderly died in droves and the mean age of the whole population dropped, arguably costing society the storehouse of wisdom that experience brings.

It was not immediately obvious, but urbanization became the way of least resistance. Controlled areas could be effectively sanitized, and infrastructure could be designed to support dense populations of people living alone. Toronto had responded by going up and up without increasing the size of the city boundary. Rural areas, with their dirt and animals, were swarming with virus, and if the disease was caught rurally there were no decent treatment facilities. The death rate in rural areas was over double that of the big, clean, well-planned cities.

Within these cities, rules were in place to control social gatherings of any kind. The short term became the long term. There was a move back towards families arranging marriages between couples that were deemed suitable. Courtship in these planned unions was physically distanced and expensive as the couple were quarantined closely and separately for a month before they were married. As the decades and generations went by, anything but virtual dating became a thing of the past; few would risk both the dangers of contracting the virus and the dangers of getting caught, which escalated as time passed. There were massive fines and even imprisonment for those found to be flouting the laws. The birth rate fell. And so it had gone for the past century.

The drones supporting the political regime had emerged as a source of fear in their role as electronic watchdogs. There had been rumours circulating that greater numbers of military men had been breaking the rules and taking their chances on finding their own women to be their lovers and the mothers of their children. There had also been a number of recent reports of men being shot for treason, although surely having a girlfriend could not be considered treason?

This was the world I had been born into, certainly new, but not very brave. I was healthy, single and intelligent, but came from a family that was not well-connected. My chances of finding a suitable and appealing husband to love were slim. My need to find a steady and well-paying job to support my aging parents was compelling.

I knocked again, with little hope, on the interconnecting door. Still no answer. My hands felt cold and numb and I stifled a little sob. Rick was my brave lover and friend whose stoic approach to the rigours of our stilted society was fulfilling our deepest needs to be touched and held. Without doubt, his support had enabled me to maintain my successful career in which I studied the impacts of our current situation and advised my superiors on a path forward. Speaking truth to power had never been trickier, and the stress of my job often tore at me. Rick was a military man to the core and had the scars to prove it. He was, conveniently, required to be at the same face-to-face top-secret meeting that I was at, once a month. Was I in love with Rick? Maybe.

My mind skimmed over the years since we had met, accidentally, at the coffee machine. With my usual grace and skill, I had allowed my coffee to overflow my cup and cascade onto the pristine counter. I turned abruptly to reach for the special cleaners that were pervasively available close by every such machine, and ran smack into physical distancing Rick, who had his back turned and was closing in on the spot that I should have vacated by now. There was a bolt of electricity between us that could have short-circuited Toronto. Fortunately, no one but us noticed it. He turned and smiled and backed off. And what a smile!

The next day, a classified e-mail had appeared, asking me for some information about numbers of cases and trends and such, and when would I be at that coffee machine again? I responded that I attended the monthly meeting regularly and would be back the following month. That month, when I arrived at the squat grey building, I was put on the 6th floor in room 632 and had been registered in that room every month thereafter. There had been a knock at the interconnecting door, I had opened it, and there stood Rick in nothing but a towel. He smiled and swept me into a much-too-close hug. I knew he felt the magic, too, as we both retreated to his room.

We talked, we showered, we tentatively touched one another. We explored, we kissed and we made passionate love for most of the night. I was afraid the next morning that when I entered the meeting room the glow would blind everyone there and announce clearly that I had had the time of my life, but it was not so. No one noticed, and so the next month we did it again, and the next, and the next, and the next. I never knew how Rick managed to get rooms 632 and 634 every month, and it seemed like the sort of question that shouldn't be asked. If Rick had a fault, and he didn't have many, it was that he would stonewall over certain questions or directions of conversation. His warm smile and open arms were all the answers I would get. I knew that he was in military security so I never pushed. For years it was enough to be in his arms one night a month.

In the small hours of the morning, I gave up. I climbed into the bed that I had never actually slept in before and sobbed myself to sleep. My mind played out every awful thing that could have happened to Rick. We had been so careful and had never given any indication of our relationship outside of these two rooms. As we approached retirement age, we had wondered what to do.

The alarm went off and I struggled out of bed to have the requisite sterilizing shower and put on my clean clothes and drink another cup of vile coffee before going to the meeting. I knocked for a last time at the interconnecting door. No answer. I threw back the curtains and took my cup onto my balcony to 'underlook' the city, with the towering buildings surrounding me on all sides except the street side to the south. I noticed that this side of the building was fitted with some sort of flying panels to protect it from the strong southern sun, scorching hot in the summer. In their midst, tangled, there was a drone.

There was a loud knock at my door as I took in the meaning of the trapped drone, antennae still very much alive, swinging gently from its entanglement above the next balcony, the one connected to room 634. As it swung south-south-west, south, south-east I knew my life would be another COVID casualty.

Quarantine 1
Betsy Hoffman

Inside
Safe
Outside
Danger
Ever
Safe
Outside?
2021
?
?
?
?

Coda

Jon Peirce

For me, the pandemic ended just as it had begun—with some heavy-duty socializing. The main difference was that while at the beginning the socializing was done with theatre people, as you may recall from my First Wave piece, this time most of it was done with fellow almanac contributors and workers.

On Saturday, July 10, co-editor Ann McMillan and I enjoyed a tasty lunch under the grape arbour of publisher Bob Barclay, the gracious host for the event along with his wife, Janet. That evening, I enjoyed a patio supper at the home of short-form poet and almanac contributor Elena Calvo, who lives just 15 minutes away from me, in the Hull section of Gatineau. The next morning (Sunday), I watched the Wimbledon men's singles finals with my landlord and next-door neighbour Joe Michel and his girlfriend, Sylvie Brunet. As we watched Novak Djokovic get past the Italian, Matteo Berrettini, we ate a sausage, pancake, and fruit cup brunch prepared by Sylvie and yours truly. Then, after a walk—needed to burn off some of those pancakes and sausages—it was out to Ann's wooded country estate in Stittsville for a scrumptious supper of vegetarian moussaka, accompanied by Greek salad and red wine and followed by cheesecake. So little time. So much good food.

I did nearly as much socializing during this two-day weekend as I had during the entire five-and-a-half months between the start of the pandemic and my departure from Nova Scotia at the end of August. I definitely had a purpose in mind when I 'loaded up' the weekend as I did: to signal both to myself and to others my return to some kind of normal life. And there was definitely something celebratory about it all. But unlike the kind of celebratory socializing that (people tell me, and I have read) accompanied the end of the Second World War, there was nothing frenetic going on here. No fireworks, no whiskey bottles, no dancing or singing or shouting late into the night. At each of my 'stops,' I drank quite moderately (or, in the case of the Sunday brunch, not at all, since we had coffee with our pancakes). I didn't feel I needed to drink all that much. Being in the company of interesting, intelligent people was stimulation enough.

Again, quite deliberately, I did virtually no work, on the almanac or anything else, for the entire weekend. About the only almanac-related work I did was to look over some sample chapters and tables that Bob had prepared, to see if I liked the format. But whatever I'd done or not done, it seems to have worked for me. In the past, when I had done this much socializing in a short period, I'd usually ended up exhausted, often having to spend all or at least part of the next day in bed. This time, instead of being exhausted, I felt energized. After returning from Ann's at around 8:00 p.m., I sat down and read the last quarter of an amazing novel by Chinese/American writer Amy Tan, *The Kitchen God's Wife*. This saga, spanning five and a half decades in the lives of a Chinese/American mother and daughter, from the mid-1930s to 1990, I've found inspirational. Indeed, I think it has a lot to offer today's readers trying to come to grips with our own situation; however bad a time any of us has had, Winnie (the novel's chief protagonist) had it 10 times worse during the war years and early post-war years in China, before finally escaping to the U.S. in 1949.

In short, the weekend had been the best of all possible bookends.

And it gets better. To my amazement and delight, though I'd stayed up quite late finishing *The Kitchen God's Wife* and then sending e-mails to friends, I awoke early this morning (before 7:00) full of ideas for new writing projects, most of which I immediately jotted down. (Could there really have been three pages of those ideas?) Since childhood, my natural rhythm has been that of the morning person, awaking full of creative energy. But during the past 16 months, when I was working all but non-stop, first on the 'Plague Journal' I kept in Nova Scotia, but since December on the almanac, I've gotten away from that natural rhythm, often staying up far too late watching televised sports, a way of winding down from the day, and then not being able to get going until 10:00 a.m., or sometimes even noon. To say that this did not do wonders for my sleep pattern is to understate things considerably.

Today, sipping my morning coffee at the kitchen table and watching three sparrows lined up on a tree limb right outside the kitchen window, shyly observing me, I felt as if I'd come home. The frenetic, almost factory-like pace I've kept up since March of 2020 can finally come to an end, with the completion of this almanac. I can write about the things I want to write about at my own pace. And yes, although I'm already starting to write about other things, I will still sometimes write about COVID, because it is still the 'biggest game in town' and is likely to be through the rest of my life, if not my children's. And I will still write very, very fast by most people's standards, because that is my natural pace when I'm writing well. But no longer will I feel *driven* to write, as I have been throughout the COVID pandemic—driven by my sense that the public needs to hear the whole COVID story, from as many different perspectives as possible, the presentation of which has been our aim throughout this project. With the pandemic apparently licked, at least in Quebec, and the almanac virtually completed, I have done my duty and can now return to 'civilian' life. All sorts of possibilities loom in the future, from new essay books and memoirs to more plays. And speaking of plays, theatre is coming back in West Quebec, and there are again plays to audition for. And there is Lac Leamy to swim in, as well as walk beside, and the restaurants are again open for indoor dining. And who knows but that by the end of the Summer it may even be possible to go down to Maine to see my aging relatives…

In this vale of tears, a person can't ask for much more. Thank you, dear readers, for sticking with us throughout this long and sometimes tortuous journey. As exciting as all this has been, I can't help hoping that in the future we may all live in less interesting times. If nothing else, this pandemic should have served to show us that normalcy does have its virtues!

J.P.
Gatineau, July 12, 2021

About our
Contributors

Peter Alexander completed a PhD in musicology at Indiana University. He is a retired staff member and adjunct assistant professor of music at the University of Iowa, where he was director of media relations for all the arts organizations on campus for 23 years. He has also worked as a music critic and church choir director. In 2009 he retired and moved to Colorado, where he plays clarinet in two community bands and writes classical music stories for *Boulder Weekly* and his own blog:

sharpsandflatirons.com

John Kevin Allen is an author and hospital chaplain living near St. Louis, Missouri with his wife Carole. His work can be found in *Broadview*, the magazine of the United Church of Canada, and in the *Chicken Soup for the Soul* series. He is an ordained minister in the United Church of Christ and a ministry partner with the United Church of Canada.

Jacqueline L. (Jackie) Amable was born in Niagara Falls, Ontario, raised in Northern Ontario, and in later years settled in Toronto. At 23 years of age, she drove transport from Edmonton, Alberta to Yellowknife, North West Territories, the only woman team driving the North at that time. For 30 years she was an Employment Standards Officer with the Ontario Ministry of Labour, investigating and resolving complaints under the Employment Standards Act, beginning in Northern Ontario and then in later years in Mississauga, Ontario, where she now resides. She retired to care for her elderly brother and mother, now both deceased, and is currently a Forex and Crypto trader.

Sally Arsove was born and raised in the U.S.A (mostly) and ended up in Ottawa in 1975, after a year of volunteer teaching in Ethiopia followed by a year studying at the London School of Economics. Sally is a citizen of both Canada and the U.S.A., and her two adult children now both live and work on the U.S. side of the border. Sally worked for many years as an Economist for the Government of Canada in the field of international development and finance. After retiring in 2007, she earned a bookkeeping certificate and now works part-time helping young companies get their businesses going. Sally enjoys the beauty of nature, gardening and outdoor exercise (especially swimming, biking, and cross-country skiing), sewing, and connecting with friends and family. Sally has continued to volunteer in the health care sector and for local poverty reduction organizations.

Robert Barclay was born in London, England in 1946. He received a Certificate in Science Laboratory Technology from the City and Guilds of London Institute (1968). After graduating from the University of Toronto with a Bachelor's Degree in Fine Arts (1975), he went on to earn an inter-disciplinary PhD at the Open University in the U.K. (1999). He has worked as a museum object restorer and musical instrument maker, and conducts trumpet-making workshops in Europe and the United States. He has published extensively in the fields of museum conservation, musical instrument making, music history and fiction. He runs a small publishing company, Loose Cannon Press, assisting first-time authors in preparing their works for publication.

Elizabeth Barnes has been writing for as long as she has been reading. She is mother to nine and grandmother to four, with another on the way. In addition to running Grandma School, Elizabeth enjoys her job at a learning centre, reading, cooking, baking, and dragon boating.

Taiya Barss immigrated to Nova Scotia in 1973 and lived in Cape Breton for 25 years. Since 1998, she has lived in Halifax. She was born in Boston, so she will always be a Come-From-Away, despite the fact that her grandfather was from Dartmouth, and one of her two sons was born in Cape Breton. Her favourite ancestor is her grandfather's great-grandfather, the notorious privateer, Captain Joseph Barss. He sailed out of Liverpool and during the War of 1812 captured Yankee ships in Boston Harbour and brought them back to Halifax as war prizes. Taiya attended Antioch College in Ohio, but after too many classes in algebra, trigonometry, chemistry and biology, she decided a career in science wasn't what she wanted. She transferred to the School of the Boston Museum of Fine Arts, where she majored in printmaking. After graduation, she turned to painting, and has been pursuing that ever since, working in oil, acrylic, and water colour.

Debra Bertrand was raised on a dairy farm in Carleton Township, living in the surrounding area for most of her life, but has settled in the town of Arnprior, Ontario for the past 20-plus years. She raised four beautiful children with her husband John, and worked as an Administrative Assistant in Arnprior for 40 years. Debra has been retired for the past four years, enjoying being part of her grandchildren's lives, and living life to the fullest by keeping healthy and active.

Valerie Buko is a teacher and writer in Ottawa. She is the author of a number of children's picture books, such as *Ella Learns English, Summer Olympic Athletes* and *Hockey for All of My Life*. She is currently focusing on writing adult fiction. Valerie is a board member of Ottawa Independent Writers (OIW).

Elena Calvo is a teacher, psychologist, writer, poet and amateur photographer who lives in Gatineau, Quebec. She started journaling and writing poetry at a very young age in her native Spain. Her writing consists mostly of Japanese poetic forms (tanka, haiku and senryu) and also includes lyric and micro-poetry, aphorisms, essays and inner sketches. Her main interest and influence is mystic writing. She enjoys languages, has collaborated in public/collective readings in Ottawa, and has done occasional articles, editing, translations and book reviews in both English and Spanish. Her work has appeared in print and online in different anthologies in Canada, England and the US, among others: *AHG-A Hundred Gourds, GUSTS-Tanka Canada, HC-Haiku Canada, In-Between Two Worlds, Inkstone, KaDo Ottawa, MB-Moonbathing, NeverEndingStory, OCWG-Ottawa Creative Writers' Group, OIW-Ottawa Independent Writers, Wah Journal;* and the following anthology books: *Gift of Silence, Harvest, Painting Sunlight, The Sea Replied* and *Sage.*

Rodney Clough lives in Sawyer, Michigan where with his wife, interior decorator, Linda Jo Clough, he owns and operates a vacation property rental. Both also maintain a residence in Chicago's Uptown neighborhood. Previously, Rodney was Adjunct Professor at Columbia College in Chicago. He is a frequent contributor to *Medium*, the online journal, where he writes on political discourse, climate justice and the media:
https://link.medium.com/HwQJKhVrifb

Brent P. D. Coates was raised in rural and smalltown settings and was first introduced to urban living in his late 20s; he now lives in the Bells Corners community of Ottawa. His academic studies in forestry, agriculture and physical geography were ideal for his career with the Canadian Federal National Parks Agency. One of Brent's passions has been the Royal Oaks tree project, which was initiated and funded by the United Nations in the late 1990s. Brent continues to support the principles of this project by planting and nurturing the tri-centennial giants of the Great Lakes forest. A number of these magnificent Red and White Oak tree species, planted by Brent, are located along the Trans-Canada Trail. Some of Brent's most pleasurable pastimes are exploring the urban, rural and woodland areas of the country. He has investigated all the Ghost towns, abandoned rail lines and navigable water routes within a 150 km radius of Ottawa. Contact him at:
brentpdcoates@gmail.com

Dianna Davison-Veber is a lifelong learner, mother of two, and retired executive administrative assistant who has a jest for life. She is a lover of music, a teller of jokes and a renowned punster. Above all, she's a perceptive observer of life, and someone who takes her own path, while caring for those around her. She is highly valued for her subtle, behind-the-scenes contributions to her local Seniors' College.

Sasha Dominique is a graduate of the National Theatre School of Canada, in the French Interpretation section. Since 1992, she has been seen in various theatre productions, mostly in French, produced in Ottawa, Gatineau and Montreal, some of which have toured across the provinces of Ontario and Quebec. She won the award *Prix d'excellence artistique de Théâtre Action* in 2004, as well as the *Prix Rideau Award Interprète féminine de l'année* in

2010. She translated and performed the solo play *The Syringa Tree* written by the South-African author Pamela Gien (*Le lilas africain*) in 2016. The play was produced by Le Théâtre de Dehors at La Nouvelle Scène Gilles Desjardins in Ottawa 2016 and 2019, and also went to Nunavut the same year. She performed at the Gladstone in the play *The Ugly One* presented by Plosive Productions, in October 2019.

Sasha has written and performed four solo shows, for both adult and juvenile audiences. During the pandemic, she has written a children's story, *La cachette de Marie-Lune*, which can be found on YouTube, and which she aims to adapt into a comic book in 2021. She is also the Artistic Director of the Théâtre AROBAS, a theatre company for elders. In addition, she is an animator, teacher, director, singer, poet, and coach for students seeking to enter specialized theatre school.

Claude Ethier, the creator of our frontpage art, is a former Canadian diplomat who now resides in North Bay, where he dabbles in art and photography.

Kathy Figueroa is a Canadian poet, photographer, freelance writer and indie publisher who resides in the beautiful town of Bancroft, in the northern part of Hastings County, Ontario. The Internet reaches all parts of the globe and, as a result, so do Kathy's often funny and irreverent poems, though some have a more serious tone. Her versified views of the world can also be found in numerous hard-copy publications, such as newspapers, magazines, dozens of anthologies, and her five published collections: *Paudash Poems, Flowertopia, The Cathedral of the Eternal Blue Sky, The Ballad of the PoeTrain Poeteer: Winnipeg to Vancouver,* and *The Renaissance of Rhyme.* (These books include her poems that have been published well over 100 times in the Bancroft newspapers.) In addition, Kathy's short play, *Conflicted About the Wolf,* was staged in Bancroft in 2012. To date, Kathy has created six literary events, including four *The Word Is Wild Literary Festivals,* and many open mic evenings. She founded the *Poets' Society of Hastings County North* in 2010, which met regularly prior to the pandemic, and continues to share poetry-related information via Facebook. For many years, Kathy was also involved with various aspects of film production, and, for two years, was Poetry Editor of the Quinte Arts Council publication, *Umbrella.* In 2018, she registered a small press, *Flowertopia Studio,* which publishes the work of Canadian poets.

Julie Fortin a étudié en Travail social à Université du Québec à Chicoutimi. Elle s'établit à Gatineau en 2019. Elle déploie ses efforts auprès de la clientèle aînée du secteur Hull avec les Logements de l'Outaouais. En tant qu'intervenante de milieu du programme ITMAV, elle tente de rejoindre les personnes âgées ayant besoin d'aide et désirant être accompagnées dans leurs démarches et soutenues pour trouver les ressources répondant à leurs besoins.

Julie Fortin is a Social Work graduate from Université du Québec in Chicoutimi. In 2019 she moved to Gatineau where she found employment as a community intervention worker for the ITMAV program (acronym of a Québec government initiative to improve the quality of life of senior citizens). Her attention and efforts are centered on providing advice and support to seniors living in the Hull sector of Gatineau, including the residents of Logements de l'Outaouais where her office is located, in their attempts to find resources and services they are in need of.

Denise Giroux is a lawyer with more than 32 years' experience as a champion for underdogs, having practiced in the areas of poverty law, family and general litigation, and labour law, with a strong focus on human rights. She recently retired from working for a federal public service union in Ottawa, and is now trying to make plans for the rest of her life in this second summer of pandemic-living. She resides in the Gatineau hills in Cantley, Québec.

Jeanette Grant was born in Nova Scotia in 1942, and now lives in Arnprior. She married in 1966 and is the mother of two and grandmother of three. Jeanette was a teacher by trade and taught in five provinces. She went back to school and graduated with her MA in 1993 from the University of Guelph. An early breast cancer survivor, Jeanette was one of the core group that initiated the Breast Cancer Survivor Dragon Boat Team, the Prior Chest Nuts. Now living with ALS, Jeanette has been thankful to contribute.

Bill Hartman retired after an extensive career in financial services. He engaged in corporate finance, investment banking, and investor relations principally at Merrill Lynch, J.P. Morgan, and Citibank where he focused on financial services companies. Years ago, he self-published *The Link*, a novel about a financial consultant saving the world. Hartman served in the United States Marine Corps and graduated from Yale University with a degree in economics. He and his wife Marilyn live in Austin, Texas. They have two sons and enjoy art.

Ruth Hawkins is a Registered Psychotherapist based in Ottawa, Ontario. Prior to starting her private practice, Ruth was a dedicated senior-level civil servant for the federal government of Canada for 33 years, retiring in 2016. As a mother and grandmother herself, Ruth approaches each client with compassion, honesty, and humour. She believes that by making sense of our past, we can all find peace in our future.

Elizabeth (Betsy) Hoffman is a professor of economics at Iowa State University, where she previously served as Executive Vice President and Provost. From 2000 to 2005, she was President of the University of Colorado System, where she is President Emerita. Her published research is in the areas of

Experimental Economics, Cliometrics, and Behavioral Economics. Hoffman was born in Bryn Mawr, Pennsylvania in 1946, the maternal granddaughter of Andre Kalpaschnikoff, who had escaped the Russian Revolution. She was raised in Wayne, Pennsylvania and in nearby Berwyn, graduating from Conestoga High School in 1964. She then attended Smith College, intending to become a music teacher, but a very low grade in music theory convinced her she would do better in another field. She wound up receiving a BA in history in 1968. An astronomy course she took at Smith had a happier outcome; it led to a lifelong passion for the subject. After graduating from Smith, Hoffman received an MA in history from the University of Pennsylvania in 1969, a PhD in history from the University of Pennsylvania in 1972, and a PhD in social science (economics) from the California Institute of Technology in 1979. While finishing her PhD at Penn, she taught history and economics at St Olaf College, Carleton College, and Macalester College. After completing her PhD in history, she was an assistant professor of history at the University of Florida, but was recruited for one of the first classes of economics PhD students at the California Institute of Technology. She then became assistant professor of economics at Northwestern University, assistant and associate professor of economics at Purdue University, and professor of economics at the University of Wyoming and professor of economics and law at the University of Arizona.

Hoffman has been a member of numerous boards, including the board of trustees of her alma mater, Smith College, the National Science Board, and a number of international astronomy boards. She is married to fellow economist Brian R. Binger and lives in Ames, Iowa.

Bill Horne was born in Windsor, Ontario and attended University of Windsor for both undergrad and grad study in Political Science and Economics. He worked for Bell Canada, Nortel, and Foreign Affairs for some 49 years. His love of English started early in life, when he was asked by his public-school principal to teach a Chinese newcomer to Canada 'Everything you know about English.' He eventually became a member of Ottawa Independent Writers, where he met Jon Peirce, succeeding him as President. For a few years he was a freelance writer and editor. He is now happily retired in London, Ontario and enjoys volunteer editing for organizations such as the Architectural Conservancy of Ontario and Turtle Guardians. Bill and his partner Elizabeth volunteer at Fanshawe Pioneer Village. Two memorable moments were establishing the Terry Fox Run in Bogota, Colombia, and travelling the world with Dr Theresa Tam of the Public Health Agency of Canada in the fight against the H1N1 pandemic. A former marathon runner, Bill now derives great pleasure from serving on the Terry Fox Run London committee and from finding typos in *The Economist* magazine.

Neven Humphrey is a Gatineau-based writer specializing in furry literature, i.e., stories where the characters are animals that walk and talk like humans. But he has other interests, too: indeed, he has written two books of editorials (with a third on the way), and is also writing a book on Canada's 100 deadliest disasters of the 20th century. And when he's not writing, he's reading, watching movies and taking long walks in Gatineau Park.

Georgia Johnson was born in Halifax, Nova Scotia. She worked as a secretary and eventually married Art Johnson, who was a member of the Royal Canadian Air Force. His career included lots of travel in Canada and a four-year posting in Germany. During their posting in Comox, British Columbia, Georgia obtained an honours certificate in Early Childhood Education and worked in that field until her retirement in 1999. After Art's retirement in 2006, they moved back to Nova Scotia, where she continues to live today. A lady of faith, she devotes herself to her church and family.

Ian Johnson retired in 2015 from the Nova Scotia Government and General Employees Union after serving 20 years as a policy analyst/researcher/communications coordinator. He has also worked with the Nova Scotia Provincial Health Council, the Nova Scotia NDP Caucus, and the City of Halifax's Social Planning Department. Outside of work, Ian served as a director with two Nova Scotia pension boards. He has also been active with the Seniors' College Association of Nova Scotia, the Nova Scotia Health Coalition, and the Nova Scotia Office of the Canadian Centre for Policy Alternatives. He is married, lives in Halifax, and has a stepdaughter and two sons.

Lee Keener was born in 1945 and received a BA from Amherst College in 1967 and a doctoral degree in mathematics from Rensselaer Polytechnic Institute in 1972. He has held academic appointments at Dalhousie University, Indiana University at South Bend, and the University of Northern British Columbia, and has also taught at the University of Waterloo, the University of Oregon and the University of Alberta. He is now retired and lives with his wife and daughter on Nukko Lake, outside Prince George, British Columbia.

Marcia Brumit Kropf, PhD, is retired after a long career in the non-profit sector as an educator, researcher, and senior executive, working to change the world for women and girls. Currently, she serves on the board of directors of the Children's Art Guild, a non-profit organization working with educators, students, and parents to create transformative learning environments where every child is able to embrace the value of their own experiences. She lives with her husband, Roger, in New York City, not far from her two adult children and their families, including four amazing and delightful grandchildren.

Jany Lavoie, native de l'Outaouais, au Québec, elle a aussi vécu à Montréal, La Pocatière et Vancouver. Elle a gagne sa vie avec les mots, comme professeure de français et correctrice d'épreuves, pour se retrouver maintenant en République démocratique du Congé, c'est-à-dire à la retraite ! Depuis le bacc. en arts visuels, Jany a toujours maintenu une pratique artistique, que ce soit en danse, en musique, en écriture, en multi média ou en peinture. En cette année de COVID, elle a trouvé beaucoup d'apaisement à fréquenter la nature, lors de randonnées qui lui permettaient aussi de voir ses ami-e-s.

Jany Lavoie is a native of the Outaouais region of Quebec, who has also lived in Montreal, La Pocatière, and Vancouver. She earned her living with words, as a French teacher and proof-reader, and is presently enjoying retirement. Since graduating with a Visual Arts degree, Jany has maintained an artistic practice, including dance, music, writing, multimedia and painting. During this pandemic year, she found peace in nature, taking long walks that have also allowed her to connect with friends.

Paul Lenarczyk is a proud Polish-Canadian teacher, writer, performer and arts advocate. Growing up in Fredericton, New Brunswick, he fell in love with musical theatre, Celtic music, and the performing arts in general. Since obtaining three degrees from the city's two universities, including one of the first ever Fine Arts Minors in Creative Writing awarded by the University of New Brunswick, he has continued to write, teach, and perform. After a 14-year teaching career in public schools in New Brunswick, he moved to Halifax, Nova Scotia with his wife Karen and daughter Daniella in 2016. Paul is an active member of the Polish community in Nova Scotia and avid performer in online kitchen parties for now, but hopefully will soon be performing live with friends and extended family around the country.

Alan Lennon is a retired trade union representative and activist. After stints teaching philosophy and then working as an immigration officer, he joined the Canada Employment and Immigration Union (PSAC) where he was on staff for about 25 years. In that role, he wrote for a variety of magazines and journals as well as developing and delivering labour education courses. In his retirement, he divides his time between Toronto and Gatineau and pursues interests in labour history and social theory. He looks forward to being able to travel and photograph the world again.

Catherine A. (Cathy) MacKenzie's writings have been published in numerous print and online publications. She has also published several short story collections, books of poetry, and children's picture books. She published her first novel, *Wolves Don't Knock,* in 2018. *Mister Wolfe* (the second in the series) appeared in 2020. *My Brother, the Wolf,* the final volume, will be available in 2022. She lives in West Porters Lake, Nova Scotia, Canada. Reach

out to her, check her website and follow her on Facebook at:
    writingwicket@gmail.com
    www.writingwicket.wordpress.com
    https://www.facebook.com/cathy.mackenzie.790

Suha (Su) Mardelli is an emerging writer from Ottawa who traded her well-trodden corporate high-heels to spend a year writing in Birkenstocks. She spent twenty-two years living in Dubai, surrounded by accents in English, and draws on her experiences as an entrepreneur, an award-winning business executive, and 'love of listening to people' to produce thought-provoking stories. She is currently photographing food for her new cookbook and writing her first novel. At one point she wrote stories about food, recipes included, on her blog:
    www.papergrape.com

Christopher Millard is principal bassoonist with Canada's National Arts Centre Orchestra. He has enjoyed a long and varied musical career as a performer and educator in both Canada and the U.S.A. He created the NAC's first classical musical podcast, writing and producing over 60 hours of eclectic programs. He is currently completing a book on woodwind acoustics. Although he can produce good sourdough bread and a reasonable demi-glace, his lifelong interest in physics is currently stalled by the confusing implications of quantum loop gravity theory.

Susan Mills lives in Arnprior and is a policy analyst in real life. She loves analyzing the pros and cons of various issues. Being an essential caregiver to her mom led her into becoming an outspoken critic of long-term care policies which separate loved ones from their support systems. Susan loves dragon boating and cannot wait for the day she is back on the water. You can follow Susan and read her views on:
    twitter @Priorhockey

Gavin Murphy is an Ottawa lawyer and legal editor of the *Commonwealth Law Bulletin* in London. He is also a member of the Rockcliffe Lawn Tennis Club and is always looking for games.

Colleen Naomi has been involved in theatre for 30 years. Her early start at the age of seven launched a life-long love of the performing arts. Over the years she has been involved as actor, director, and script writer, and has toured two of her original shows. In 2010 her focus became offering theatre camps for children and youth. Colleen has been Artistic Director for South Shore Players since 2016 and now teaches regular online theatre workshop for adults. She lives in Nova Scotia with her children, her partner, his children, and seven adorable pets. You can read more about Colleen and her theatre projects at:
    PlaysOnStage.ca

457

Bill Newmann as a child liked to take splinters out of his family members' fingers, so naturally he wound up pursuing a career in family medicine. However, this route was a crooked one in that his college experience directed him more toward the liberal arts, given the competitive nature of those grinding away with pre-med courses. So, he joined the Peace Corps serving in Côte d'Ivoire (during the late 60s) on a mobile health education team, hoping someday to return as a 'real doctor.' Then, when his brother's kidneys failed, gritting his teeth, he took pre-med courses, intending at first to become a dialysis technician, but then got his medical training at an enlightened university in Ohio that valued his work experience and became a 'womb to tomb' family doctor. After 40-plus years practicing in Olympia, Washington, he 'retired' and now assists the terminally ill who wish to have the choice of medical aid in dying under that state's Death with Dignity Act. He maintains his interest in the French language and his friends and family, from North America to Europe and Africa.

Fran Ota is an ordained minister with The United Church of Canada. Born in Canora, Saskatchewan in 1946 into a minister's family, she grew up in the church, and in many parts of Canada. In 1970 she received a Bachelor of Music Performance from the University of Manitoba, and went to Japan as Overseas Personnel with The United Church of Canada. In 1971 she married her language teacher, Norio Ota. Together they travelled and worked in Việt Nam, New Jersey, Australia and Michigan, and in 1984 settled in Toronto. Fran has worked in refugee services, medical research, administration, and as a church musician. In 1995 she received a Master of Divinity from the University of Toronto, and has served in various churches in Ontario, as well as in Corner Brook, Newfoundland. She is currently taking a joint Master's Degree at the University of Iceland and University of Oslo, in Viking and Medieval Norse Studies. Fran and Norio have four grown children and four grandchildren, and love looking after their homes in Toronto and in Kamakura, Japan as well as partial retirement in Portugal.

Donald Oluf Peirce, an identical twin, was born in 1939 in Boulder, Colorado. His parents moved to the Philadelphia area in 1945, residing in Wayne, Pennsylvania for his growing-up years. He graduated from Radnor High School in 1958, and in 1960 attended Drexel Institute of Technology. After a stint in the Marine Corps from 1963 to 1968, Mr Peirce matriculated at Temple University and graduated with a BS in Elementary Education. In 1978 he received his MEd in Elementary Education as well as certification as a Reading Specialist to teach K-12. After teaching at Bartram High School from 1975 to 1980, he obtained a job at Locke Elementary School as Reading/English Language Arts teacher, remaining there from 1980 through his retirement in 2001.

On his retirement, Mr Peirce entered the Bryn Mawr Music Conservatory to pursue studies in composition, theory, and performance. During his seven years there, he was able to compose 20 classical music compositions and have two of them performed locally. A CD was made of other live performances at the Conservatory. Now in his 80s, he is pursuing various writing projects, one of which is a memoir of his teaching career. He hopes to have the 300 page-plus book completed this year.

Jim Pellegrin is a retired family practice doctor who lives in Point Reyes Station, California with his wife, Sally Jones, and five chickens, a lucky rooster and four hens. Dr Pellegrin has turned to quackery in recent years, and doles out idiotic advice to gullible hypochondriacs under the appropriate *nom de plume* of Dr Quackinthebush.

Camille Pellerin-Forget est physiothérapeute en réadaptation pédiatrique au CISSS de l'Outaouais, Gatineau. Elle a été délestée en zone chaude d'une ressource intermédiaire pour aînés en mai-juin 2020, afin de prêter main forte l'au moment d'une éclosion massive.

Camille Pellerin-Forget is a pediatric physiotherapist at CISSS Outaouais, in Gatineau. In May to June 2020, she was sent to an intermediate resource for seniors, in the red zone, where there was a massive COVID outbreak.

Jim Petrie is a versatile, soon-to-be 63-year-old who follows his passions. Lately he has been dabbling in Stand-Up Comedy at the *Comedy Cove* in Dartmouth, Nova Scotia, and he absolutely loves to hear people laugh at what he says. He is part of a growing demographic, the working retired, by driving an Access a Bus, delivering challenged adults to their jobs. He lives with his beautiful wife Cheryl and their golden retriever Lily, in Middle Sackville, Nova Scotia.

Teresa Patterson is an adult graduate of the Theatre Studies Program at Acadia University and has been involved with live theatre for many years and has worn all the hats. Most recently, Teresa started taking part in on-line courses conducted in lieu of being able to partake in live theatre due to COVID. In one of these courses, Playwriting was the topic and Teresa was hooked. She appreciates the opportunity to have contributed in some small way to this anthology and looks forward to seeing it published.

Paul W. Pickering is one of those quiet folks who happen to have great stories. He listens, appreciates and tries to make the world a more compass-sionate place by relating instances where our humanity shines through. Employed by Immigrant Services Association of Nova Scotia, Paul co-ordinates the Workplace Culture Program, working with employers to attract, retain and promote immigrants while addressing racism and other forms of discrimination. He has worked on filmsets, provided voiceover for documentaries and ads, sung amateur opera in the USSR, lived, worked and traveled through Asia, Europe and North America and 'performs' regularly through his online and onsite workshops. He shares his life in South Shore Nova Scotia with his partner (also in this almanac), her children, his children and various mini creatures they call pets. 'Long-Term Perspective' in this almanac is his first script.

Yves Rochon lives in Gatineau, Québec. He worked for close to 24 years as a labour relations officer and union educator for federal public service employees' unions, until his retirement in 2017. In June 2019, he resumed working for a not-for-profit organization, Logements de l'Outaouais, which provides affordable housing to approximately 150 elderly persons. At the time of writing this note, the end of March 2021, he still worked, part-time, for Logements de l'Outaouais, where to that point, none of the residents had been diagnosed with COVID.

Résident de Gatineau, Yves Rochon a travaillé pendant près de 24 ans à titre d'agent de relations de travail et de formateur pour le compte de syndicats de la fonction publique fédérale jusqu'au moment de sa retraite en 2017. En juin 2019, il a recommencé à travailler cette fois pour un organisme sans but lucratif, Logements de l'Outaouais, qui offre des logements abordables à environ 150 personnes âgées. Au moment d'écrire cette note, aucun-e des résident-e-s n'avait obtenu un diagnostic de COVID.

Jagjeet Sharma, a Kemptville resident, is a freelance journalist, poet and author. She hosts a weekly radio show in Ottawa along with her team of dedicated volunteers on CKCU 93.1fm. She has three collections of poems to her credit, including *Nature's Subtle Seductions* (2018) and *Fragments* (2019). *Raindrops*, her third collection, was launched in June 2020. The limited edition *COVID-19 Chronicles: Reflections on the 2020 pandemic* was published in November 2020 and launched the following month. Jagjeet has also contributed to several publications, including the Ottawa Independent Writers' anthology, *Short Stories for a Long Year* (2020); Broken Keys publishing anthology, *Love & Catastrophē Poetrē*, (June 2021); *The Glebe Report*; and *Canadian Literature: A Quarterly of Criticism and Review* (UBC, June 2021).

David Shaw graduated from the Ontario College of Art in 1969. He worked at McClelland & Stewart as a book designer and illustrator. In 1977, he started his own design company, which continues to this day. In 1985 he designed the first edition of Hurtig Publishers' *Canadian Encyclopedia*. He will be getting his second Pfizer shot later this June.

Ralph F. Smith has had a lifelong interest in writing historical literature. He wrote MA and PhD dissertations on Charles Dickens, the latter on Dickens's representation of epidemics. He also completed a two-year novel-writing certificate program from Stanford University. He has had numerous poems and prose pieces published, including the fantasy novel *Bright Deep*

(2013) and a mystery novel set in 1868, *Concession Street Secrets* (2019). His current project is a novel about the Trek to Ottawa and the Regina Riot of 1935. He lives in Ottawa with his wife, Dr Fionnuala O'Kelly and family.

Jo-Anne Stead grew up in Thunder Bay, but is now an Ottawa-based writer, who started her career as a newspaper reporter before moving on to explore other career paths in the construction industry and the federal public service. Recently retired, she's spending more time on writing in a variety of formats, including short stories, memoir and freelance articles. She likes the outdoors (when it's nice) and enjoys skiing, biking, and kayaking.

Harold Tausch is a professional actor, voice actor, and dancer and an amateur singer/songwriter based in Toronto. He is also a Feldenkrais practitioner and maintains a parttime practice, helping people to improve the quality of their movements. You can follow his performing arts adventures here:
https://www.imdb.com/name/nm10674878/?ref_=fn_al_nm_1
You can find out more about his Feldenkrais practice here:
https://www.feldenkraisintoronto.ca

Rowena Torrevillas is a Filipina poet, essayist and fiction writer who lives in Iowa City, Iowa with her husband, Lemuel.

Elizabeth Zimmer writes, mostly about the arts, teaches writing wherever she is invited, and edits manuscripts of all sorts. She practices the Feldenkrais Method, reads voraciously, and works as a standardized patient in hospitals and medical schools. Her ambition is to keep people laughing.

Ann McMillan is a retired scientist who loves to write, but often gets asked to edit. Ann lives on 10 acres near Stittsville where she can think about words while she pulls weeds. Ann transitioned from working life by editing *Air Quality Management: Canadian Perspectives on a Global Issue,* with Eric Taylor in 2014. It dawned on her that although she had been working in science policy for the government for a very long time, what she was really being paid for was the two-minute elevator briefing, and writing. Finding the former stressful, but loving the latter, she has explored her softer side with *The New Devil's Dictionary* and *Naked in Time.* Ann happily takes all the credit for the idea for this current almanac, and is pleased to have exploited this vehicle for story-telling, verse and essay-writing. Now this project is complete, she is looking for more writing and editing and can be reached at:
mcmillan@storm.ca

Contributor

Jon Peirce is a writer, actor, writing mentor, teacher, and sometime improvisational dancer, singer and progressive political activist who plies his many trades—with varying degrees of success—in his cozy half-duplex by the banks of the Gatineau River in Gatineau, Quebec. His favourite writing subjects include education, technology, theatre, the world of work, love and romance, food and drink, popular culture or the lack thereof, the Canadian and American political scenes, and the ever-changing mores of the English language. Twice-divorced, he has two daughters, one son, and one grandson. He holds a bachelor's degree in English from Amherst College, a Master's Degree and a Doctorate in English from Dalhousie University, and a Master's degree in industrial relations from Queen's University, in addition to parts of another doctorate in industrial relations and another master's degree in history. His interests include tennis, cooking, swimming, bird-watching, train travel and going for long walks. He is a board member of Ottawa Independent Writers.

Jon began his writing career in boarding school, where for three and a half years he singlehandedly put together a weekly debate society review. At Amherst, he wrote for the college paper and served as assistant editor. After his graduation, he was a reporter for the *Springfield Union,* and then spent two years in Baltimore working for that city's welfare department as a social worker in lieu of service in the American military. Brief stints as a mover's helper, prep school English teacher, bartender and daily newspaper editor punctuated his lengthy graduate school career at Dalhousie, at the conclusion of which he taught English composition and literature at Susquehanna University, Central College, and Queen's. Tired of moving from one short-term gig to another, he switched fields, changing over to industrial relations at age 39. There followed a five-year stint as researcher-writer at the Economic Council of Canada, a shorter and unhappier stint as a policy analyst at the Canadian federal Department of Energy, Mines and Resources, and three years as an assistant professor of industrial relations at Memorial University of Newfoundland in St John's.

For two and a half years he valiantly attempted to maintain a freelance writing and editing business in Ottawa, while teaching industrial relations and human resource management part-time at Carleton University and the University of Ottawa. He then did an 18-month stint as research director for the Fryer Commission on Labour-Management Relations in the Canadian Federal Public Service before landing his final gig, with the Professional Institute of the Public Service of Canada, a public service union known to the cognoscenti as PIPSC. After nearly 11 years as a researcher, labour relations officer, and all-around policy wonk, he retired from PIPSC in 2011, devoting himself since then primarily but far from exclusively to writing. (His eight-year post-retirement stay in Halifax saw him appearing in ten community theatre productions and teaching numerous Nova Scotia Seniors' College courses.)

Jon's publications include: *Canadian Industrial Relations,* an introductory industrial relations textbook which ran to three editions, an essay collection, *Social Studies,* and a novella, *Love and Love.* He has published four pieces in the *Chicken Soup for the Soul* series, several research papers on subjects related to the world of work, and over 200 articles, op-ed pieces, and book reviews; these have appeared in such publications as *The Globe and Mail,* the *Ottawa Citizen,* the *Toronto Star,* the *Christian Science Monitor, Books in Canada,* the *Kingston Whig-Standard,* the *Winnipeg Free Press,* the *Halifax Chronicle-Herald,* and *Halifax* magazine. Jon believes that the present almanac represents the culmination of his lengthy writing career and that, like it or not, the COVID pandemic, like the Second World War before it, is something people will be talking, arguing and writing about for many decades after it finally ends. That said, he will be glad to start writing about other things once this almanac has been 'put to bed.' Most of the time, he's grateful to Ann McMillan, the co-producer of this almanac, for having suggested he undertake the project. Jon may be contacted at:

www.jonpeirce.ca

Acknowledgements

In the words of W.B. Yeats, '…my glory was I had such friends.'[1] This almanac is a tribute and a testimony to the friends I have made throughout a long and active life. Without you, my dear friends, this almanac would not exist.

Initially, when we put out our call for contributions, Ann and I thought we would be lucky to get 30 pieces. In the end, we got more than 70. Friends from almost every phase of my life eagerly sent in pieces. Best of all, some of them told *their* friends about the book, and some of *those* friends sent in pieces. It was almost as if I were a modern-day Tom Sawyer, re-enacting the scene in which he gets his friends to whitewash his aunt's fence. Within a month after we had put out our call, the collection process had taken on a momentum of its own.

My first cousin, Don Peirce, I have known since early childhood. But only recently did I discover he's a writer as well as a musician. From my boarding school days at Andover came classmate Bill Hartman. From my college days came Amherst classmates Rodney Clough, Lee Keener and Bill Newmann, as well as Betsy Hoffman (Smith '68), who I often saw over at Amherst. It is thanks to Bill Newmann that we have the humorous piece by Jim Pellegrin (Dr Q). From my graduate school days at Dalhousie came Elizabeth Zimmer, a fellow student in the first modern dance class I ever took, just half a century ago. Also from those graduate school days came David Shaw, who I met in Toronto, the friend of a mutual friend. Many years later, David would become a Facebook friend and fellow Trump basher.

From my time in Toronto came my dear friend Harold Tausch, who I met at a 'Barefoot Boogie' dance and from whom I learned about the Feldenkrais method, which has helped keep me at least relatively flexible into my mid-70s.

From my previous stint in Metro Ottawa came fellow writers Elena Calvo and Ralph Smith, with whom I spent many joyous hours at critique group sessions, as well as fellow Ottawa Independent Writers (OIW) board member Bill Horne. And Neven Humphrey I remember from Bill's famous mid-summer OIW pool parties. Also from that stint, Denise Giroux and Yves Rochon were valued and beloved colleagues from the Professional Institute, the public service union where I spent the final 11 years of my working life. In addition to contributing some excellent pieces of his own, Yves brought on board his partner, Jany Lavoie—who is French language editor of the almanac as well as a contributor—actor and poet Sasha Dominique, Toronto writer Alan Lennon, and Logements de l'Outaouais co-workers Julie Fortin and Camille Pellerin-Forget. A friend indeed!

From my post-retirement years in Halifax came Ian Johnson, a tennis partner who became a good friend, fellow St Margaret's Church member and chorister Georgia Johnson, and Seniors' College students Taiya Barss and

Dianna Davison-Veber. From those years as well came poet Cathy McKenzie, at whose home I once offered a writing workshop.

Other Nova Scotia friendships came from my time in community theatre in that province. Jim Petrie I first met when we 'trod the boards' together in two Bedford Players productions. And from the South Shore came Colleen Naomi, Teresa Patterson and Paul Pickering. Colleen cast me in a play, then put up with me in at least half a dozen of her online workshops, in one of which (*Scriptease*) I came across fellow playwrights Patterson and Pickering.

My final Nova Scotia connection, Paul Lenarczyk, is someone I've never met, but whose weekly musical 'kitchen parties' provided virtual entertainment and companionship at a time when both were sorely needed.

OIW, where I learned how to be a professional writer during my previous stint in Metro Ottawa, was once again the source of a number of contributions to the almanac, including those of poets Valerie Buko, Kathy Figueroa and Jagjeet Sharma, memoirist Jo-Anne Stead, and short-story writer Su Mardelli. Special mention should be made of essayist Bob Barclay, who in addition to being a contributor, is the book's publisher. In working with me to put together an almanac in, essentially, three different languages, and comprising five literary genres, Bob has gone far beyond the call of duty and the specifications of our initial agreement. His technical prowess has enabled us to overcome many difficulties. While the difficulties have been numerous, I believe that the final product—a COVID almanac like no other—is something we can all be proud of.

Memoirist John Allen I 'met' at a virtual launch party for a *Chicken Soup for the Soul* anthology to which we had both contributed. My remaining friends, I know primarily or entirely from Facebook. They include essayist Peter Alexander, memoirist Jackie Amable, artist Claude Ethier, memoirists Marcia Brumit Kropf and Fran Ota, and poet Rowena Torrevillas. I hope to have the pleasure of meeting all of them in the future.

Reading through all the pieces as I prepare them for the press, I feel truly blessed and honoured at the wealth of material with which we've been presented. My glory is that I have such friends.

J.P.
Gatineau, Quebec
July 26, 2021

As so articulately stated by Jon, this book's creation has taken on a life of its own. When the waves of contributions started breaking over us, my reaction was to back off. Not so, Jon. Nevertheless, contributors presented themselves from several of my 'walks of life.'

The largest chunk of them are members of the Prior Chest Nuts, a dragon boat team for breast cancer survivors. Interestingly none of them spoke much about their cancer or the team. Thus, Jeanette Grant, Susan Mills, Deb Bertrand and Elizabeth Barnes are my Sisters from another Mother from the boat.

I also approached my friends including Sally Arsove, who has now walked and talked with me for years, interspersed with the odd swim or snowshoe as the season demanded. Gavin Murphy, who I had met in a career long ago and a place far away, stepped up to contribute as well.

My long-time yoga co-student and more recent arborist, Brent Coates stepped up when he heard about the project. Who knew he could write?

We agreed that we needed someone to talk more deeply about mental health. After racking my brain, I remembered Ruth Hawkins, who I had worked with in the federal government and who I knew from policy circles was an excellent writer. I knew she had left government to retrain as a mental health professional, but could I find her and would she be willing? I did and she was, and the result is remarkable.

I also had set my heart on a Canadian piece on music and thought that it would be easy for me to find someone through the Friends of the National Arts Centre Orchestra (FNACO). After several attempts, I was introduced to Chris Millard, who delivered what was requested and more.

Jon is talking about a sequel. Fortunately, I do have some friends out there who have not yet been asked. I hope they don't run when they see me coming.

A.M.
Stittsville, Ontario
August 3, 2021

---

[1] The Municipal Gallery Revisited